Rival Truths

It is common sense that our survival as individuals depends on the survival of our physical bodies. However, common sense has been medicalised. Terms such as 'road rage' and 'premenstrual syndrome' sound like medical problems and suggest that it is affected individuals, rather than experiences or circumstances that require treatment.

Without denying their importance, *Rival Truths* challenges four basic common-sense views of health and illness and offers rival social psychological explanations. The primacy of biological facts is challenged by looking at the effects of social psychological influences, such as those mediated by stress. The assumption that medical practices are scientific is challenged by evidence that they also reflect and recreate social constructions. The assumption that medical advances are the most effective way to combat disease is questioned as their success may rely on changes in beliefs or behaviour, and finally, critical analyses suggest that medical treatment can sometimes be to the disadvantage of patients.

Lindsay St. Claire has helped to raise awareness that health problems might be caused by social arrangements, not biological dysfunction. Thus social psychology might suggest new ways to enhance health status which do not depend on medical breakthroughs. This book will be of interest for health psychology students, medical students and anyone involved in caring professions.

Rival Truths

Common Sense and Social Psychological Explanations in Health and Illness

Lindsay St. Claire

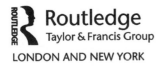

LONDON AND NEW YORK

First published 2003
by Psychology Press

2 Park Square, Milton Park, Abingdon, Oxon OX14 4RN
711 Third Avenue, New York, NY 10017, USA

Routledge is an imprint of the Taylor & Francis Group, an informa business

First issued in paperback 2016

Typeset in Times by Keystroke, Jacaranda Lodge, Wolverhampton
Cover design by Anú Design

British Library Cataloguing in Publication-Data
A catalogue record for this book is available from the British Library

Library of Congress Cataloging-in-Publication Data

St. Claire, Lindsay.
   Rival truths : common sense and social psychological
   explanations in health and illness / Lindsay St. Claire.
      p. cm. — (International series in social psychology)

     ISBN 978-1-138-87686-6 (pbk)
     ISBN 978-0-415-18858-6 (hbk)
   1. Clinical health psychology.   2. Social medicine.
   3. Social psychology.   I. Title. II. Series.
   R726.7 .S72 2003
   610'.1'9—dc21   2002015080

For John, Jack, and Harry

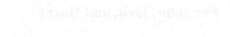

Contents

Figures

Tables

Activities

Acknowledgements

I would like to thank Peter Robinson for his patience, kindness, and constructive comments. I would also like to thank John Telfer, Steve Arnott, Kyra Neubauer, Mo and Jim Milne, Mike Pugh, Nick Ambler, and Norman Freeman.

1

Introduction and Overview

The first aim of this chapter is briefly to introduce the key concepts and perspectives that underpin the chapters that follow. Its second aim is to explain their overall purpose and structure. In the first section "common sense" is defined, and the relationship between common sense and a particular way of thinking about health and illness, known as the "medical model", is discussed. In the second section four common sense views of health and illness based on the medical model are identified and challenged, in order to outline four of the main purposes of this book. In the third section the biopsychosocial model of health and illness is introduced. As its name suggests, social psychological influences play an important role in this model. Their importance justifies the social psychological bases of this book. In the fourth section the focus is on social psychology itself. From the diversity of approaches in social psychology, four levels of analysis will be described in order to explain both the order of chapters and the emphasis of their content.

1. Common Sense and the Medical Model

To state the obvious, human beings have physical bodies. By means of our bodies we move around in our world and interact with others. Our bodies influence how others perceive and interact with us and how we feel and think about ourselves. Indeed, our very survival as individuals depends upon the survival of our physical bodies. Most of us rejoice when we feel fit and healthy; most of us fear threatening pathological processes when we feel ill. The importance of the physical reality of our bodies is common sense in our society.

The *Oxford English Dictionary* defines "common sense" in two relevant ways, which focus on individuals and communities respectively. In the first, common sense is "the endowment of natural intelligence possessed by rational beings; ordinary, normal or average understanding; the plain wisdom which is everyman's [sic] inheritance;" or "more emphatically, good, sound practical sense; combined tact and readiness in dealing with the everyday affairs of life; general sagacity" and "ordinary or untutored perception". In the second definition, common sense is defined as "the general sense, feeling or judgement of mankind [sic] or a community".

In the chapters that follow, "common sense" will be used in both of these senses. Most often, a common sense view will be described in order to identify a familiar, rational starting point for theorising about an issue of health or illness. In these cases, the term will simply reflect the views of friends, acquaintances, students, media, or myself. These will be taken to reflect an everyday understanding of the issue. Occasionally, (particularly in Chapter 6) the term "common sense" will be used in the second sense, in which case it will more formally describe empirical studies of lay beliefs.

There is an interesting paradox inherent in the nature of common sense views of health and illness: healers who can relieve suffering and postpone death acquire power, wealth, and status in most societies (Stainton Rogers, 1991). Furthermore, within each society, one system of healing generally develops an official status, which gives it precedence over the others. In Britain (as well as most Western and many other countries) biomedicine is the healing system that enjoys this status (Helman, 2000). Medical professionals not only control access to many resources, but also have the power to construct public knowledge about health and illness. The result is that medicalised clichés and ways of seeing the world are often taken for granted as common sense (Bartlett, 1998; Stainton Rogers, 1991).

For example, Cornwell (1984) interviewed 15 women and 9 men in the East End of London in order to gather common sense ideas about health and illness. She found that their theories seemed (or tried) to be medical in form and content. Prefixes such as "They [i.e. doctors] say" frequently showed a deference to medical authority and there was a general acceptance that health is a matter for experts. A glance at current media paints a similar picture. Terms such as "road rage", "stress", "premenstrual syndrome", and "false memory syndrome" sound like medical problems that people have. In turn, this gives the impression that it is they, as opposed to their social experiences or circumstances, that require treatment. A similar, but funnier, example is the representation of liking to be fed chocolate by a handsome man as a menstrual symptom! (See Figure 1.1 and Section 2.4, below, where the example will be developed along more critical lines.) My argument is that common sense, or what everybody "knows" already about health and illness, has been medicalised. Therefore, it is appropriate briefly to describe the key characteristics of the medical model.

The medical model is based on scientific rationality which emphasises objective reality, precise measurement, and the elucidation of cause–effect laws, generally by means of hypothesis testing and experimentation (Helman, 2000; Still, 1996b). Since the scientific attitude is that individual opinions are unlikely to be objective because of interpretative bias, the interpretations of scientists are backed up by data which are open to public scrutiny and which can be (dis)confirmed by others. The assumption is that scientific explanations describe reality and therefore, have the authority of "truth" (Devalle, 1996).

The essence of the medical model is a scientific paradigm within which abnormalities of the structure and function of body organs and systems can be identified and named (Helman, 2000). Although there is an acknowledgement

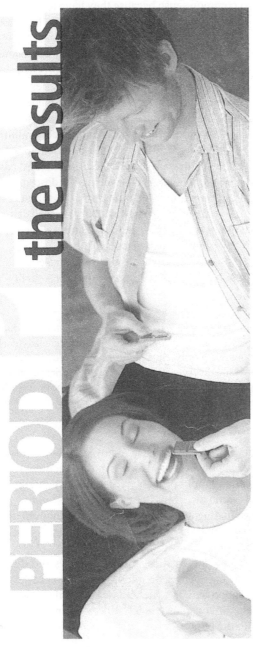

PERIOD PEACE

the results

You, him and your period. How do blokes react to it?
Our national survey reveals all...

Your boss, your lover,
your dad... In our July
issue, Company and
Feminax asked how these

ALL BECAUSE THE LADY LOVES...
Chocoholics, move to Scotland this minute. We asked what happened when you'd eaten the last bit
of chocolate in the house, then burst into tears. Nearly 60% of Scots girls reported that their brilliant
boyfriends would rush straight out for more chocolate – 10% more than average. But sadly nearly half
the blokes just say patronisingly, 'you've got PMT', and Irish guys in particular should take some
hints from the Scots.

FIGURE 1.1 Craving chocolate can be represented as a menstrual symptom caused by hormones.
Article from *Company* with permission.

that appearances can mask it, it is assumed that an underlying reality exists and can be discovered. However, the knowledge and methods by which this can be achieved stand in contrast to common sense because they have to be taught over a long period to a carefully selected group of hard-working and intellectually gifted individuals.

One of the great strengths of the medical model is its foundation in accumulated knowledge of clinical facts and general laws concerning the cause, course, and treatment of disease. Since this knowledge is untouched by the vagaries of individual experience, it is possible to make accurate estimates of the incidence and severity of a given disease. In populations these take the form of morbidity and mortality rates. Knowledge of these characteristics allow (for example) communities to be compared and resources to be diverted where they are most needed. In individuals, diagnosis confirms the incidence of a disease, and in the case of breast cancer, for example, "staging" is a way of representing its severity; T1 describes tumours of 2 centimetres or less, T2 tumours are 2–5 centimetres; T3 tumours are over 5 centimetres; and T4 tumours are fixed to the chest wall or skin, and can be of any size (Clark, 1991). Knowledge of a patient's stage at diagnosis means that her treatment plan can be guided by accumulated wisdom.

However, this approach tends to result in the disease, as opposed to the patient becoming the focus of attention. Moreover, the disease and its "personality" become reified (Baron, 1985):

> In general, modern medicine takes disease to be an anatomicopathologic fact. We tend to see illness as an objective entity that is located somewhere anatomically or that perturbs a defined physiologic process. In a profound sense, we say that such an entity "is" the disease, thus taking illness from the universe of experience and moving it to a location in the physical world. We use object words to describe illness—lesion, tumour, infiltrate and rely on pathologists reviewing diseased tissue to define disease for us.

As an example, Baron notes that comprehensive nosographies of the 18th and 19th centuries did not include peptic ulcer as a disease, but rather included a variety of symptoms and situations that would probably come under that label today. It was not until the 1830s that peptic ulcer was "born" as a disease entity, when "it" was observed as an objective finding at post-mortem that was thought to correlate with patients' symptoms. Thus, the disease was defined by anatomical fact, as opposed to experienced symptoms.

Similarly, treatment based on the medical model employs the discourse of biological reductionism because it focuses on micro-level biological events. This has led to a "factor analytic" approach, in which it is assumed that one factor may be treated, while others remain constant (Engel, 1980). Helman (2000) neatly caricatures the approach with the phrase "spare-part surgery", which suggests that analogous to car repairs, components of people may be replaced, without psychological and social implications.

To summarise, the gist of the medical model is captured in four common sense assumptions: "the facts are the facts"; "given time and resources, science will accumulate a full understanding of the facts about disease"; "medical advances offer the most effective way to combat disease"; "medical treatment is the best remedy for ill people".

Recently a great many challenges to the medical model have been articulated (e.g. Engel, 1980; Taylor, 1995). Just four, which directly address the above assumptions, will be developed.

2. Four Challenges to Common Sense, Biomedical Ways of Thinking about Health and Illness

2.1 The facts are the facts

The phrase, "the facts are the facts" represents the common sense idea that objective, publicly verifiable biological facts are what matters in health and disease. However, the presence of a potentially serious disease can be of surprisingly little consequence, because it is frequently impossible to pinpoint its onset. For example, breast cancer is likely to have been caused by events 20 to 40 years before its onset, and once begun, it can take up to 16 years for a breast tumour to grow large enough to be detected (Clark, 1991). Such a state of affairs not only undermines the validity of morbidity rates, since the "true" incidence of disease is likely to be unknown, but it also shows that psychological experiences and management of disease can be more important than its presence or absence.

One of the strongest challenges to the phrase, "the facts are the facts" is to be found in a study of the interpersonal dynamics within a family of four (Minuchin, 1974). In the family, there were two daughters who were both diabetic and the study was carried out in an attempt to understand why the elder of the two appeared to suffer much more; for example, experiencing many emergency hospital admissions. During the study, the levels of free fatty acid in the bloodstreams of family members were continuously measured. These provided a measure of stress, because free fatty acid is liberated from body tissues and carried by the blood to the liver, to be converted into energy for flight or fight during stress reactions (e.g., Cassidy, 1999). In phase one of the study, the parents were interviewed while the two daughters, aged 17 and 15, were watching from behind a one-way mirror and the free fatty acid levels in both daughters rose, even though they were only observing from a different room. After an hour, the daughters were invited to join the parents and their free fatty acid levels rose further. Those of the older daughter however, rose almost twice as much and after the session they remained raised for over an hour whereas those of the younger daughter quickly returned to normal. Minuchin (1974) observed that each parent appealed for support to the older, but not the younger, daughter during disagreements. He reasoned that she experienced stress as a result of conflicting loyalties, and that the stress exacerbated her disease.

Minuchin's (1974) study shows that disease processes are not determined by physical facts alone. On the contrary, it suggests that the social world permeates the physical boundaries of humans and that different personal experiences lead to different anticipations of a common physical world so that the same objective facts cause different biological events.

Further intriguing examples of the interaction between social meanings and biological events are case studies of "Voodoo Death" (Cannon, 1942). In one, a young man was invited to a feast and given chicken. He was assured that it was not wild hen, which was a taboo food for him, so he ate it. Much later, he discovered that it was in fact wild hen. He "immediately began to tremble", returned to his lodgings and died.

Without denying the importance of biological facts, I believe that a tight focus on them is frequently misleading in the quest to understand health and illness. It is one purpose of this book to challenge the primacy of biological facts by tracing the permeability of human biology to social psychological meanings and influences.

2.2 Given time and resources, science will accumulate a full understanding of the facts about disease

Helman (2000) identifies an increasing public conviction that biomedicine is failing to solve health problems. Since lack of resources is seen as its cause, the common sense solution is to increase funding and Health Minister Dobson, for example, announced an additional £40bn for UK Health and Education Budgets in July 1998, in order to pay for an extra 7000 doctors and 15,000 nurses. Extra funding for the National Health Service was set at £60bn in the first budget of the new millennium. In the USA, healthcare services have been estimated to consume 11% of US Gross National Product (GNP) (Taylor, 1995) and at least one long-term projection identifies the year 2055 as a kind of Armageddon for modern medicine. This is because 2055 is the year in which healthcare costs in the US are expected to reach 100% of GNP (Sheridan & Radmacher, 1992).

Such figures suggest that resources to fund scientific understanding of disease cannot continue to grow steadily in the future. Irrespective of whether resources and progress are positively correlated, the related assumption—that there has been steady growth in the past—may also be challenged. This is the common sense idea that the medical model stands on a smooth accumulation of truths about our biology. Moreover, since these truths are objective, the idea is that they are impervious to fashion and bias (Lupton, 1994). This assumption may be challenged by historical analyses, which reveal that the medical model evolved out of its social context. According to Beattie and Jones (1992) an important reason for its emergence was the Reformation in the 16th century, which had the effect of reducing the church's power to police ideas and prevent practices such as carrying out post-mortems. A second reason was colonialism and the growth of capitalism, which together helped to change the view of the position of humans in the universe. As part of this movement, scientists began to suggest that the world was rational and mechanistic and that there was a split between divine intelligence and the mechanical body. Subsequently, "the sick man" [sic] with his idiosyncratic symptoms disappeared from Europe and a new hospital-based medicine led to a focus on objectively defined diseases, diseased organs, and impersonal cases. Furthermore, these changes were supported by many other events, including the invention of the microscope and medical instruments such as forceps (Jewson, 1976).

Interestingly, Armstrong (1983) argues that human bodies had been seen as undifferentiated flesh before this time and it was changes in attitudes and beliefs, as opposed to a gradual accumulation of facts, that led to the recognition of specific organs. These only became visible once scientists "knew" them to be there. Such analyses suggest that the medical model is a way of thinking, which is socially constructed like other ways of thinking. It also suggests that the idea that truth has been steadily accumulated is part of that construction.

Without denying the reality and importance of medical advances, a second purpose of this book is to argue that the beliefs and practices of medical practitioners as well as lay people often reflect social constructions even though common sense assumes they are based on science and/or objective reality. I hope that social psychological analyses of beliefs and practices might help to encourage the development of new ways to enhance health status that do not depend on medical breakthroughs (and which might be quick, effective, and cheap!).

2.3 Medical advances offer the most effective way to combat disease

Perhaps the most important common sense assumption beneath a medical approach to health and illness is that it offers the most effective way to combat disease. This assumption may be challenged because there is no guarantee that advances in understanding, preventing, or treating a disease effectively reduce its incidence.

To illustrate, McKeown (1979) famously plotted the annual incidence of various acute diseases in the UK. Figures showed that marked and steady declines had begun in the mid-19th century and correlated with improvements in sanitation, housing, and other social changes. To focus on TB, a key medical breakthrough in the mid-20th century was the BCG vaccination, but this barely makes a "blip" in the already downward trend.

Whereas acute diseases such as pneumonia, 'flu, and TB were the most virulent causes of death at the turn of the century, First World citizens at the dawn of the third millennium are likely to fall victim to cardiovascular diseases or cancer (e.g., Taylor, 1995). Since their incidence depends greatly on human behaviour, Becker (1976, cited in Stroebe & Stroebe, 1995) argues provocatively that most, if not all deaths from these are "suicides", in the sense that they could have been postponed, had the victims adopted healthier lifestyles. Salovey, Rothman, and Rodin (1998) cite American statistics that vividly illustrate the point. If Americans stopped smoking, there would be a 25% reduction in cancer deaths and 350,000 fewer fatal heart attacks each year, and a 10% weight loss would decrease coronary artery disease by 20%.

Without denying the effectiveness of medical advances, a third purpose of this book is to challenge the assumption that they are always the most effective way to combat disease. It will be argued that changes in beliefs or behaviours might be essential to their success or even more effective in their own right. Moreover, it will be argued that relevant changes might also need to occur in the beliefs and behaviours of medical practitioners and politicians, since as well as being suicides, some premature deaths might be manslaughter!

2.4 Medical treatment is the best remedy for ill people

A famous memoir is that of a doctor who was captured during the Second World War and put in charge of medical care for his fellow prisoners (Cochrane, 1971). Although he had virtually no medicine, to his surprise, most of his patients made a full recovery.

This story is only a weak challenge to the assumption that medical treatment is the best remedy for ill (or injured) people because, of course, the patients might have recovered better if they had been treated. Statistical analyses of British childbirths (Tew, 1990) present a stronger and more distressing challenge. First, Tew notes that the two exceptions to the fall in mortality rates during the 1870s were women and babies. Still more bizarre, records kept by lying-in charities during the mid-19th century showed that maternal death rates among urban poor, who were often half-starved and diseased, were frequently less that those of better-off patients who were attended by male accoucheurs with the latest instrumental interventions. Next, Tew (1990) cites an analysis carried out by the Registrar General for the years 1930–32 which revealed an "unexpected advantage of being poor": the maternal mortality rate for classes I and II was 4.44 per 1000 whereas for social class V, it was 3.89. For all causes of death except abortion and post-partum haemorrhage, it was the relatively advantaged mothers who were more likely to die. In particular, the increased risk of dying from puerperal sepsis as a result of less hygienic living conditions, lower fitness, and poorer nutrition was "apparently more than offset by reduced risk as a result of fewer contacts with doctors". Ironically, the reduction in maternal mortality that heralded current times was not achieved through a better understanding of obstetric medicine, but through the introduction in 1936 of drugs that enabled iatrogenic infections to be treated.

Tew (1990) continues that the years 1964–1975, which are the only ones for which data were published, show that maternal deaths were significantly higher for mothers booked for hospital delivery (.190 as opposed to .165 per 1000). Clearly, it might be that hospital figures were inflated by the inclusion of more high-risk cases, but figures dealing separately with these groups show the same pattern. This and a corpus of further evidence suggests that obstetric intervention only rarely improves on the natural process, yet by the 1980s most of the world had accepted as common sense that birth should be planned and controlled by medical experts. In Britain, hardly 1% of births occur in the family home, which previously had been the traditional birthing place.

Tew (1990) develops the critical argument that medical intervention is responsible for *decreasing* the well-being of a majority of women during childbirth. She describes dreadful cases from the 19th century in which practitioners deliberately and unnecessarily used dangerous instruments to hasten birth in order to save time, impress the family, and justify a higher fee. She also condemns the apparent contemporary imperviousness of the obstetric profession to evidence that discredits its practices and philosophy. Finally, she notes that the increasing hospitalisation of birth advocated by doctors for the benefit of mothers and babies also resulted in a competitive advantage, which reduced the status of midwives and confirmed the ascendancy of male-dominated medical obstetricians.

Such critical analyses challenge the idea that medical treatment is the best remedy for ill people and raise questions about the "real" beneficiaries of medical treatments. Frequently they reveal a fallacious representation of social norms as laws of nature. This diverts attention away from the changeability of social conditions and towards the treatment of individuals who do not conform. The net result is maintenance of the status quo, and this might be of more benefit to high-status doctors than to their patients (Sapsford & Dallos, 1996). A striking illustration is *draeptomainia*, a disease of Negro slaves. Its main symptom was trying to escape, its causes included over-indulgent treatment, and its treatment included punishment (Jones, 1997; Stainton Rogers, 1991). To return to the example of childbirth, a critical analysis questions why normal, well women become patients, and why, only a generation ago, they were given treatments such as enemas and had their pubic hair shaved "for their own good".

It is the fourth purpose of this book to attempt some critical analyses. The aim is not to accuse medical professionals of deliberate attempts to impose their explanations upon the public in order to advance themselves. Although issues related to power always lie at the heart of health debates (Beattie & Jones, 1992), personal blame of (powerful) scientists is rarely appropriate because most believe themselves neutral and objective. Second, lay people often adopt medicalised common sense ideas about health, which are to their own disadvantage (Sapsford & Dallos, 1996). Rather than to blame, my aim is to help raise awareness that the root of health problems might sometimes lie outside patients' biology and inside social arrangements. To the extent that patients endorse and accept these arrangements, they are holding beliefs that justify the system and militate against improvements in their own health status. However, it need not be so. Large-scale social change or perhaps a small-scale change in personal beliefs or self-concept might provide a therapy to promote health and alleviate handicap.

3. Introduction to the Biopsychosocial Model

To help answer challenges to the medical model, Engel (1980) suggested a biopsychosocial model of health and illness in which, as its name makes clear, biological, psychological, and social factors are all-important determinants of health and illness. The model, which is shown in Figure 1.2, accommodates the common sense observation that nature is ordered in hierarchies, with simpler systems nested within more complex ones.

In the model, two main hierarchies may be distinguished, with the person at the highest level of the organismic hierarchy and simultaneously at the lowest level of the social hierarchy. The constituent systems of the person are the focus of the biomedical model, but in the biopsychosocial model, the person is not considered in isolation. Rather, "hospital", "school", "family" and so on represent social systems in which s/he is nested, and category labels like "patient", "pupil", "mother" and so on describe the person's role in such systems. Although each system has distinctive qualities and demands its own level of study and explanation, its stability is maintained not only by its internal dynamics, but also by those of the systems above and below it. In other words, the systems transact such that disruption of one level can change other systems. Moreover, resultant changes can feed back to affect the original disruption of the first system.

To contrast biomedical and biopsychosocial approaches to illness, a seminal paper (Engel, 1980) describes the case of a man who has suffered a threatened heart attack, been admitted to hospital, is stabilising and feeling better. Unfortunately,

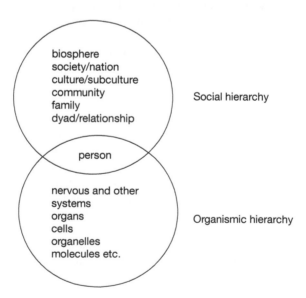

FIGURE 1.2 Systems of the biopsychosocial model (after Engel, 1977, 1980).

Casualty staff have difficulty in administering an injection and after several attempts, they leave the patient and go for advice. While he is alone, he suffers a cardiac arrest about 30 minutes after he was admitted.

An evaluation based on a medical perspective focuses on changes in the organ system, and attributes the cause of the cardiac arrest to initial myocardial injury. This leads to congratulating the patient on his good luck, because he might not have survived if he had been admitted half an hour later. An evaluation based on the biopsychosocial model however, focuses on the interplay between systems, and questions whether the cardiac arrest would have happened at all had the man not been admitted and stressed by his experiences. In this latter evaluation, the "trouble" was located in systems outside the heart.

It follows that the "critical flaw" (Engel, 1980) of the biomedical model, is that it under-represents what it is to be a person. Thus, unlike the medical model, the biopsychosocial model poses no clear boundaries to mark the end of the individual and no exclusive emphasis on physical factors. On the contrary, psychosocial systems not only present additional sources of information for the understanding of the individual's health and illness, but also present additional loci for intervention.

In order to build a more detailed impression of the systems that "constitute" a human and his or her ecology, the nature of the two hierarchies of the biopsycho-social model, and the way they interact need further elaboration. Stevens (1996a) identifies three dimensions that help to characterise what it means to be a person, which usefully suggest more about systems below the level of the person in the biopsychosocial approach. These are depicted in Table 1.1.

Stevens (1996a) notes the importance of emotions in characterising human experience and points out that their causes and precise nature might sometimes be unconscious. In addition, he emphasises the importance of conscious experience and argues that to be a person is to be aware not only of the world around us, but also of a multiplicity of inner worlds. Beyond that, humans are aware that they (and others) are aware. Third, he points out that to be a person involves experiencing oneself as a coherent entity in time, with a continuous past, present, and future. Moreover, people construct consistent, unifying narratives, although events themselves might be haphazard and aspects of the self fragmented. Emotions, cognitions and awareness, and the active construction of narratives provide examples of systems within people and offer alternatives to common sense sites

TABLE 1.1 *Five aspects of being human (after Stevens, 1996a)*

To be a human involves:

Having a physical body
Living in a social context
Sometimes being unconscious of reasons for personal actions
Living in a private world of experience
A sense of existing continuously for a finite time

such as organs and other biological systems, in terms of which both "trouble" and positive influences for an individual's health status may be conceptualised.

To turn to the hierarchy above the level of the person, common sense conceptualisations include "hospital", "school", "family", "community", and "culture", which exist physically in the real world, and which can be operationalised. For example, someone who has an "extended family" may be compared with a member of a "nuclear family" or people from different cultures might be contrasted with each other. However, such operationalisation is vague about the ways in which the human ecology is internalised, that is, how it gets under our skins.

Bronfenbrenner's (1979) ecological model of human development helps to clarify this issue. The model is broadly similar to Engel's (1980) biopsychosocial approach but the crucial difference is Bronfenbrenner's insistence on the importance of the way individuals perceive the systems in which they are nested, rather than on the importance of the systems *per se*. This means that the environment is filtered through the individual's expectations, which are themselves socially constructed. In fact, Bronfenbrenner sees the human environment like a series of Russian dolls in which the individual is nested. At the first level is "the microsystem", which consists of face-to-face environments such as the individual's perception of his or her workplace, family, or friends. At the second level is the inter-related system of microsystems, which is called the "mesosystem". Thus, an individual might enjoy a range of positive microsystem experiences, but conflict between some of these—for example between the relationship with his or her mother and the relationship with his or her father—might be a source of stress, which springs from the mesosystem level.

At the third level is the exosystem, which refers to perceived environments that affect the individual, but into which he or she does not actually go. For example, parents are likely to be profoundly influenced by their perceptions of an operating theatre in which their child is to undergo surgery. Finally, the macrosystem refers to perceptions of wider cultural influences, which are built up over generations of human activity. These include ways of thinking and communicating, social settings, and institutions. Examples are the perceived attitudes of healthcare personnel, or beliefs about the "proper" behaviour of men, which might influence a man's pain experiences or his decision to seek help. Thus, the approach emphasises that many systems of the human ecology do not consist of physical entities but are made up of shared meanings and practices into which perceivers are born (Helman, 2000; Still, 1996b; Wetherell & Still, 1996). For example, the perceiver's nuclear family does not simply consist of a few other individuals. It also consists of "inherited" normative expectations concerning the proper behaviour of mothers, fathers, sons, and daughters, mutually constructed meanings, including made-up words and family jokes, together with a shared family history.

The emphasis on perceptions as opposed to the environment *per se* also means that individuals living in the same physical context might be subject to non-shared influences, because the environment might mean something different to each.

ACTIVITY 1.1 Key systems and contexts of well-being

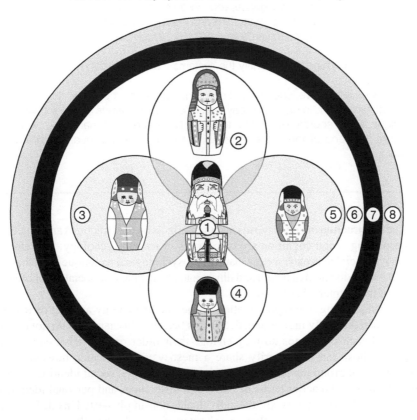

1 Internal systems
2–5 Personal relationships
6 Balance between personal relationships
7 Influential contexts not entered by the individual
8 Wider institutions

1 is intended to represent systems internal to you, including for example, your cardiovascular system or your emotional system. For simplicity's sake, no further attempt has been made to represent systems nested within these, but you can note any that are salient to your own well-being.
2–5 are intended to represent a selection of key friendships or personal relationships including face-to-face relationships within your family.
6 is intended to represent the harmony—or otherwise—between the relationships you have depicted from 2 to 5. Are they mutually supportive or, for example, does your family disapprove of some of your friends?

7 is intended to represent influential contexts that you don't usually enter yourself, such as your partner's workplace, your children's school, or your boss's office. 8 represents wider national institutions and ideologies such as "the government" ideologies or "attitudes towards women" in your workplace.

Annotate the diagram to identify the systems that are of importance to you in your life.

When you have identified important systems, consider how they affect each other. In particular, pay special attention to areas of conflict, which might be a source of stress to you. Note areas of harmony, where more than one of the systems combine to promote your health and well-being.

The construction of social norms and their effects on the structures and processes underpinning social cognition are core topics in social psychology. Therefore, a biopsychosocial approach means that social psychological techniques and theories are relevant to the field of health and illness and this justifies the social psychological basis of the chapters that follow.

Notwithstanding, the representation of the human ecology as a set of Russian dolls is paradoxically individualistic. This is because Russian dolls do not expand to engulf each other, nor do they change their order or even visit each other, so that a host can temporarily share a mesosystem. Humans, however, "are psychological group members who act in terms of shared social identities as well as individuals who act in terms of individual differences and personal identities" (Turner, 2000). In other words, the individual is not simply nested inside his or her family, hospital ward and other social categories—s/he has the psychological capacity to be a family member or a patient, or to act in terms of what Turner (2000) calls "higher-order" selves. Clearly, such a change is likely to recalibrate not only the systems of an individual's social ecology, but also the meanings through which s/he perceives them. Moreover, such changes do not occur in isolation. They might be synchronised with equivalent or complementary changes in other individuals, who are acting in terms of the same shared higher-order self. Alternatively, such changes might affect or be affected by changes in the social context, which is not static, but a pulsating universe of others' ecologies. An emphasis on the capacity of humans to act in terms of social categories is at the heart of the social identity approach and this approach will shape much of the theorising to come, which, especially in the later chapters, will attempt to consider the impact of "we-ness" on health.

However, in order to overview the way in which the coming chapters are structured, it is necessary to describe a little more of the concepts and approaches in social psychology that will be used to underpin them.

4. Structuring Diversity in Social Psychology and Overviewing the Book

Social psychology is relevant to the field of health because the reflexive individual, who embodies and experiences health and illness, is embedded in a range of social and psychological systems. Experiences are directly or indirectly shared with, influenced by, and have influences on others, and it is the interaction between intra-individual psychology and the social that is at the core of social psychology. To describe social psychology more precisely is difficult, because it is characterised by diversity. However, brief histories of the discipline provide insights into this diversity and help establish a basis on which to structure the coming chapters.

Still (1996a), for example, sees two "ancestors" of modern social psychology which he traces back through two millennia to the writings of St. Augustine, in which a split was described between what is pure and unchanging in humans and what is subjective, changeable, and mortal. Today, Still discerns the former line beneath the experimental and cognitive emphasis of "psychological social psychology", which seems to seek eternal, abstract, and general truths, detached from the hurly-burly of everyday life and which is firmly centred on intra-individual structures and processes. On the other hand, he discerns the latter line beneath the constructivist and hermeneutic emphases of "sociological social psychology", which seeks to build an understanding of human experience bounded by space and time and which is centred on the interaction between the individual and the social. Although Graumann (2001) constructs a different "ancestry" which locates the origins of individual-centred approaches in Aristotelian schools and those of socio-centred approaches in the Platonic school, he agrees with Still (1996a) that tension lies at the heart of current social psychology: as a branch of psychology it deals with intra-individual structures and processes, and as a social discipline it focuses on the role of the social context. This tension means that social psychology is characterised by debates about definitions, approaches, and perspectives which reflect core disagreements about the nature of the individual and society and even about the type of knowledge that is possible (Wetherell, 1996a).

To stereotype briefly, one major contender in the debate is psychological social psychology, within which key assumptions are that social behaviour may be objectively described and measured, and is subject to general causal laws that may be discovered, chiefly through experimentation (McGhee, 1996). This perspective is emphasised in American social psychology, which tends to be relatively individualistic, ahistorical, ethnocentric, and laboratory-oriented; its key foci include social cognition and information processing and how these are modified by social factors (Graumann, 2001). From this perspective, definitions of social psychology are likely to emphasis its scientific basis (Wetherell, 1996a).

Criticisms of this perspective and of scientific methods in social psychology are well known (Gergen, 1985). They emphasise the ways in which what is truly social—such as cultural meanings and interactions between people—tends to be ignored, or operationalised as the presence of a few strangers in a laboratory, for example. Other critics point out that scientific methods guarantee neither truth nor understanding, since alternative interpretations of empirical data are always possible and to establish the cause of an action is not to understand it (Banister, Burman, Parker, Taylor, & Tindall, 1994).

A more *social* social psychology addresses such criticisms and characterises the second main contender in the debate, which is labelled sociological social psychology. Its core subject matter is the interplay between society and the unique meanings and other experiences of individuals. These can be actively constructed, rather than caused by external variables. However, they are not amenable to objective measurement, since they are not observable, and are constantly changing or "becoming" (Stevens, 1996a, 1996b). This perspective tends to be emphasised in European social psychology and its critics focus on the unreliability of shifting intersubjectivity (Graumann, 2001; Wetherell, 1996a).

More recently, a third contender, known as critical social psychology has been proposed (Wetherell, 1996a). This takes as its subject matter the ways in which the social world has been structured over time by inequalities in the power of individuals and social groups. Of particular interest is how these social structures construct the individual, influencing his or her self-image, life choices, and other experiences. Wetherell (1996a) continues that critical social psychology is moral and political in the sense that it identifies what could and what should be.

Each of these social psychologies has already been mentioned in the challenges to the medical model. For example, psychological social psychology underpinned the idea that a person's beliefs about a disease might be more important determinants of behaviours than its presence *per se*. Sociological social psychology on the other hand, underpinned the idea that the medical model and related ways of thinking are socially constructed, as opposed to reflecting a gradual discovery of "the truth". Third, critical social psychology underpinned the idea that scientific "facts" concerning diseases and their treatment, often turn out to be socially, as opposed to biologically, constructed and often happen to be to the advantage of the healers, rather than the healed.

Each of these social psychologies will be met again in the coming chapters, which consequently, are epistemologically diverse. However, because health psychology is dominated by social cognition models (Lowe, 2001, personal communication) an attempt will be made to emphasise more social and critical social psychologies.

Diversity in social psychology is increased because there is a range of different perspectives from which these types of social psychology are approached and an even wider array of methodologies, which are shared by some perspectives but not others. To make sense of such diversity in social psychology, several classification systems have been suggested (e.g., Stevens, 1996c). The one suggested by Doise (1978, see also Sapsford, 1996) will be used to structure the coming chapters.

4.1 Overview of the book

Doise (1978) identified four levels at which explanations and activity in social psychology might be located. Sapsford (1996) prefers to use the term "domain" in order to avoid implying that higher and lower levels differ evaluatively. However, the earlier term will be retained here.

The intra-individual level focuses on structures and processes within individuals. Much literature in the health field is located at this level, since it encompasses biological, cognitive, emotional, and other systems that exist within individuals. A key argument in social psychology at this level is that we can only know the world (including our own part in it) through our cognitions and senses. Thus, we act on what we know, and whether or not there is an objective reality "out there" is a matter of debate. Important questions to arise at this level concern the ways in which the social world is represented in the cognitive systems of individuals and how these representations are acted out in the social world. The type of social psychology most likely to be encountered at this level is psychological social psychology, and experimental methods are also likely to feature.

The second level of analysis in social psychology is the interpersonal level, which deals with structures and processes that exist between individuals. A key contention at this level is that relationships can only be understood through understanding the shared meanings developed by participants, and that these meanings are not apparent to outsiders. Important questions at this level concern the influence of the expectations that individuals bring to new relationships or how power differentials and levels of intimacy vary, and interact with the meanings communicated. The hermeneutic approaches of social social psychology are likely to be especially relevant at this level and experimental methods are likely to play a relatively minor role.

Third, the intragroup level of analysis focuses on structures and processes that exist within groups. Key issues in social psychology at this level are conformity among group members and the ways in which group decisions and behaviours differ from those of individual group members. Important questions concern the ways in which an individual's beliefs and behaviours change as a result of the salience of different group memberships. There is a rich seam of experimental research on groups dating from the 1930s (see H. Brown, 1996, for a review) but more recently other methods such as discourse analysis have emphasised the ways in which group identities can be constructed during conversations and interwoven into personal histories (Wetherell, 1996b).

Fourth, the intergroup level focuses on structures and processes that exist between groups. A central topic in social psychology at this level is the nature of interactions between people who are acting in terms of their group memberships, and important questions concern the effects of stereotypic perceptions. At this level, critical social psychology is likely to be especially relevant, raising awareness of differences in social status and other "arrangements" that have become self-fulfilling.

With reference to levels of analysis, the structure of this book makes sense. Each of the coming chapters begins with a common sense, biomedical view on a selected health issue, which (with the exception of doctor–patient communication) is grounded at an intrapersonal level. The second section of each chapter challenges common sense with case studies and empirical evidence that contradict what is taken for granted. The third and subsequent sections of each chapter attempt to evaluate social psychological influences to make better sense of the issue. These are rival truths to common sense explanations. The final section of each chapter tentatively suggests a more social social psychological approach to the issue. However, although social psychological explanations at all levels of analysis contribute to each chapter, the issues have been selected and ordered so that the emphasis moves from intrapersonal through to an intergroup level as the book progresses.

Thus, Chapters 2 and 3 especially emphasise the intrapersonal level, although other levels of analysis are briefly considered. Chapter 2 considers how the individual knows that s/he has a symptom. The intra-individual world of perception and cognition offers a rival explanation to the common sense idea that symptoms are caused by bodily signs. Chapter 3 focuses on responses to symptoms, specifically on how individuals understand or appraise them. In this case, intra-individual cognitions, specifically schema-based appraisals, offer a rival explanation to the common sense idea that symptoms form the building blocks of rational illness appraisals. However, Chapter 3 also makes an important transition to more social social psychological influences, in arguing that the individual's appraisals might be constructed by forces outside his or her own cognitive structures.

Chapter 4 focuses on the plans individuals make to remedy their symptoms. In particular, it focuses on the decision to seek professional medical help. Since this decision is enacted in the individual's social world, the chapter moves away a little from the emphasis on private worlds. Social psychological influences at all four levels of analysis offer rival explanations to the common sense idea that people seek medical help when they think they have serious symptoms.

Chapter 5 considers what happens if the individual visits a doctor to seek help with symptoms. The common sense level of analysis of doctor–patient communication is interpersonal, and common sense assumptions are that the patient tells the doctor about his or her symptoms; the doctor listens and works out what to do; the doctor advises the patient; the patient takes the advice. Challenges to each of these assumptions are discussed and subsequently all levels of analysis in social psychology contribute to rival explanations. In particular however, group-level analyses trace how conformity to patient and doctor roles might influence communication. The critical argument is that intergroup-level influences provide a backdrop to the relationship between doctors and patients even though only two people might be engaged in a private and confidential consultation. These might subtly transform individually tailored patient care into rituals that reinforce expectations for his or her behaviour.

Chapter 6 considers what happens when the individual feels well again. The focus is on how s/he makes this decision. Common sense assumes that an individual's self-assessment is an intrapersonal matter. It assumes that health status is judged rationally with respect to health beliefs that are like a medical model of health, or perhaps like a more positive model of health as mental, physical, and social well-being. Common sense is challenged by the fact that people often say they are well even though they have serious signs and symptoms. Next, social psychological influences on health beliefs are reviewed. These offer rival views of the cognitive model people might use when evaluating their health, and although all levels contribute explanations, group levels of analysis suggest that relevant health beliefs might belong to situations and groups, as opposed to individuals. Subsequently, social psychological influences on the process of evaluation are considered and a social identity approach is used to understand how a person's judgements about his or her own health might vary according to changes in self-categorisation and creative strategies to protect self-esteem.

The tone of Chapter 7 is different from the rest of the book because it focuses on a single topic, menstruation, and attempts to integrate themes that have been met in previous chapters. A common sense model assumes that menstrual pathology causes disabilities in women's performances and that these disabilities, in turn, cause social disadvantages. Each of these assumptions is challenged with logic and empirical evidence. In the third section social psychological influences on menstrual experiences are reviewed. Although all levels of analysis contribute to the discussion, the emphasis is on group- and cultural-level influences, which suggest that menstrual symptoms, deficits, and consequences are often socially constructed. A critical analysis of menstrual experiences questions who benefits from the assumption that menstrual pathologies cause women to be unable to perform normal roles, and whether the status quo can be resisted. In the fourth section of Chapter 7 a social psychological model is suggested in order to deconstruct the common sense causal relationship between menstrual pathology and its consequences on women's performance and social status.

Chapter 8 ends the book with a review and some suggestions for future directions.

5. Summary

This chapter defined, introduced, or otherwise discussed key theoretical concepts and themes that underpin the chapters that follow.

In the first section, common sense and the medical model of health and illness were defined, and the relationship between them was discussed.

- It was argued that common sense ways of viewing health and illness are often medicalised.

In the second section, four common sense views of health and illness, which are based on the medical model, were challenged in order to outline four purposes of this book and introduce the biopsychosocial model

First, the phrase "the facts are the facts" represented the common sense idea that the medical model deals in objective reality and biological facts. This was challenged by the demonstration that social conflicts can trigger pathological processes, and by the argument that beliefs about a disease can sometimes be more relevant than its presence.

● The relevant aim of the book is to show that human boundaries can be permeated by social psychological influences.

A second common sense view is that given more resources and time, scientific progress will lead to a full understanding of disease. This was challenged by the fact that medical resources cannot continue to be increased indefinitely, and in any case do not guarantee that more advances will be made. Moreover, historical analyses revealed that the medical model evolved out of its social context, and does not represent a progressive accumulation of objective truth.

● The relevant aim of the book is to explore the ways in which beliefs of medical carers are social constructions and how these together with lay beliefs might influence health outcomes. Since these are potentially open to interventions by health psychologists, new ways of alleviating suffering and promoting health might be identified.

A third common sense view is that medical advances are the most effective way of combating disease. This was challenged by evidence that secular changes and people's lifestyles, as opposed to medical advances, often hold the key to health and longevity.

● The relevant aim of the book is to show that social psychological therapies might sometimes be the most effective weapons against diseases.

A fourth common sense view is that medical treatment is the best remedy for ill people. This was challenged by critical analyses which suggested that medical treatment is sometimes more beneficial to doctors than its recipients, whose illnesses may reflect social deviations as opposed to biological dysfunction.

● The relevant aim of this book is to attempt critical analyses to raise awareness that changes in attitude or social arrangements might promote health.

In the third section of this chapter, the biopsychosocial model of health and illness was introduced. What it means to be a person, the importance of shared traditions and beliefs to the human ecology, and the human capacity to act in terms of shared group identities were described in order to justify the social psychological approach of the book.

In the fourth section, the focus was on social psychology itself. From the diversity of approaches in social psychology, four levels of analysis were described, and although all levels will be picked and mixed as appropriate in each chapter, the emphasis moves from intrapersonal to intergroup as the book progresses:

- Chapters 2 and 3 emphasise the intrapersonal world of symptom perceptions and appraisals but show that these are influenced by social psychological factors.
- Chapter 4 considers what individuals do when they have a serious symptom, in particular, why they are likely to delay seeking medical help.
- Chapter 5 considers doctor–patient communication and although the common sense level of analysis for this topic is interpersonal, group-level influences emerge as likely to impede it.
- Chapter 6 considers what happens when the patient feels well again. In particular, the focus is on how s/he knows s/he is well. Again, all levels of analysis contribute to an answer, but the emphasis is on (1) intergroup differences in beliefs about health which provide individuals with social cognitive structures on which to base their judgements; (2) strategies to protect self-esteem, which influence in individuals' judgements of health status.
- Chapter 7 attempts a critical analysis of the consequences of menstruation on women's health, behaviour, and social standing, which integrates all four levels of analysis.
- Chapter 8 provides a brief review and suggests a few future directions.

2

Do I Have a Symptom?
How Do I Know What I Feel?

"Does it hurt when you get shot?"
"I sense injuries. The data could be called pain."
Arnold Schwartzenegger in the film *Terminator II*

This chapter is about the ways in which people perceive symptoms, or how they know what they feel. Throughout it, the example of pain will be given special emphasis because pain has been described as the symptom of most concern (Taylor, 1995). The chapter focuses predominantly at the intrapersonal level of analysis, because it deals with sensations, experiences and decisions that take place within individuals.

In Section 1 key concepts are outlined together with a common sense model in which the symptoms we perceive are a reasonably accurate reflection of bodily signs. In Section 2 this common sense model is challenged by empirical data and a case study, which indicate that people are generally inaccurate in perceiving events in their bodies. In Section 3 types of inaccuracy are briefly identified and laboratory studies are outlined in order to explore the nature of inaccuracy in symptom perceptions. Subsequently some implications of this inaccuracy for measuring pain are noted.

In Section 4 the role of social psychological influences in building a rival explanation of the relationship between bodily signs and symptom perceptions is discussed. Most of this section builds on information-processing approaches which complement rather than rival common sense explanations, but other intrapersonal factors, including personality traits, attitudes, and emotions are briefly considered. Subsequently, interpersonal and group-level influences are also mentioned.

In Section 5 a more social social psychological approach to symptom perception is suggested. In Section 5.1, the Gate Theory of pain is introduced and in 5.2 some initial ideas for a more general model of symptom perception are sketched. A rival to the common sense model of symptom perceptions will be tentatively suggested, in which symptoms can be functional or accurate in the individual's social ecology even if they do not map onto the material world.

1. Introduction and a Common Sense Model of Symptom Perception

---

ACTIVITY 2.1 Consider whether you are currently experiencing any of the symptoms on the checklist below.

Lack of appetite or craving for food	Nervous twitches
Tiredness	Nausea
Indigestion or heartburn	Cramps or muscle spasms
Insomnia	Fainting
Constipation or diarrhoea	Breathlessness without exertion
Chest pain	Impotence or frigidity
(Unexplained) sweating	High blood pressure
Cough	Stomach pains
Headaches	

When you have made your decision, reflect on how you "knew".

In Activity 2.1, it is likely you answered "yes", since Pennebaker and Skelton (1978), for example, found 80% of 1000 healthy students were currently experiencing at least one common symptom. If you are an older adult, female, unmarried, or unemployed, a range of large-scale surveys suggest you are even more likely to be experiencing symptoms (Pennebaker, 1982). This chapter concerns the structures and processes underpinning symptom perceptions, or how you know what you feel. How the individual interprets and responds to symptoms once they have been perceived will be the topics of the next two chapters.

A common sense model of symptom perception is depicted in Figure 2.1. The model is entirely intrapersonal and it has two core assumptions. The first is that bodily signs (which can be measured and verified) are reflected in symptom perceptions, (which are apparent only to the affected individual). A symptom perception can relate to a state, for example a steady heart-rate of 70 beats per minute, or a change, for example an accelerating heartbeat. Pennebaker and Brittingham (1982) use the term "symptom" to mean the subjective experience of physiological events, regardless of whether these are thought to be caused by pathological processes, and the term is used in this way throughout this chapter. Thus, as depicted in Figure 2.1b, the common sense model can be projected to include disease as the cause of signs, where this is appropriate.

The second assumption is that there is a lawful correspondence between signs and symptoms. Thus, the epistemology on which common sense is based is a cognitivist theory of meaning in which objective physical reality takes precedence (Still, 1996b; Wetherell & Still, 1996).

Similar assumptions to those of the common sense model of symptom perception are reflected in Descartes' theory of pain, which was published in 1664. In this,

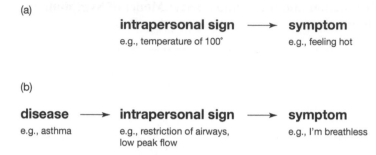

(a)

intrapersonal sign ⟶ **symptom**

e.g., temperature of 100°   e.g., feeling hot

(b)

disease ⟶ **intrapersonal sign** ⟶ **symptom**

e.g., asthma   e.g., restriction of airways,   e.g., I'm breathless
             low peak flow

FIGURE 2.1 Common sense models of symptom perception.

Descartes hypothesised that pain results from injury or damage and the larger the injury or damage, the more intense the pain. Essentially, he conceptualised pain as a system that operates straight from the skin to a pain centre in the brain. Impulses from this centre quickly travel to the site of the injury, which consequently is rapidly withdrawn (see Melzack & Wall, 1988). This highlights a third assumption of common sense models of symptom perception, namely that pain is a reaction of defence that puts individuals on guard against risk of further injury or damage from disease.

Case studies and research both show that common sense models of symptom and pain perception fall short.

2. Challenges to a Common Sense Model of Symptom Perception

2.1 Empirical studies

The common sense model of symptom perception predicts that a disease such as asthma, for example, causes signs, such as restriction of airways and reduction of peak air-flow, which are perceived by the individual as symptoms, such as tightness in the chest and breathlessness. In one relevant study however, Kendrick et al. (1993) studied 255 asthmatic patients from Bristol general practices. Participants were trained in the use of peak flow meters to measure signs of asthma. They were asked to do this regularly and record the result in a diary. They were also asked to complete a visual analogue scale to rate symptom severity at the time of the recordings. Meters were carefully designed to produce a coded answer, so that patients' ratings would not be biased by actual peak flows, but would reflect their own perceptions. Contrary to common sense, the results showed no significant correlation between signs and symptoms of asthma for 155 or 60% of participants.

The field of pain can present challenges to each stage of the common sense model. First, the assumption that pain results from injury or damage is challenged by migraine, which causes pain in the absence of underlying signs. Furthermore, up to 75% of people who have had limbs amputated experience phantom limb pain.

Moreover, causalgia describes an intense burning pain, which can persist after a wound has healed (Melzack & Wall, 1988). Second, the assumption that pain is proportional to the severity of the injury was challenged by a famous early observation that about 25% of soldiers requested morphine for severe battle wounds, whereas about 80% of peacetime patients requested morphine for comparable surgical wounds (Beecher, 1959, cited in Taylor, 1995). Moreover, passing a kidney stone, which is relatively trivial in terms of physiological signs, is said to be "disproportionately painful" (Melzack & Wall, 1988).

The third element of the common sense model is that pain is a reaction of defence that puts the individual on guard. Melzack and Wall (1988) challenge this with the observation that many dangerous diseases such as cancer rarely produce pain in their early stages, when a warning might have adaptive value. Likewise, the pain of a heart attack is paradoxically referred to (i.e. felt in) the left arm.

2.2 Case study

After a restless and disturbed night, the alarm wakes me just after I got to sleep. I drag myself out of bed, not feeling too well. My head hurts; my mouth suddenly waters profusely and my stomach churns. I start the day in the usual manner. I've got a lot of work to do. But cannot face the toast I've just made. I feel sick and shakey. I think I've got a temperature. I look in the mirror. I appear solemn but I don't think I'm pale, or flushed. I ask my partner to feel my forehead. I ask the kids if I look odd. I don't feel right. I return to the bed I just left. I feel guilty about my work, change my mind and get up again. My partner says I'd be irresponsible to go to work. He says he'll phone in for me. He seems concerned. The thermometer shows the decision is not unreasonable . . .

(Anonymous, 2001)

Case studies vividly challenge a common sense model of symptom perception. Surprisingly, physical changes are not necessarily clearly experienced as symptoms. Rather, a range of diffuse feelings seem to transpire out of a negatively oriented context and the individual has to think hard, perhaps enlisting outside help to working out what, if any symptoms s/he feels.

In summary, there is plenty of evidence of a mismatch between signs and symptoms, which challenges the common sense model of symptom perception.

3. The Nature and Implication of Inaccuracies in Symptom Perception

3.1 Types of inaccuracy

Apart from challenging common sense, the mismatch between signs and symptoms has serious implications. To illustrate, treatment for asthma in general practice is

TABLE 2.1 *Types of inaccuracy of symptom perception*

Type of error	Consequences
Type 1 False alarms	• People will perceive many symptoms when changes are few • If so, people who report many symptoms are likely to be less accurate • Services will be over-utilised
Type 2 Misses	• People will perceive few symptoms when changes are many • If so, people who report few symptoms are likely to be less accurate • Services will be under-utilised

guided by patients' symptoms and therefore, poor accuracy in symptom perception might lead to receipt of inadequate treatment (Kendrick et al., 1993). More generally, two types of inadequacy may be distinguished and these are shown in Table 2.1. First, inaccuracy might be characterised by Type 1 errors, (false alarms), in which case individuals will perceive symptoms that are not underpinned by levels of, or changes in, signs. These correspond to "medically unexplained symptoms" or "somatisation" (Deary, Clyde, & Frier, 1997) and related inadequacies of treatments are likely to include suffering the side effects of unnecessary therapies. Knock-on effects at a personal level might include iatrogenic disease. At community levels, they might include the presence of oestrogens and antibiotics in the food chain and the wastage of health resources. Solutions would involve encouraging patients to adopt more stringent criteria and doctors to check signs more closely.

On the other hand, if inaccuracy is characterised by Type 2 errors (misses), individuals will perceive few if any symptoms when physical signs are present. In this case, treatment is likely be inadequate or more likely, non-existent because the individual fails to seek help, or self-regulate. Solutions would involve encouraging individuals or groups to adopt more lax criteria or to take screening tests. The latter, in particular, might be hampered by political concerns about resources.

Kendrick et al. (1993) found both types of inaccuracy, but their study was not designed to explore them further. Pennebaker and his team, on the other hand, investigated more systematically the nature of inaccuracy in symptom perception. Their findings are discussed in the next section.

3.2 Exploring the nature of inaccuracy of symptom perception: Laboratory studies

To examine baseline accuracy in symptom perceptions, Pennebaker and Brittingham (1982) adopted a within-subject approach as the preferred method, since between-subjects designs are particularly vulnerable to individual differences in use of scales and variation in baselines, which can mask other evidence. They asked 15 male and 15 female first-year psychology students to carry out 20 tasks, separated by 2-minute rest periods. Tasks were intended to manipulate physiological states and emotions and included running on the spot, relaxing, and watching gory, sexually arousing, or boring slides. During each task and rest period, three sets of symptoms and signs were measured: (1) self-reported pulse, the concomitant sign being heart-rate; (2) self-reported warm hands and finger skin temperature; and (3) self-reported sweaty hands and galvanic skin response (GSR). As there were 20 tasks and 20 rest periods, it was possible to compute within-subject correlations for the three sets of self-reports and physiological readings. Results showed that the mean correlation between self-reported pulse and actual heart-rate was .2 (ranging from .67 to −.21). For self-reported warm hands and finger skin temperature it was .17 (ranging from .68 to −.49), and for self-reported sweaty hands and GSR it was .05 (ranging from .82 to −.44).

These laboratory studies supported the findings of case and field studies, by suggesting that baseline accuracy of symptom perceptions is low. However, the wide range of correlations shows that some individuals perceived some symptoms accurately, but interestingly, accuracy was not unidimensional. Thus, the common sense idea that some individuals at least are "in touch with their feelings" also did not hold true.

One methodological possibility that might account for such inaccuracy was that the kinds of verbal judgements required in these experiments are unreliable in comparison to a mechanism that is linked directly to action. Such verbal reports might be constrained by language or might reflect inferences about symptoms, rather than direct symptom perceptions. An analogy would be evaluating subjects' verbal descriptions of a spiral staircase. Poor descriptions might not reflect inaccurate knowledge so much as a requirement not to use their hands! To test the theory, Pennebaker (1982) devised a paradigm in which subjects tracked their heartbeats, by means of finger tapping. Again, results showed that the mean within-subject correlation between estimated and measured heart-rate was low and variable. It was only .12 and it ranged from .7 to −.43. On average, estimates deviated from measured heart-rate by 22 beats per minute. Furthermore, self-reported assessments of accuracy did not correlate with calculated accuracy, and a replication allowing subjects more time, more practice, and the opportunity to feel their pulses for 20 seconds, yielded essentially the same results.

Next, Pennebaker and Brittingham (1982) focused on the nature of inaccuracy. A total of 15 male and 15 female first-year psychology students completed the Pennebaker Inventory of Limbic Languidness (PILL), a checklist designed to measure the frequency with which 54 common symptoms are experienced. Subsequently, the participants were assigned to high or low PILL groups and asked to complete a heart-rate tracking experiment. The rationale for the experimental hypothesis (which has already been met in Table 2.1), was that if inaccuracy is characterised by Type 1 errors, *high* PILL scorers should be less accurate, but if inaccuracy is characterised by Type 2 errors, then *low* PILL scorers should be less accurate.

The results showed no difference in accuracy between high and low PILL scorers. Thus, no light could be shed on the typical nature of inaccuracy. However, the experiment did provide a couple of important leads (Pennebaker, 1984). In spite of no difference between the actual heart-rates of high and low PILL scorers, high scorers *thought* their heart rate was higher and more variable. This was taken to indicate that people who experience more symptoms are responding more to external information, irrespective of accuracy levels and although physiological events in their bodies are no more varied than those of people who report few symptoms. Consistent with this interpretation, Pennebaker (1982) describes an earlier study in which participants reported increased stomach contractions or skin temperature as a function of viewing revolting or sexually arousing slides, but not as a function of concurrent physiological measures. Hence, Pennebaker (1984) concluded that although symptom perceptions might not be predictable from physiological signs, they might still be predictable.

Before reviewing some relevant social psychological predictors, the paradoxical question of accuracy in the field of pain will be briefly considered.

3.3 Exploring the nature of inaccuracy of symptom perception: Measures of pain

From the common sense model of symptom perception, it follows that an objective measure of pain could be developed and used to investigate individual differences in the accuracy of pain perception. To develop just such a measure was a goal that occupied many early researchers (Sarafino, 1998; Skevington, 1995). Of course, ethical considerations precluded systematically inflicting injuries of varying type and severity on volunteers (one hopes!), so the typical paradigm employed psychophysiological techniques, exposing volunteers to painful but not destructive stimuli, such as electric shocks, beginning at very low levels and progressively increasing. Participants would be asked to indicate a number of perceptions, the most common being the moment at which they perceived any stimulus at all and the moment at which stimuli became painful. Averaged across a series of trials, these two stimulus intensities would express the individual's sensation and pain thresholds, respectively. The moment at which the participant asked for the stimulus to be withdrawn, together with the latest moment he or she would accept after being encouraged to go on, could also be used to calculate pain tolerance and encouraged pain tolerance thresholds. However, since these latter two measures imply a predominantly interpersonal rather than an intrapersonal level of analysis, they are of little relevance here, and the focus will be on the first two.

Common sense predicts a reliable relationship between the magnitude of stimuli and pain perceptions but in her review, Skevington (1995) remarks that sensation thresholds are relatively reliable, but pain thresholds are characterised by variation and unreliability. Moreover, both ethical standards and ecological validity of relevant studies were frequently dubious because researchers might deliberately confuse participants about procedures, in order to maintain secrecy, outwit malingerers, or eliminate subjectivity. Although more recent approaches have been made more objective by incorporating variables such as activity in muscles in order to reflect tension associated with pain, Skevington (1995) concludes that there is still no objective measure of pain.

A comparison with an imaginary measure of perceived heart-rate sheds further light on some of the reasons why this is so. First, a researcher interested in the accuracy of perceived heart-rate, has actual heart-rate as the common sense objective sign. A pain researcher, on the other hand, has no consensual objective sign of pain and might use voltage, size of wound, or redness of pimple (!) among other variables. Second, the heart-rate researcher can use perceived heart-rate as the concomitant symptom. A further advantage of this variable is that it can be measured in terms of a ratio scale, (such as beats per minute), thereby allowing statistical analyses and comparisons. In addition, 150 beats per minute "is" 150 beats per minute, whether it was caused by jogging or by fear. Pain researchers, on the other hand, have no clear-cut dependent variable, and traditionally had to be content with subjective ratings although more recently they have been able to use measures such as muscle tension. However, they cannot be sure that "excruciating" uttered by a cancer patient is equivalent to "excruciating" uttered by a laboratory volunteer undergoing an electric shock, a coalman who has been off work for 2 weeks with back pain, or a 13-year-old with an outbreak of spots.

Third, it is common sense that the heart-rate researcher will measure both actual and perceived heart-rate in terms of the same scale (i.e., beats per minute) and will assess accuracy according the correspondence between the two, taking the objective sign as the benchmark. The pain researcher, however, has to use different scales (e.g., volts and perceived pain), there is no calibration system to indicate how much pain should accompany a given stimulus level, and no objective benchmark as to where pain "should" begin.

It would be wrong to conclude that researchers into perceptions of measurable bodily signs have an easy life, as Pennebaker (1984) raises a number of additional methodological difficulties. These were designed to help account for the inaccuracy of symptom perceptions in his laboratory studies but can also be extended to the present discussion of pain. For example, he notes that subjects were estimating near baseline rates and speculates that accuracy might be better when physiological signs differ significantly from usual. Alternatively, rather than the absolute levels measured by experimenters, perceivers might encode changes. If so, common sense variables such as beats per minute would need to be replaced by second-order variables such as acceleration in heart-rate (e.g., beats per minute per 5 seconds). Another possibility is that normal perceptual processes entail a "window" of error, and that the magnitude of these windows depends on the level of the sign under consideration. For example an error of 10 beats per minute heart-rate means something different for a person with an average heart-rate of 60 than for a person with an average heart-rate of 120. If so, accuracy becomes a relative concept (Pennebaker, 1982).

Although perception and reporting are conceptually distinct, another potential problem is that it has to be assumed that reported symptoms accurately reflected perceived symptoms. After many debriefings, Pennebaker (1982) was convinced that subjects honestly believed what they reported and his conviction was further justified by the minimisation of differential reinforcement for reporting and self-presentation concerns. In the field of pain, Skevington (1995) similarly remarks that it is extremely unlikely that ethically recruited people in chronic pain or volunteers would systematically attempt to falsify their reports.

In the face of these and other difficulties, observational methods of measuring pain were developed by some researchers who abandoned the search for an objective measure. For example, a range of measures was based on impaired walking, distorted postures, or other such visible behaviours (see Skevington, 1995, for a review). With trained observers, these measures reach acceptable levels of reliability, but they share a problem with observational methods in general, in that events "picked-up" for consideration and the way they are interpreted might say more about the observers than what is being observed (see Banister et al., 1994). Moreover, individuals might feel the same pain but show it differently.

Such problems are circumvented if entirely subjective measures of pain are used, because in these, the individual's experience is paramount, without a need to verify it with reference to some objective benchmark. An example, currently used in a Pain Clinic in Bristol, is depicted in Figure 2.2. Patients use the figures to indicate the site of their pain and then they can use verbal and written descriptions to convey its nature and intensity. Another example is the Visual Analogue Scale (Scott & Huskisson, 1976, cited in Skevington, 1995), which provides an early example. Participants using this simple and reliable method are asked to indicate their level of pain along a line, (optimally 10–15 centimetres in length). The line is anchored at each end by labels such as "no pain" to "worst ever pain". However a serious criticism of the technique is that it represents pain as a unidimensional experience, and Skevington (1995) goes on to question the ecological validity of unidimensional and affect-free approaches to pain measurement in general. She explains that during the 1980s more interest grew in psychometric techniques, which included dimensions of meaning instead. She also argues critically that their development had been retarded by the unfounded concern that they might be manipulated by malingerers (although there was little concern that they might lead to *under*-estimated levels of pain).

The best known psychometric measure of pain, which acknowledges both its subjective and its multidimensional nature, is the McGill Pain Questionnaire. In developing it, Melzack and Torgerson (1971) began by differentiating aspects of pain experiences, by sorting 102 words describing pain into piles. Three general classes of meanings—sensory, affective, and evaluative—emerged. Below these were a number of subclasses. For example, sensory aspects of pain included subcategories concerning its pressure and thermal qualities. Following many additions and refinements, the McGill Pain Questionnaire consists of words from each category, grouped into 16 subclasses together with 4 additional subclasses, making 20 in all.

BODY CHART

Surname–	First names–	Age–	Unit No.–
Consultant–		Ward or Outpatient Clinic–	

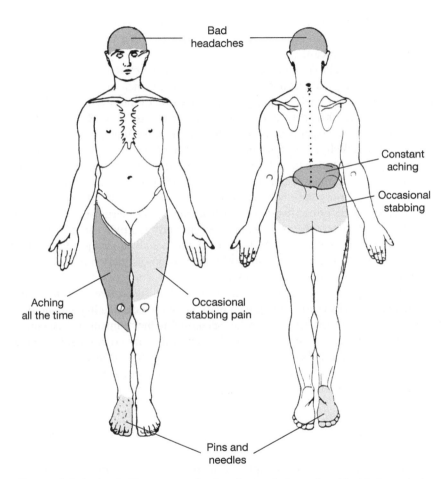

FIGURE 2.2 A visual aid to communication about pain (reproduced by kind permission of the team at the Pain Management Centre, Frenchay Hospital).

To use it, a subject selects the most appropriate descriptor from each subcategory and goes on to rate its intensity. In addition, the measure includes a current Pain Intensity scale and the opportunity to describe its temporal and spatial qualities.

Skevington (1995) notes that the measure is not without problems. One is that the original words were chosen by the researchers, not by patients in pain. Thus, terms such as "lancinating" are included, but not "stiffness" which is a common descriptor given by arthritis patients. Second, it was the researchers and not patients who derived the categories of meaning. Third is the philosophical question of whether pain experiences, or culture-bound words about pain, are being measured. Fourth is the fear that use of the measure might socially construct the experience of pain for respondents in a way that reflects the beliefs of the researchers. Notwithstanding, Skevington (1995) continues that the McGill questionnaire is generally acknowledged as the best to date. Its key strength is that it represents pain as something that is experienced and communicated, rather than something that may be objectively measured.

In fact, the pivotal role of human experience plays a key role in assessing pain in contemporary clinical practice, and multidimensional measures span the impact of pain on the patient's life including his or her views of the way in which others respond (Ambler, 2001, personal communication; Kerns, Turk, & Rudy, 1985). The focus on human experience is also reflected in recent attempts to define pain, but Melzack and Wall (1988) argue that research simply has not progressed enough for an adequate definition to be formulated. They suggest that of Merksey, Abbe-Fessard, Bonica, Carmen, Dubner, Kerr et al. (1986) is the best so far devised: "An unpleasant sensory and emotional experience associated with actual or potential tissue damage, or described in terms of such damage." The merits of this definition include the looseness of the association between injury and pain and the emphasis on negative human experience, which means that pain is always subjective. In other words, within the victim's personal world, there is no distinction made between the misery of actual and potential damage.

What is important for present purposes is that subjective measures and experiential approaches to defining pain mark not only a change in methodology, but also a change of perspective, from the "scientific" to the "humanistic". Accuracy assessed with reference to an objective reality, and with it the common sense model of symptom perception, belong to the scientific perspective. Hence, to the extent that a humanistic perspective is employed in the field of pain, the common sense model has been challenged and found not only wanting, but also irrelevant.

3.4 Conclusions

Contrary to common sense, symptoms, including pain, frequently cannot be predicted from bodily events. This does not mean that they are entirely haphazard. Laboratory studies of external influences on symptom perceptions, together with the acknowledgement that it is the victim's experience that is paramount in pain perceptions, suggest that social psychological structures and processes might provide some useful ways of predicting them. According to Pennebaker (1982) three general psychological approaches have been employed in such studies. These are information processing, labelling, and a third which derives from early interest in emotion. All are at an intrapersonal level of analysis and provide a convenient rough structure for the next subsection (4.1) after which interpersonal and group-level influences will form much shorter subsections (4.2–4.4).

4. Social Psychological Influences on Symptom Perceptions

4.1 Intrapersonal influences

4.1.1 Information-processing approaches I: Stimulus characteristics and attention

In order to investigate intrapersonal predictors of symptom perceptions, recent research most frequently adopts a scientific information-processing paradigm, in which it is assumed that individuals encode, process, and represent physiological stimuli in essentially the same way as other stimuli (e.g., Pennebaker, 1982).

A key feature of information-processing approaches is that individuals have limited capacity and therefore can attend to and encode only a portion of available stimuli. Questions naturally follow, concerning the characteristics that influence the likelihood with which a given bodily event as opposed to another internal or external stimulus will be "picked up" (Pennebaker, 1982). These include dimensions such as complexity, uniqueness, and change, but Pennebaker (1982) remarks that the number of competing cues present is also important. According to cue-competition theory, the probability of encoding a given sign (such as a racing heart) is a function of the ratio of internal to external events. Thus, for a given set of bodily events (such as a racing heart, dry mouth, and cold extremities) the probability of perceiving the racing heart as a symptom will be lower when the individual is in an information-rich environment than when his or her environment is constant or unstimulating (e.g., Pennebaker & Brittingham, 1982).

Cue-competition theory was supported by a significant correlation (–.57) between the number of coughs emitted by an audience and rated interest during each 30-second segment of a film (Pennebaker, 1980). Interestingly, debriefing sessions suggested bodily information was processed at a low level, since participants had not been more aware of tickly throats or coughing during sequences of low content.

More formally, Pennebaker and Lightner (1980) hypothesised that joggers would be less likely to notice internal symptoms of fatigue when running an interesting cross-country course compared with running the equivalent distance in laps around an oval track. In a within-subject, counterbalanced design, 13 inexperienced joggers ran 1800 metres ten times over a 2-week period: five times were cross-country and five times were in laps. Results showed mean running times of 9.2 and 10.1 minutes, respectively, and no difference in reported symptoms or relevant physiological measures. These findings were interpreted as supporting cue-competition theory. It was reasoned that joggers had slowed down in the minimal environmental condition because they had paid greater attention to internal sensations, and consequently had adjusted their speed according to perceived fatigue. However,

Pennebaker (1982) acknowledges that he was simply unable to tell whether differential processing of internal and external information had really occurred and as running time rather than symptom reports had varied, the cue-competition model of symptom perception had not *really* been tested.

For these reasons, Pennebaker and Lightner (1980), conducted a second study in which experimental conditions manipulated whether participants attended to internal or external stimuli, and a treadmill was used in order to control walking time and hence physiological events. On day 1 of the experiment, 56 male participants completed a treadmill walk. On day 2, a week later, they completed a second walk wearing headphones, randomly assigned to one of three conditions. In Condition 1 they heard their own breathing relayed; in Condition 2 they heard moderately interesting street sounds; and in Condition 3 nothing was played. A range of physical signs and symptom perceptions was measured and indicated that symptom perceptions did not differ between groups on day 1. However, on day 2, participants who were forced to process internal information, (i.e., listened to their own breathing) tended to report more symptoms, whereas those who processed external sounds, and to a lesser extent control subjects, reported less. Since data confirmed that potential physiological information was consistent, differential processing must have accounted for the observed differences and this was interpreted as support for cue-competition theory. However, support seems somewhat indirect for at least two reasons. First, to "force" the participants to focus on a given source of information is not a property of the relative number of internal and external stimuli present. Second, the "internal" status of the breathing condition is questionable, since breathing relayed over headphones has been (at least partly) externalised.

In a similar study, Fillingim and Fine (1986) also attempted to manipulate whether internal or external information was processed. They assigned 15 experienced joggers to jog one mile at their normal pace under each of three conditions. In Condition 1 participants listened to a tape under instructions to count the number of times they heard the word "dog". In Condition 2 they were to focus on their breathing and heart rate, and in Condition 3, the control condition, no special instructions were given.

After each jogging session, participants completed a mood and symptom checklist. Each item could range from 1 to 7, with higher scores indicating more symptoms or worse moods. Interestingly, results showed significant differences between conditions on mood and exercise-relevant symptoms, but not on other items. For example "Shortness of breath" was rated 3.60 in Condition 1 (word cue), 4.20 in Condition 2 (internal focus), and 4.33 in Condition 3 (control). Relevant figures for self-reported fatigue were 2.67; 3.93; and 4.00, and for "being pleased" they were 1.87; 2.73; and 2.80, respectively. Planned comparisons showed that the differences were due to the instruction to focus on external words, since internal focus and control conditions did not differ.

Fillingim and Fine (1986) concluded that they had found no evidence for cue-competition theory, since it was the instruction to focus on external information rather than the number of stimuli present that determined decreased symptom perceptions. One might comment that this is not surprising, since to find support for cue-competition theory requires a different design in which the number of external stimuli for a given internal environment *is* manipulated! Notwithstanding, Fillingim and Fine suggest that distraction and mood, which were not systematically explored in the studies so far reviewed, might offer an alternative to cue-competition theory. These might have been overlooked because an information-rich external environment is also likely to be distracting, and it may well be pleasant too.

In a subsequent study Fillingim, Roth, and Haley (1988) therefore set out to investigate the effects of distractors requiring different amounts of attentional capacity on symptom perceptions and performance. More specifically, they hypothesised that the effect of a distractor ought to depend, at least in part, on the amount of attention it requires. In addition, they ensured that differing amounts of attention were not confounded with differences in mood.

In their between-subjects design, 40 female students of rather low fitness rode a bicycle ergometer while performing a distracting task of high or low demand. A further 20 participated in a control condition in which there was no systematic distraction. Results showed no differences in reported symptoms or measured performance as a function of the different experimental conditions. Because there were many methodological differences between this and previous studies, it was not possible to explain the null result and Fillingim et al. (1988) maintained that distraction is a useful strategy for reducing symptom perceptions even if its mechanism is not understood. Once again, however, cue-competition theory does not seem to have been directly tested, because as stated earlier, it depends on stimulus properties, not perceivers or their cognitive strategies.

Overall, therefore, cue-competition theory yields curiously little information about the likelihood with which internal symptoms as opposed to external stimuli will be perceived. A first reason is that it concerns *ratios* between internal and external stimuli, not the amount of external information present. In other words, the intuitive appeal of the stereotypical individual who reports many symptoms because of an unstimulating life, cannot be supported unless it is known that s/he has the same number of internal stimuli as comparative individuals in busier worlds. However, Norretranders (1998) gives the astounding statistic that the brain receives 11 million bits of information from its senses in any given second. Of these only 16 are consciously processed. Against such a backdrop, the idea that cues are scanned, partitioned into external and internal categories, and compared on the basis of their dimensions in order to identify the 16 seems a bit unlikely.

A second criticism of cue-competition theory is that, in spite of its characterisation as an information-processing approach, it depicts the human as an entirely passive receiver of inputs. In this respect, it resembles the common sense model, since what is to be processed, and hence the key determinant of outcomes, is defined in terms of objective reality as opposed to any characteristics of the perceiver. In the field of symptom perception, this would mean that characteristics of signs, such as their size or degree, would determine whether a symptom is felt and this of course, was precisely the position that was challenged earlier in Section 2.

More recent approaches within the information-processing paradigm, however, emphasise more the role of the perceiver. In particular they focus on his or her cognitive structures in guiding attention to and structuring of perceptions. These approaches form the topic of the next section.

4.1.2 Information-processing approaches II: Introduction to schema theory

At medical school, it is well known that learning about a disease results in a proportion of the class perceiving that they have its symptoms (e.g., Taylor, 1995). The cause of "medical student's disease" is a new knowledge structure, which guides the information students encode, and biases the perception of symptoms.

Many terms for such structures are employed in the literature, including sets, expectancies, or working hypotheses (Pennebaker, 1982); illness representations (Leventhal, Nerenz, & Steele, 1984); explanatory models (Helman, 2000); illness prototypes (Lalljee, 1996); and more recently, personal models (Hampson, Glasgow, & Strycker, 2000). The general term "illness schema" is adopted here, in order that convenient use of cognitive literature might be made.

Schemata are unconscious mental structures that underlie the molar aspects of human knowledge and skill (Brewer & Treyens, 1981). They contain abstract generic knowledge that has been organised to form qualitative new structures. Since schemata represent knowledge, not objective fact, they are built on experience, acculturation, communication, and many other social psychological influences. This is why they are relevant here and in subsequent chapters.

Schemata may be envisaged as frames that link elements of knowledge into organised structures, and during information processing incoming experience is incorporated into the elements, and therefore assimilated into what the individual already knows (e.g., Greene & Coulson, 1995). Schemata are hypothesised to operate as unified masses, the whole structure being activated on an all-or-nothing basis (Brewer & Treyens, 1981). This is important because an individual who is attempting to interpret information about bodily signs might find a range of schemata into which that information potentially fits, but at any moment only one schema may be active. Thus, a different symptom should be perceived according to which schema is triggered, and this provides a useful way of understanding variation between symptoms perceived in response to a given sign.

This effect, which is equivalent to what Pennebaker meant by labelling, was illustrated in a study in which an ambiguous stimulus was experienced according to manipulated schema salience (Anderson & Pennebaker, 1980). Participants were 49 first-year psychology students who were assigned to a pain, pleasure, or control condition, according to the experimental instructions they received. The task was simply to place a middle finger on a vibrating board for 1 second. Although it was "dressed up" in technical-looking apparatus, the board was simply a harmless emery board. Subsequently, subjects rated their perceptions on a 13-point scale (scored from −6 "painful" to +6 "pleasurable"). Results showed highly significant differences between conditions. Subjects in the pleasant schema condition averaged about +1 as opposed to about −1 for those in the painful schema condition.

Once active, schemata guide perceptions, since schema-relevant stimuli are perceived more quickly and accurately (e.g., Fiske & Taylor, 1984). A fascinating study of perceived temperature (Pennebaker & Skelton, 1981) demonstrated this effect on the perception of bodily information. Subjects who expected an elaborate placebo (ultrasonic noise) to raise their finger temperature reported raised temperatures. Paradoxically, their reports were generally correct, although overall their temperatures were not raised. This puzzle is resolved if it is hypothesised that signs vary around a mean value and that the schema guided perceptions so that individuals selectively searched for consistent physical sensations and ignored inconsistent ones. Thus, they simply failed to notice (and report) instances when their temperatures fell.

The implication is that symptom perceptions often follow the patient's schemata about bodily structures and processes, rather than anatomical "facts". Helman (2000) reviews early studies which have found the distribution of numbness, weakness, tremor, hysterical pain, and paralysis to follow lay beliefs about body regions and nerves, rather than anatomical science (Waddell, McCullock, Kummel, & Venner, 1980; Walters, 1961). From these and other studies, Helman estimates that two-thirds of lay ideas about organ location are incorrect. Thus, "non-factual" symptom perceptions might be the rule, rather than the exception. Other potential, if unlikely, consequences are illustrated in the politically incorrect joke in Figure 2.3.

In another fascinating study that is also relevant to this issue, Fields and Levine (1981) studied patients who had had impacted wisdom teeth surgically removed under anaesthetic. Two hours later, as their anaesthetics began to wear off, they were given an injection and three hours later still, a second injection. Participants were randomly assigned to one of three double blind conditions: in Condition 1 they received a placebo, then naloxone (a drug that acts as an antidote to opiates and opioids); in Condition 2 participants received naloxone followed by a placebo; and in Condition 3 two placebo injections were received. A second independent variable manipulated the schema participants were likely to use in interpreting their symptoms. This also had three levels (i) they were told that the injections would increase their pain, (ii) they were told that the injections would decrease their pain, or (iii) they were told that the injections would have no effect on their pain. The dependent variable was, of course, perceived pain which was measured after each injection.

From this complex study, many interesting results accrued. The most relevant for present purposes are from Condition 1. Not all of this group reported relief after the first (placebo) injection. However, the important point is that those who *did* report relief, reported increased pain after the second (naloxone) injection, whereas those who did not, reported no change on receipt of naloxone. These results suggest that the placebo effect is schema-based and is mediated by endogenous opioids because, like morphine, they are blocked by the chemical naloxone. Assuming that the experimental instructions were effective, instantiation of a

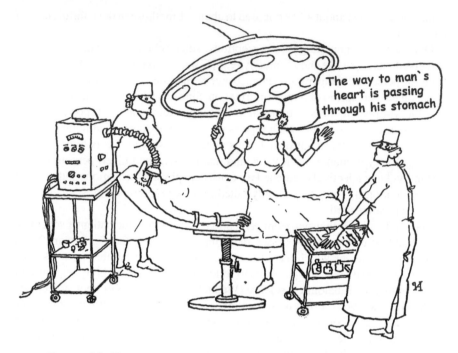

FIGURE 2.3 The way to a man's heart . . . Reproduced with permission from
CartoonStock www.CartoonStock.com

"pain-free" schema does not achieve this effect in all individuals. Clearly, research
to illuminate these individual differences could be of great benefit.

Such studies promote the possible strategic use of pleasant schemata to relieve
pain. For example, a day on a beach could be imaged in order to make an
individual's "beach schema" salient. In this context, painful sensations could be
reinterpreted, say, as cold sensations by imagining that the affected area is resting
against a can of iced drink. One meta-analysis found that cognitive strategies
attenuated pain in around 85% of studies (Fernandez & Turk, 1989; see also Tennen
& Affleck, 1997).

Since schemata are knowledge, they have to be learned, and a final issue concerns
this process. As the present emphasis is on intrapersonal issues and most learning
takes place in a social context (e.g., Durkin, 1996) only a few pointers about the
maturation of pain perception will be raised. Horn and Munafo (1997) describe a
"sorry tale" of underestimation of pain and under-medication in studies of
hospitalised children. Surgery or other procedures, such as circumcision, were
performed on babies without pain relief because it was thought that they had not
yet developed the cognitive structures necessary to experience pain (Bush, 1987).
Bush goes on to cite an early study of the responses of 75 infants to pinpricks
(McGraw, 1963). A few hours after birth there was no apparent response. By

1 week, babies responded with diffuse body movements, crying, and reflex withdrawal. By 1 month, however, they showed increasing organisation, including localisation of response, deliberate withdrawal of the pricked area, and anticipatory avoidant behaviours. According to Bush, the evidence suggests that infants feel less pain only for a short period and that pain perception follows a fixed sequence as cognitive development unfolds.

For ethical reasons, few experiments have investigated children's pain, but existing evidence suggests that pain ratings grow higher until children reach the age of about 12 (Skevington, 1995), and this highlights the importance of both maturation and experience and is consistent with the idea that pain perceptions are underpinned by developing cognitive schemata.

Taken together, the studies so far reviewed suggest that perceived symptoms are an outcome of an interaction between cognitive schemata and signs, and sometimes, of cognitive schemata *per se*. Since schema theory offers a means of accounting for the lack of a common sense link between signs and symptom, it offers a rival truth to the common sense model of symptom perception.

Schema theory will be revisited in Chapter 3 (Section 3.1). However, to return to the present focus the role of many other cognitive variables in symptom perception has been examined. Two of the best known are cognitive dissonance and perceived control, and these will be briefly noted in the next section.

4.1.3 *Other cognitive variables: Dissonance and control*

Cognitive dissonance (see Festinger & Carlsmith, 1959) arises when an individual experiences inconsistency between his or her cognitions. It is an aversive state, which motivates attitude, behaviour, or other changes to relieve it. In one relevant study, Trabin, Rader, and Cummings (1987) investigated 75 men attending an in-patient rehabilitation programme for low back pain, of whom 50 who were receiving disability compensation were compared on a range of dependent variables with 25 who were not. There were no significant differences between groups at the start of the programme, and both groups improved as it went on. At its close however, the compensation group reported a significantly higher level, and the non-compensation group a significantly lower level of pain than was predicted by pre-programme levels.

These results support the idea that compensation might have hidden disadvantages because it needs justification, perhaps in the form of pain, if it is not to create cognitive dissonance. Because this might sabotage pain relief, some therapeutic programmes refuse to accept people involved in litigation (Trabin et al., 1987). Clearly, however, a critical question is who really benefits from such refusal?

Like cognitive dissonance, perceived control has received much attention in the field of pain. Irrespective of objective control, this has many implications for symptom perceptions (Lazarus & Folkman, 1984), and in her excellent review Thompson (1981) attempts to answer the question "will it hurt less if I can control it?". This turns out to have a very complex answer, because there are many conceptions of perceived control and levels of pain. In brief, Thompson found that perceived control over an aversive stimulus (so-called "behaviour control") seems to reduce anxiety, and increase pain tolerance, but does not seem to reduce the amount of pain perceived. Cognitive control, such as denial or relabelling, on the other hand, seems to have more uniformly positive effects on reducing pain experiences. Information control, or knowing when pain is coming, can reduce or increase both anxiety and pain, depending on the situation, whereas retrospective control, or changing the meaning attributed to a painful event, has been relatively successful in reducing pain.

Clearly, these and other cognitive variables further help to explain why a given sign might be associated with a range of different symptom perceptions. As such they contribute to explanations that might rival common sense.

4.1.4 Personality, attitudes and mood

Both professionals and lay people frequently explain human behaviour in terms of stable underlying dispositions such as personality traits and attitudes (Ajzen, 1988). For example, Pennebaker (1982) notes that a propensity to perceive (and report) symptoms may be viewed as a stable personality construct, which is correlated with a range of individual differences including self-consciousness, Type A behaviour, anxiety, repression, self-esteem, and other variables. In addition, studies have focused on the influence of stress and emotions on symptom perceptions (see Lazarus, 1999). Indeed, there seems to be an "embarrassingly rich" (Deary et al., 1997) choice of overlapping psychological constructs, which potentially help to fill the gap between a given sign and the symptom perceived by an individual. Only a few examples will be mentioned here but many more are to be found in Ajzen (1988), Golub (1992), and Lazarus (1999), for example.

4.1.4.1 Personality

Early attempts to predict individual differences in pain perceptions sought to use psychometric techniques in order to identify a "pain personality" and Skevington (1995) describes several such profiles. One of these characterised pain sufferers as high on hysteria, hypochondriasis, and depression. The idea was to use this profile to diagnose individuals who might be more disabled by their pain. Similarly, links between psychological problems and menstrual symptoms were readily interpreted as support for the idea of a psychogenic factor in the aetiology of dysmenorrhea (Golub, 1992). From this perspective, lack of a common sense link between a given bodily state and perceived symptoms could be explained because certain individuals with personality problems simply perceive worse symptoms in response to a given sign or even in the absence of one.

However, such explanations were problematic because the direction of causality could not be isolated. While a "pain personality" might predispose individuals to experience more pain, it was also possible that more pain experience might change personality (Sarafino, 1998). In fact, the bulk of recent research suggests that it is pain that causes personality to change. In the long term, it leads to helplessness and depression, which are exacerbated by interference with the victims' work, social, and family life (Skevington, 1995). That causality is in this direction is supported by observations of chronic pain patients who are cured, whose psychological status rapidly improves once they are pain-free (Skevington, 1995).

There are a number of additional criticisms to make about the idea that certain personality traits can cause pain. For example, the assumption that depression in pain patients is equivalent to depression found in psychiatric patients is incorrect, because it is not so much an enduring trait as an appropriate and realistic response to a disrupted life (Skevington, 1995). Similarly, although depression is often associated with menstruation, it is far less intense than that experienced by psychiatric patients (Golub, 1992, see also Chapter 7, Section 2.3).

4.1.4.2 Attitudes

Research has also sought a causal link between attitudes and symptom perceptions. To distinguish this from the studies already reviewed, it is worth briefly considering differences between attitudes and personality traits, some of which are summarised in Table 2.2.

According to Ajzen (1988), the main difference is that attitudes concern evaluative responses whereas trait-related responses may or may not concern evaluation. A second difference is that personality traits are "outside-in" in the sense that they describe a wide range of an individual's responses in terms of a single (or a small number of) internal dispositions. In turn, such dispositions conveniently classify individuals into personality types. In contrast, attitudes are "inside-out" in that they focus from the person to external targets and conveniently differentiate between behaviours directed at different targets. A third difference is that compared with traits, attitudes are hypothesised to be relatively changeable.

A typical hypothesis about attitudes and symptoms was that career women with a negative attitude towards traditional feminine roles would suffer more menstrual

TABLE 2.2 *Comparisons between attitudes and personality traits (after Ajzen, 1988)*

Similarities	Differences	
	Personality traits	Attitudes
Intrapersonal	Evaluative or neutral responses	Evaluative responses only
Hypothetical	Describe the holder's responses	Describe the holder's disposition
Manifest across	in a relevant domain towards	towards an object, a person, an
a wide variety	the person with the trait, i.e.,	institution, or an event, i.e.,
of observable	inwardly directed	outwardly directed
responses	Less malleable	More malleable

distress (Golub, 1992). Correlations between negative attitudes and menstrual distress were readily interpreted as support for this view (Lyus, 1999). Again, more recent work has discredited this interpretation. For example, comparisons of patterns of correlations suggest that traditional or religious attitudes about women's roles are more closely related to menstrual distress than "modern" attitudes (Paige, 1973). Moreover, cross-cultural evidence shows huge variation in attitudes to menstruation, but relatively small variation in symptoms, which suggests that culture may shape attitudes towards menstruation, but neither culture nor negative attitudes cause dysmenorrhea (Golub, 1992).

In general, research into the causal effects of both personality and attitudes on symptom perceptions has been abandoned, since it was fraught with methodological problems and in any case, failed to predict anything useful, such as suitable treatment (Skevington, 1995). (Notwithstanding, a few exceptions in the field of menstruation will be reviewed in Chapter 7.)

Although individual differences in personality and attitudes might not cause symptom perceptions, they might still moderate the relationship between signs and symptoms so that the extent to which a sign is reflected in a related symptom is different for different individuals. For example, an anxious person might perceive more pain in response to the prick of an injection than his or her non-anxious neighbour. Ajzen (1988) warns against this approach because it is possible to generate an inferential explosion of possible moderators, limited only by the creativity of the researcher. Thus, a self-conscious, self-monitoring, depressed, female anxious person might perceive even more pain, and so on. The resultant proliferation of higher-order interactions quickly becomes unmanageable and the application of moderator variables in order to specify an ever more select subgroup for whom a given relationship applies, means that the group for whom it *does not* apply, grows ever larger. In other word, as Ajzen (1988) points out, the use of moderator variables in order to shore up common sense consistency in this case, between objective signs and symptoms, ultimately leads to a theoretical dead end.

4.1.4.3 Mood

The relationships between moods and symptom perceptions are also complex and have stimulated much research. For example, Levine, Krass, and Padawer (1993) found that perceived failure increased pain reports. They reasoned that the mediator was negative affectivity. In another example, 34 male and 46 female psychology students at an American university were studied over 7 weeks in order to test the hypothesis that people report more symptoms when they suffer from bad moods (Watson, 1988). Many measures were taken, including subjective and objective assessments of physical complaints and "negative affect", a general factor that subsumed a broad range of aversive mood states, including: distressed, nervous, afraid, angry, guilty, and scornful. Over the 7 weeks of the study, the correlation between reported physical complaints and negative affect was .34, suggesting an enduring relationship between bad moods and symptom perceptions. Interestingly, negative affect was not correlated with objective signs, which meant that these could not have caused both negative moods and increasing symptoms and so account for the observed correlation. To explain the observed relationship, Watson (1988) suggested that negative affect leads to an "unsettled and vigilant cognitive mode", which causes the individual to "scan the environment with uncertainty and apprehension". From this point of view, negative affectivity can become a nuisance variable because it leads to the perception of symptoms that are not underpinned by signs (see Salovey et al., 1998, for a more recent discussion).

Interestingly, Watson's (1988) interpretation suggests that schemata mediate the influence of affect on symptoms by biasing individuals to scan for, and hence perceive, more symptoms, as discussed earlier (in Section 4.1.2). However, this still does not mean that the direction of causality is settled. Golub (1992) reviews three studies, which show that women who have experienced stressful life events report more menstrual symptoms. If Watson's interpretation is right, increased symptoms should be experienced because these stressed women have become hypervigilant and anxious, which predisposes them to search for and find negative stimuli such as symptoms. Golub (1992) points out, however, that stress hormones might have a direct physiological effect on menstruation. Thus, more signs might after all underpin the perception of more symptoms, and both schema-based and physiological explanations of the link between negative affect and symptoms might be true. However, even this does not exhaust possibilities, because in the context of chronic fatigue syndrome, Ray, Wier, Cullen, and Phillips (1991) note that psychological distress has variously been described as a part of the syndrome, a risk factor for it, a result of it, or a cause of it!

Thus, although variation in personality, attitudes, moods, and emotions help explain why a given sign might result in different symptoms for different people, the suspicion begins to arise that seeking an explanation to fill the gap between signs and symptoms is to seek an answer to the wrong question. This is because the question itself has not escaped from the strong gravity of the common sense model, in that it begins with a given sign and assumes a lack of correspondence between it and a related symptom *demands* an explanation. This point will be explored a little more at the end of the chapter.

In summary, the probability with which an individual will perceive a given bodily event is influenced by a complex pattern of schema-based processes and other intrapersonal variables. Hence, it is important to consider where these come from and how the social world shapes or changes them. Such more social influences will be briefly considered in the next section.

4.2 Interpersonal influences on symptom perceptions

In a famous early study, Valins (1966) showed men photographs of semi-nude women. While they were viewing, they were given false feedback concerning their heart-rates. The dependent variable was the rated attractiveness of the women, but results were directly relevant to symptom perceptions, since the men's ratings followed the feedback, rather than their actual heart-rates. Thus although the study seems ethically dubious and politically incorrect by current standards, it suggests that information supplied by others can override bodily signs, when perceiving symptoms. Such findings highlight the importance of doctor–patient and other relationships, and in support of this idea, Hyland, Finnios, and Irvine (1991) found that symptoms experienced by asthma patients during asthma attacks were not related to pulmonary function but correlated with steroid prescribing and physicians' judgements of severity. Similarly, an over-solicitous spouse can inadvertently reinforce and exacerbate pain (Horn & Munafo, 1997; Sarafino, 1998).

A study in the field of pain warns that the influence of family relationships on perceptions is likely to be extremely complex. In a comparison of four ways of assessing pain, Gill, Shand, Fuggle, Dugan, & Davies (1997) studied 25 children with sickle cell disease and 25 normal controls aged 7 to 16. Participants kept diaries that assessed a number of health-related experiences including duration, intensity, and frequency of pain. In addition, they and their parents were inter-viewed. Concurrent measures of the total impact of pain included disruption of daily life, days off school, and for the children with sickle cell disease, the number of days in hospital.

Results suggested parent and child interviews were both poor methods of assessing pain because they failed to correlate with other measures, seemingly underestimating pain compared with diaries. Parents underestimated more than children and, paradoxically, controls reported more pain over the previous month than the children with sickle cell disease. Gill et al. (1997) were unable to offer an explanation for these findings but suspected that parents might underestimate their children's pain in order to help themselves cope with it. However, they noted that diary measures did correlate with impact scores, days off school, and days in hospital. Thus, this intriguing study suggests that the experience of pain might be influenced by parents' responses to it, but that the parents' responses are moderated by differences in coping strategies and might not reflect symptom severity.

Similarly, some dentists give pain-killing injections for dental fillings, in order to relieve their own stress at the prospect of hurting the patient! Moreover, patients who have to pay for injections often consider them entirely unnecessary (St. Claire, 2000).

Overall, variations in interpersonal relationships can help explain why a given sign might result in different symptoms for different people. Once more, these explanations often do not rival common sense. Rather, they seem to explain away challenges to it by showing how a symptom does after all map onto a related sign. However, the suspicion begins to arise that causality might sometimes be in the opposite direction.

4.3 Intragroup influences on symptom perceptions

Intragroup-level influences on symptom perceptions are shown in another famous seminal study in which subjects were given injections of ephedrine, which causes sympathetic nervous system arousal. Injections were administered under one of three conditions: (i) correct information concerning side effects of the drug was given, (ii) misleading information concerning side effects of the drug was given, or (iii) no information was given (Schacter & Singer, 1962). After the injection, participants were asked to wait with a confederate of the experimenter while it took effect. There were two waiting conditions. In the first, the confederate behaved in an euphoric manner, for example, launching paper planes into the room. In the second, the confederate behaved in an aggressive manner, for example, kicking the waste bin. When asked about their feelings, there was a tendency for subjects who were misinformed or uninformed to report symptoms that conformed to the behaviour of the confederate, even though all participants experienced essentially the same physiological arousal. As an aside, it is worth noting that this process might underpin so-called mass psychogenic illness, a phenomenon in which many individuals appear to perceive the same symptom(s) in the absence of any known physiological concomitants (see Suls, Martin, & Leventhal, 1997, for a recent discussion).

The studies so far reviewed concern relatively short-term influences. However, there is evidence that family interactions have long-term influences on symptom perceptions. For example, Pennebaker (1982) reviews three other hypotheses, which link socialisation experiences with later symptom reporting. The first simply proposes that children learn their parents' strategies for interpreting signs. Thus, children who experience many symptoms should have parents who show a similar pattern. Second, children in aversive family environments experience more symptoms, both as a result of stress-related autonomic arousal and as a result of increased attention, which serves directly to reinforce symptoms and indirectly reinforces them by reducing family conflict. Third, a number of related proposals emerge from psychoanalytic theory. These revolve round the notion that increased symptom perceptions arise because anxiety-provoking sexual experiences, worries, or other conflicts have been converted into physical sensations. Overall, however, Pennebaker (1982) concludes that the higher prevalence of symptoms in individuals who experienced a troubled childhood is consistent with any of these interpretations but there is only weak empirical support for any one of them.

Thus an alternative approach might prove more successful. Seminal work on the formation of norms suggested that once formed, norms provide the individual with long-lasting frames of reference (Sherif, 1936). To recap on the original paradigm, subjects were placed in a darkened room and observed short displays of a pin point of light for about 2 seconds. Their task was to state out loud how far the light moved. In fact, the light was stationary, but since conditions were right for an optical illusion known as the autokinetic effect, it seemed to move. Some subjects performed the task in isolation first and they soon developed a characteristic individual range within which their judgements fell. Second, they repeated the task in groups of three or four, and a mutual convergence in estimates reflected the development of a group norm. The point is that this persisted even when individuals made further judgements in isolation. Thus, the interesting question is whether analogous frames of reference for symptom perceptions emerge during development and are internalised to exert long-term effects.

A longitudinal study of 350 mother–child pairs (Mechanic, 1980), suggests that they do. Initial data were gathered in 1961, when children were 10 and 14 years old. Sixteen years later, their reports of 15 common physical complaints (such as headaches, coughs, aches and pains, constipation, diarrhoea, vomiting, and skin problems) in the last 3 months were assessed and eight groups of social, psychological, and physical variables were measured as predictors. In the first stage of analysis, results showed that subjective reports of poor health and psychological distress explained most variance in the number of reported symptoms. However, further analyses suggested that these were in turn influenced by family interactions, especially their mothers' reactions to their childhood illnesses. Consistent with Watson's (1988) conclusions (see paragraph 4.1.4.3 above) high levels of attention and keeping the child off school were thought to contribute to a pattern of internal monitoring and increased attention to bodily sensations. This, it was argued, increased the detection and reporting of symptoms.

In summary, there is plenty of evidence that intragroup influences help build rival explanations to the common sense ones of the gap between signs and symptoms, and that an important part of these explanations is likely to involve the internalisation of norms.

4.4 Intergroup- and cultural-level influences on symptom perceptions

The common sense model of symptom perception predicts that large-scale intergroup differences in symptom reporting reflect genetic differences, variations in diet, access to medical facilities, exposure to pathogens, or other objective variables. A challenge to this model is posed by Pennebaker (1982, 1984) who cites a conglomeration of survey data demonstrating that women report more symptoms than men, while shorter life expectancies and higher morbidity suggest that more pathological signs exist in men. Since his studies demonstrated no systematic differences in accuracy (e.g., Pennebaker and Brittingham, 1982), the possibility arises that intergroup-level social psychological influences, including cultural differences, account for differences in symptom perceptions.

One suggestion concerning the way in which cultural differences in symptom perceptions might be mediated, is the possibility that social circumstances may underpin negative moods which result in increased symptom perceptions for a given set of signs. Another is that cultural differences in relevant health beliefs and practices exist and influence schema development (e.g., Helman, 2000; Pennebaker, 1982). If so, the schema concept can also provide an explanation for the ways in which social psychological influences "get inside" symptom perceivers.

More generally, Helman (2000) conceptualises culture as a meta-system of implicit meanings and explicit rules that individuals inherit by virtue of their membership of society. These rules are present in a society's language, symbols, and rituals, and they inform its members how to view and experience the world. An example is an individual's body-image which not only includes his or her intrapersonal attitudes, feelings, and wishes, but also reflects cultural influences that shape the ways in which s/he has learned to organise and integrate bodily experiences and the ideal shape to which s/he aspires.

In yet another famous early study, Zola (1966) set out to test the hypothesis that such cross-cultural differences in meanings, as opposed to signs, could account for cross-cultural differences in symptoms. Over 200 new hospital patients were interviewed before they had seen a doctor. Patients were from three ethnic groups, (ethnic group being taken as a measure of culture), and were carefully matched according to diagnosis and a range of social variables in order to control for signs. The idea was to observe whether cultural differences in symptoms remained after signs had been controlled. Results supported the "culture" hypothesis. For example, Irish participants tended to focus on specific bodily complaints and understate their difficulties, whereas matched Italians described more symptoms and saw them in more general terms, such as energy or emotions. Such differences were hypothesised to reflect cultural roles and literature. Thus, for the Italians, the large number of symptoms were understood in terms of "cultural expressiveness". For the Irish, on the other hand, the main cultural outlet was thought to be alcoholism and the relevant attitude was "the less said the better".

Cross-cultural differences in meanings might also explain differences between cultures in responses to pain, which to Western eyes appear most vivid in societies where the pain of mutilation is tolerated because it represents an initiation or a religious honour (Horn & Munafo, 1997). Indeed, Helman (2000) comments that cultural norms may sometimes act against the direct biological needs of the individual.

4.4.1 Conclusion

Plenty of evidence suggests that culture can influence an individual's perception of a given sign. However, little has been said about the ways in which the relationship might be mediated. In fact, the implicit explanation has been individualistic in nature, since it has simply been assumed that members of a given culture or group have been exposed to the same meanings, assimilate them into their schemata, and go on to replicate them. A rival explanation can be gleaned from an interesting study of equal numbers of men and women who were tested by attractive male and female experimenters in a factorial design (Levine & De Simone, 1991). Results showed that women reported higher levels of pain, but of more interest was a significant interaction in which men reported less pain to female experimenters. This was interpreted as indicating that conformity to a tougher male stereotype had occurred and this implies that strategic conformity to cultural norms as opposed to exposure to them is the important factor. It is important to note that the study concerned pain reports as opposed to pain perception, however the authors note that other studies either show no sex differences in pain thresholds or that men have higher thresholds. They also point out that previous studies have not enhanced the salience of gender identity. The intriguing possibility arises therefore that conformity to cultural norms might also affect pain perception.

In the field of pain, Gate Theory suggests a physical basis for cultural influences, and therefore it will be briefly introduced in the next section before some suggestions for a more social psychological model of symptom perceptions are made.

5. Towards a More Social Social Psychological Model of Symptom Perception

5.1 Introduction to the Gate Theory of pain

A paradigmatic shift in the understanding of pain was made with Gate Theory, which was first suggested by Melzack and Wall in 1965 (Melzack & Wall, 1988). The visionary aspect of the approach was the move from a linear to a synergistic pain transmission system which incorporated physiological and psychological influences with "only limited specificity to noxious stimulation" (Horn & Munafo, 1997).

Briefly to outline the approach, Melzack and Wall (1988) describe two general classes of afferent fibres which are involved in conveying sensations to the spinal column from the skin, internal organs, joints, and muscles. The first class comprises A-delta and A-beta fibres, which are myelinated and therefore allow impulses to travel quickly. A-delta cells are associated with sharp, localised "first pain" experiences, and A-beta cells seem to inhibit pain experiences, unless they are exposed to higher levels of stimulation in which case they facilitate A-delta activity and exacerbate pain. The second class of afferent fibres comprises smaller, unmyelinated C fibres. These seem associated with diffuse, dull pains, perhaps reflecting the tissue chemistry of inflammatory responses to burns or arthritis (Melzack & Wall, 1988; Skevington, 1995). According to the theory, the relative inputs from these fibres are processed in so-called T cells (transmitter cells) which are located in the grey matter of the dorsal horns of the spinal column. The output from these transmitter cells travels to the forebrain, and from there it is relayed to the sensory cortex.

The important point for present purposes is that, as its name suggests, the theory postulates that a gate-like mechanism is involved in the experience of pain. This is thought to be located in, or at least mediated by, the T cells (Melzack & Wall, 1988; Skevington, 1995). When the gate is closed, afferent fibres transmit information about bodily movements and other sensations to the T cells, and thence on to the brain. If the gate is open, however, the sensations are experienced as painful.

One of the strengths of Gate Theory is that the flow of information is not one-way. On the contrary, once the gate is open and pain is perceived, a number of descending central control systems tend to close it. The most likely mediators of these effects are opioids that inhibit T cell activity (Horn & Munafo, 1997; Melzack & Wall, 1988; Skevington, 1995) and under some situations, such as extreme stress, pain might not be felt at all. Conversely, central control mechanisms can also facilitate the level of stimulation in afferent fibres and this accounts for the effect of anxiety and attention on pain.

A schematic representation of Gate Theory is depicted in Figure 2.4 which emphasises that whether pain is felt depends on what happens at the gate, not what happens at the site of an injury or pain location. What happens at the gate in turn depends on the overall patterning of ascending and descending inputs.

The complexities of current physiological pain research are beyond the scope of present chapter, but are reviewed by Skevington (1995) who notes a number of unresolved weaknesses in Gate Theory. For example, neither the location of T cells nor the relevant neural processing systems have been conclusively identified. In addition, the presence of multiple multi-synaptic systems means there is ample opportunity for pain signals to be further modified between the thalamus and the cortex, where they are likely to be combined with social psychological and other

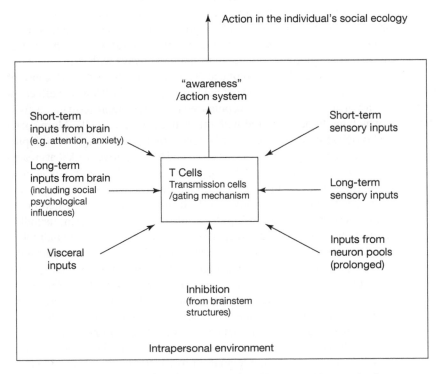

FIGURE 2.4 A schematic representation of the Gate Theory of pain
(after Melzack & Wall, 1988).

information. Notwithstanding, Skevington (1995) concludes that the Gate Theory of pain is the best available to date because it does not conceptualise pain as a direct result of stimulation from nerve endings, but as a gestalt that emerges from the whole person. Because part of this gestalt includes long-term inputs from the individual's brain, social psychological influences such as culture, intragroup expectations, family relationships, and so on are also accommodated.

5.2 Towards a more social psychological model of symptom perception

A model of general symptom perception needs to accommodate the "unreliable" correspondence between a given physiological sign and the symptom perceived by incorporating a range of intra-individual cognitive variables and wider social psychological influences. Thus, a sensible beginning is to borrow Gate Theory as a basis of symptom perceptions in general. A consideration of graded pain control (Melzack & Wall, 1988) shows that this is nothing new, since Gate Theory already accommodates other symptoms. To explain, the end goal of pain control is that the person should feel nothing in the area that once hurt. However, for chronic pain patients who have been unable to reach this goal, alternative goals might be identified. For example, the person might learn cognitive coping skills, such as distraction or guided imagery so that, although s/he still feels something, it is no longer pain (Taylor, 1995). That something might be "tingling" or "throbbing" and this means those symptoms are likely to share pathways with pain.

Gate Theory is essentially physiological (Horn & Munafo, 1997). Because of this, it is pitched entirely at an intrapersonal level of analysis. Thus, the effects of distraction and such variables are conceptualised in terms of short-term inputs from the brain, which are to be processed with other inputs in the T cells. More social social psychological influences are simply conceptualised as longer-term inputs from it. However, these inputs are taken as given and the cognitive work that created them does not receive further consideration. In a more social social psychological model the possibility arises that the individual's own cognitive structures and processes have not done this cognitive work. It might have been created in the context of an interpersonal relationship. It might reflect a group norm, including perhaps a family tradition that was created by a grandparent whom the individual never even met. It might even have been created by politicians and go against the interests and purposes of the perceiver. Moreover, it might not be cognitive *per se*, but coloured by hot emotions which themselves might not be the work of the individual. In a more social social psychological model of symptom perception, the nature and operation of such social influences needs to be accommodated.

A great strength of Gate Theory is that it does not define sensory inputs in terms of the characteristics of external signs. Thus, it accommodates the suspicion raised earlier (in 4.1.4) that seeking an explanation to fill the gap between signs and symptoms is to seek an answer to the wrong question. This is because this question assumes that a lack of correspondence between a sign and a related symptom *needs* an answer. In turn this means it is underpinned by the common sense assumption that the objective sign "should" determine what is to be perceived.

To consider the issue in more depth, it is helpful to digress for a moment and think about photographs instead of signs as stimuli for perceptions. Recent research has made progress in defining universal facial characteristics that result in a human face being perceived as attractive. An example is facial symmetry. This can be calculated with respect to the "golden ratio" of 1.618 which is to be found throughout nature. Because symmetry is a visible marker of fertility, to find a symmetrical face attractive is evolutionarily fit and this is why the preference is universal (e.g., Archer, 2001). To facilitate such research, objective measurements can be made of a photographic image, and its attractiveness determined. To flip back to the field of symptom perception, this is analogous to determining the objective properties of a physical sign.

Individual differences in the rated attractiveness of a given image could be explained by variation in information processing and the addition of moderators, such as personal tastes, attitudes, and emotions. If the parameters are known, attractiveness scores for a given image might be calculated for an individual. This is analogous to attempting to explain the gap between measured and perceived heart-rate with intrapersonal variables.

It is easy to see that a perceived attractiveness score calculated to take such intrapersonal variables into account might miss the mark, since the attractiveness of an image is likely to change if the person depicted is known to the perceiver. Indeed, it might vary dramatically according to ups and downs in their relationship! This is analogous to acknowledging that interpersonal influences might overlay and modify intra-individual influences on the gap between signs and symptoms.

Finally, normative fashions, markers of wealth, or political events such as terrorist attacks might influence perceived attractiveness of an image and this is analogous to acknowledging group-level influences.

To expand Gate Theory (or adopt another approach) in order explicitly to incorporate all these levels of social influences in a model of symptom perception is a tall order, but even this does not go far enough. To picture what is missing requires some magic. What it has to achieve can be understood by considering one of the most charming ideas in the current Harry Potter books (e.g., Rowling, 1997), namely "wizard photographs" in which the images smile and wave at viewers. The images have been bewitched so they maintain some characteristics of the people depicted. Thus, they respond to viewers and events, for example, smiling vigorously at a loved one, tut-tutting at overheard conversations, or showing offence at a disliked viewer. Thus, an image in a wizard photograph would *make* itself more attractive to a loved one, or even compete with other images to get his or her attention. Wizard photographs offer a better analogy than normal images for symptom perceptions because symptoms can demand attention according to their relationship with the perceiver. For example, a racing heart is not simply an additional 50 beats per minute. It is something that grabs attention because of what it means to the person. In addition, it might arise or change as a result of the attention it has elicited.

Thus, in a more social social psychological model of symptom perception, stimuli and perceivers have a synergistic relationship, so that stimulus characteristics that lead to stimuli being processed are likely to be a joint function of both.

Against a backdrop of multiple social influences, and non-linear and even "reversed" causality, questions of accuracy with respect to objective benchmarks seem irrelevant. Perhaps a more relevant question is whether symptom perceptions might after all be "accurate" if judged according to the social world in which perceivers live.

To illustrate the point, Pennebaker (1982) describes an early study in which physiological measures of arousal and perceptions of fear were measured in parachutists. Correspondence between measures and self-reports was low, but interestingly the novices were relatively more accurate than the experienced jumpers. This suggested that the experienced jumpers had learned to suppress awareness of their physical states. However, this was likely to be highly adaptive, perhaps by releasing capacity to process information about the jump or otherwise increasing the ability to cope with it. Furthermore, it is interesting to note that symptoms have the potential to become self-fulfilling, in the sense that a low rating of anxiety might feed back to reduce arousal. Indeed, this should not be surprising for, as Scherer (2001) argues, an important function of emotional feelings is to allow monitoring and control of the self.

This leads us to question why symptom perceptions should be expected to be accurate with respect to a physiological analogue, devoid of social meaning. These truths were unknown to men and women in previous ages, and only emerged to challenge their accuracy in a world of stethoscopes, galvanic skin response monitors, sphygmomanometers, and so on. Likewise, even "useful" pain such as appendicitis pain presumably was of no use before May 1880 when Lawson Tait became the first surgeon to perform deliberate appendectomy for acute appendicitis (Rains & Capper, 1968). More especially, its usefulness might be said to have evolved between then and the advent of antibiotics and anaesthetics. Interestingly, it might even be of more use to the doctor than the patient, since it "may be said to have served its purpose as soon as the doctor has been sent for and has satisfied himself [sic] of its presence" (Roberts, undated). In other words, the expectation that symptom perceptions should be accurate with respect to a physiological analogue reflects the dominance of a common sense, scientific view of reality, in which the "real" truth is the one that can be measured with scientific instruments and even confirmed by doctors.

The overall conclusion is that the "inputs" for a more social psychological model of symptom perception are meanings, in the sense that stimuli that are experienced as symptoms are those that are more meaningful to the perceiver. This means that what people think about their symptoms and what they plan to do about them needs to be included as top-down influences in a model of symptom perception. Thus, a more integrated social psychological model of illness in which such meanings and decisions interact with symptom perceptions will be suggested at the end of the next two chapters, which consider thinking about symptoms and deciding whether to seek professional help for them, respectively.

6. Summary and Conclusions

This chapter was about the ways in which people perceive symptoms.

In the first section, key concepts were outlined together with a common sense model of symptom perception in which the symptoms we perceive are depicted as a reasonably accurate reflection of bodily signs.

In the second section, this common sense model was challenged by a case study and empirical data, which indicated that people are generally inaccurate in perceiving events in their bodies.

In the third section, the nature of inaccuracy in symptom perception and some of its implications were discussed.

- Two types of inaccuracy were briefly identified.
- In inaccuracy characterised by Type 1 errors (false alarms); individuals perceive symptoms, which are not underpinned by levels or changes in signs. Possible results include wasting health resources and suffering the side effects of unnecessary therapies.
- In inaccuracy characterised by Type 2 errors (misses), individuals will perceive few, if any, symptoms when physical signs are "remarkable" or changing. Possible results include failing to seek help, or to self-regulate, both with possible life-threatening implications.
- Laboratory explorations of inaccuracy in symptom perceptions suggested that both types of inaccuracy abound.
- A useful finding was that inaccuracy might not reflect random error, but greater responsiveness to external stimuli.
- The search for an "accurate" measure of pain was discussed.

In the fourth section the role of social psychological influences in building rival explanations to common sense of the relationship between bodily signs and symptom perceptions was discussed.

- Most of the section was pitched at the intrapersonal level of analysis and concerned information-processing approaches such as cue-competition theory and schemata, although other intrapersonal factors including emotions were also briefly mentioned.
- Interpersonal and group-level influences on symptom perceptions were briefly touched upon.

In the fifth section, a more social social psychological approach to symptom perception was suggested.

- The Gate Theory of pain was introduced. This theory began a shift in perspective because it suggested that pain perceptions depend on the processing of a range of psychological and physiological inputs and not on events at the site where pain is felt.
- A more social model of symptom perception could usefully build on Gate Theory, but such a model needs to incorporate the socially constructed nature of the stimuli.
- It was concluded that the inaccuracy of symptom perceptions with respect to the material world might not need explanation in a rival framework to common sense, in which the accuracy of symptom perceptions is evaluated with respect to the individual's social ecology.

Overall, the question of accuracy in symptom perceptions seems to have created more heat than light because it is divorced from the world of human meaning and experience. Pennebaker (1982) makes a related point that humans might be better adapted to perceive more global and meaningful states such as fear, hunger, stress, and illnesses rather than specific symptoms. It is patently the case that most people do self-regulate adequately most of the time, and in spite of the idiom, few would really "shop till they drop"! These perceptions involve integrating and interpreting a range of physical and other information. Thus, the next chapter moves from symptom awareness to the wider issues of interpreting and understanding symptoms.

3

I've got a Symptom. Am I Ill?

Distension, rigidity, vomiting, pain,
Are actors abdominal, which often deign
To act on behalf of the chest, spine or brain,
Or general ills of which typhoid's the main.

> From *The Acute Abdomen in Rhyme* by Zachary Cope, undated,
> cited by Rains and Capper (1968)

"—the trouble is, humans do have a knack of choosing precisely those things
which are worst for them."

> Professor Dumbledore in *Harry Potter and the Philosopher's Stone*
> (Rowling, 1997)

This chapter begins where the last chapter ended, that is with a symptom perception. Thus, it begins when the individual knows s/he feels hot, cold, itchy, sore, hurt, or whatever. Rather than dealing with the question of accuracy and the intra-individual processes leading up to this moment, the focus of this chapter is on what people think next. More specifically, the focus is on how people organise and understand, or appraise their symptoms.

In Section 1 key concepts are discussed and a common sense model suggests that people appraise symptoms rationally. This predicts that a symptom appraised as painful, debilitating, or bothersome will be further appraised until the individual understands or otherwise resolves it.

In Section 2 this model is challenged by empirical studies and a case study, which demonstrate that delay characterises appraisals of even life-threatening symptoms.

In Section 3 social psychological explanations for such delays are suggested as rivals to the common sense model of symptom appraisals. Section 3.1, which is pitched at an intrapersonal level, draws further on schema theory, and in Section 3.2 interpersonal influences on symptom appraisals are briefly examined. Section 3.3 makes the important transition to more social social psychological influences. In it, social factors are not just conceptualised as external influences on an individual's symptom appraisals. Rather it will be argued that appraisals might be created in social interactions, which take place outside the individual's cognitive structures and processes. Alternatively, the individual might be acting as a group member when s/he appraises a symptom.

In Section 4 some suggestions for a more social social psychological model of symptom appraisals are suggested. It is argued that the common sense model reflects a scientific or medicalised perspective, which assumes that symptom perceptions are the building blocks of later cognitions. Rather than this unidirectional influence, it is concluded that social cognitive influences not only colour symptom appraisals but also contribute to the creation of the symptoms themselves.

1. Introduction and a Common Sense Model of Symptom Appraisals

Illness has been defined as "the subjective response of the patient and of those around the patient to his or her being unwell; particularly how the patient and they interpret the origin and significance of this event; how it affects his or her behaviour and relationships with other people; and the various steps taken to remedy the situation" (Helman, 2000).

According to the definition, an individual can have some undetected disease without being ill or can be ill in the absence of any physiological abnormality, a circumstance which, incidentally, pertains to 40% or 50% of patients (Skevington, 1995). Thus, in the context of illness, the question of accuracy with respect to underlying signs is not an issue. The focus of this chapter is on the early stages of illness, that is, on the ways in which individuals interpret the origin and significance of symptoms that make them feel unwell. In other words, the focus is on how individuals understand or appraise their symptoms. The focus of the next chapter is on later stages of illness, namely on the steps taken to remedy the situation. Of course, this distinction is artificial, since understanding a symptom is likely to shape later decisions about it. Notwithstanding, it is worth keeping for two reasons. First, to deal with both stages together would result in an unmanageably long chapter. Second, there is an important theoretical distinction between symptom appraisals and planning what to do, since the former concerns intra-individual thought and the latter concerns turning thought into action in the external world.

A common sense model of symptom appraisal is depicted in Figure 3.1. It begins with symptom perception (without addressing underlying signs). The model is based on a scientific, information-processing perspective. Thus, its major assumption is that symptom perceptions form the building blocks of later appraisals, the information flowing through ever more elaborated stages until a rational under-standing is achieved. An early stage of processing is a cognitive representation, in terms of which symptom perceptions are organised. On its basis, the individual evaluates whether s/he is ill, that is to say, whether a problem is indicated or whether the symptoms can be ignored. When illness is appraised, the model predicts that the symptoms will be further appraised, until they are understood or resolved in some way.

Rationality is defined in terms of the fit between the symptoms and the ways in which they are appraised. Thus, symptoms appraised as painful, debilitating, or

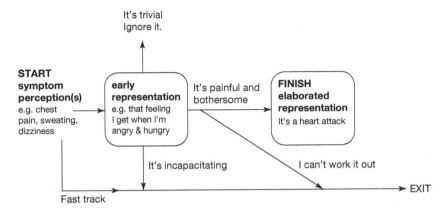

FIGURE 3.1 A common sense model of symptom appraisal.

in some way bothersome should lead to an appraisal of illness. Likewise, there should be a match between the characteristics of the illness and the way in which it is understood. Thus, common sense predicts that symptoms appraised as intense and disruptive should be identified as serious and resolved quickly.

Only one early and one late stage are shown in the model. This is for the sake of clarity. In real life, there are likely to be many stages, which are not distinct but which mature out of each other.

Appraisals may not be possible for people who are rapidly overcome by extremely severe or incapacitating symptoms and a pathway for these is represented by the fast track exit of the model. This simply represents a resolution, such as seeking urgent help, without deliberation. This could even be organised by others if the individual is incapable. If an individual is unable to achieve an understanding of his or her symptoms, the model predicts that s/he will recognise this, cease further appraisals, and in effect join the fast track.

The model is not at all relevant for those who suffer mental delusions or who are otherwise unaware of problems that cause them to be appraised as ill by others. Likewise, it does not apply to very young children or anyone for whom appraisals are made by others.

Overall, empirical and case studies show that the common sense model of symptom appraisal falls short.

2. Challenges to a Common Sense Model of Symptom Appraisal

2.1 Empirical studies

DiMatteo and Friedman (1982) estimate that up to 70% of the people who die from a heart attack, die *before* receiving any medical treatment. For half of these, it was probably the delay rather than the heart attack that was fatal, because deaths usually result from ventricular fibrillation, which can often be reversed provided that treatment is administered within about an hour. Typically, however, almost 50% of heart-attack victims arrive at hospital at least 4 hours after they first perceived their symptoms (see Cacioppo, Andersen, Turnquist, & Petty, 1986). Although it is not possible to conclude with certainty that it is symptom appraisals that account for this delay, this is the most likely interpretation because it seems beyond belief that an individual, having appraised that s/he is in mortal danger, would take so long to obtain help.

Consistent with common sense, people do try harder to understand unexpected, serious, pains (Skevington, 1995). More challenging, however, is the fact that individuals often do not cease appraisals (and seek help for example) if they are unable to understand worrying symptoms. On the contrary, many continue to try to explain them unaided, and the more they fail, the more likely they are to become depressed (Cacioppo et al., 1996). Consistent with this picture were the results of a study in which 55 patients with rheumatoid arthritis were asked to explain what they thought caused their disease. Eight were unable to give an explanation, and these were more anxious, depressed, and hostile than those who could (Lowery, Jacobsen, & Murphy, 1983).

2.2 Case study

Case studies offer vivid challenges to the common sense model of symptom appraisals.

Jim Milne, 58, looked forward to a weekend's relaxation after 3 months of unusually gruelling work. The first night's highlight was to be a sumptuous dinner with some new friends. After a few mouthfuls, Jim felt some minor dyspepsia, but was determined not to let it disturb his good time or embarrass the guests and he pointedly ignored it.

After the starter, Jim cleared the dishes and excused himself, on the pretext of wanting a cigarette. He paced about in his back garden, feeling short of breath and experienced gastric pain . . . he believed it to be nothing more than indigestion and again ignored the symptoms. He thought a few drinks would relax him, and rejoined the dinner party. However, during the main course, he felt worse—still tired and a bit stressed, with increasingly painful indigestion. The main course was consumed but he could not face dessert and had to abandon his plan not to disrupt the evening in front of the guests because he began to feel very ill. He excused himself and went for a brisk walk. On his return, he had severe pain in his chest and his left arm. In the kitchen, he asked his wife how she felt as they had eaten the same. She felt fine, so he excused himself once more and went to bed. He was distressed and worried that something was wrong.

When his wife came to bed, she looked at him and called the neighbour who worked at the local hospital. It was the neighbour who decided the situation was serious. Later, it was confirmed that Jim had suffered a heart attack.

This case shows that appraisals of incapacitating, bothersome, or painful symptoms are not necessarily quick or rational.

2.3 Summary

Empirical and case studies show that common sense, rational appraisals of symptoms do not necessarily occur. On the contrary, individuals seem to ignore symptoms or iterate through many irrational appraisals. This phenomenon has been labelled "appraisal delay" (Safer, Tharps, Jackson, & Leventhal, 1979). It challenges common sense.

3. Do I Need to Do Something About This Symptom? Social Psychological Influences on Appraisal Delay

The first (logical) stage of illness is an appraisal that a symptom cannot be dismissed as trivial, but indicates a problem that needs further cognitive work in order to understand and resolve it. The second stage is this understanding. This section is concerned with social psychological explanations for delay in making such appraisals.

3.1 Intra-personal influences on appraisal delay: More about schemata

Many researchers have studied the social psychological underpinnings of delay in appraising a symptom as indicating a problem, using a general attributional framework known as Psychophysiological Comparison Theory. According to Andersen and Cacioppo (1995), this framework postulates four major groups of social psychological principles.

First, it is postulated that people are motivated to explain unexpected events, such as the perception of symptoms, because unexplained states are aversive. Second, the motivation to understand and evaluate symptoms is a function of their unexpectedness, salience, personal relevance, and perceived consequences. Third, the psychophysiological comparisons themselves are hypothesised to involve four classes of variables: (i) situational factors, such as recent behaviours and social contacts; (ii) cognitive processes, especially the extent to which a relevant illness schema is accessible; (iii) heuristics and biases, such as optimism; (iv) the symptoms themselves. More diffuse symptoms, for example, lead to more comparisons and greater likelihood of error and change.

The fourth major group of principles in Psychophysiological Comparison Theory considers what will happen if a person fails to interpret the symptom(s). Essentially, the idea is that comparisons will continue, but will undergo qualitative changes, as continued failure diverts attention from searching for relevant schema, and optimism changes to pessimism and later depression.

Psychophysiological Comparison Theory usefully indicates heuristics and biases and other influences, which are missing from the common sense model depicted in Figure 3.1. Since these are likely to influence the search for, as well as the selection and elaboration of, relevant illness schemata, the decision time that underpins appraisal of a symptom may be conceptualised as the time taken for the individual to activate and assimilate information into a relevant schema. Schemata were introduced in Chapter 2 (Section 4.1.2) as a way in which the cognitive structures underpinning symptom perceptions may be conceptualised. Schemata are thought to be embedded in each other (Fiske & Taylor, 1984; Greene & Coulson, 1995). This means that the schemata concerning bodily organs and systems that guide symptom perceptions are likely to be subsumed by more complex schemata that contain everything a thinker knows about illnesses, and which provide higher-order structures to underpin symptom appraisals. In turn, these might be embedded in schemata dealing with more general beliefs, such as health locus of control (Lau, Hartman, & Ware, 1986). This "nesting" is another reason why the focus of Chapter 2 on perceiving a symptom *per se*, without considering its meanings, was artificial (and why indeed, there is overlap between this chapter and the next).

3.1.1 Schemata, illness identity, and symptom information

Early symptom appraisals are likely to construct a cognitive representation, in terms of which perceptions are organised. This schema might not be sufficiently organised to have a verbal label or overall identity. Evidence in support of this idea is that pain patients often have detailed memories of the location, intensity, and nature of pain (Skevington, 1995) which suggests that schema slots might contain sensory or muscular information as opposed to higher-level language-based codes or labels. In addition, Pennebaker (1982) found people reliably experienced constellations of symptoms without giving them a label more precise than "that feeling I get when . . .". In such instances, delay in appraising symptoms as indicating a problem might arise because a schema has not yet been sufficiently elaborated.

To make a rational decision at this stage might not be as easy as common sense suggests. This is because common sense reflects a logical fallacy identified by Pennebaker (1982) as endemic among professionals, that the symptoms of a disease are common to all its victims. In everyday life, and as illustrated in the earlier case study (Section 2.2) it is rare to experience a single "pure" symptom. Rather, a matrix of symptoms of varying intensities is typically experienced. To weight them appropriately and synthesise them even into an early appraisal can require a great deal of cognitive work and this can contribute to delay.

As illness schema become more organised, information about the physical nature of the symptoms is likely to be clarified and perhaps given early labels, and this introduces more room for variability in appraising that a problem exists. For example, Pennebaker (1982) found individual differences in low-level labels used to represent similar bodily experiences—some individuals calling shallow panting "shortness of breath", and others calling it "laboured breathing". Furthermore, Pennebaker and Skelton (1978) observed that mood labels can be used instead of physical labels, such that an individual who is unusually quiet might be suspected as sickening for something or sulking! Interesting in this respect is "alexithymia" which has been mooted as a potential new paradigm for understanding why some individuals report many somatic symptoms unrelated to disease (Deary et al., 1997). The literal meaning of the term is "lack of words for emotions" and the idea is that people with limited emotional vocabulary and understanding use physical schemata to evaluate their emotional arousal instead, and that this results in somatisation of emotional problems. In present terminology, this would mean that an individual who cannot access the rational or appropriate schema in which to understand an emotional experience such as anger, might access an inappropriate schema, such as a heart schema and consequently make an appraisal that s/he has palpitations. By inference, a similar process might mean that symptoms that "ought" to be appraised as indicating illness are simply appraised as indicating a bad mood or another emotion, and this is likely to lead to delay.

Taken together, the evidence suggests that different early labels used to organise symptom perceptions might be triggered for the same symptoms. Choice of the "wrong" early label might sabotage later decisions about overall illness identity or otherwise delay the appraisal that a problem is indicated—this is the position caricatured in Dumbledore's quotation at the start of this chapter.

Much research has been designed to discover what elements exist in more elaborate illness schemata and what happens when different values fill their "slots". The most important two elements are thought to hold information about (i) symptoms, or the short-term consequences of an illness, and (ii) a label, which gives an illness its identity (Fortune, Richards, Main, & Griffiths, 2000). These are equally important because symptoms provide the information upon which the name of an illness is decided and vice-versa. Their joint role is fundamental because the nature of the symptoms or the label of an illness set the default values for many other slots and therefore guide understanding. Thus, the moment an identity is assigned to a symptom set defines the moment an illness is understood. Persuasive evidence of the importance of these two elements is that 49% and 37% of respondents spontaneously named their disease and described their symptoms when asked about their most recent illness (Lau & Hartman, 1983).

Figure 3.2 suggests some values that might fill the label slot in a schema used for appraising a chest pain. The subsequent activity (3.1) is designed to show how inferences about seriousness and many other variables depend on the choice and therefore should highlight its importance. Because of its importance, a key research question is how an individual decides on an overall illness identity or label for his or her symptoms.

Based on Rosch (e.g., 1975), Bishop and Converse (1986) hypothesised that people classify symptom sets according to their degree of fit with stored disease prototypes, or typical examples of diseases. In terms of schema theory, typicality

IT IS:
- a heart attack
- indigestion
- stress
- that feeling I get when I eat sardines late at night
- overdoing it
- nerves

FIGURE 3.2 Some examples of labels (identity information) for a schema used to process chest pain.

ACTIVITY 3.1 Consider how actions and appraisals of the chest pain will vary according to its identity.

might be represented in at least two ways. First, a typical value is simply the default value for a given element. This is the value that will be inferred on the basis of the schema, in the absence of information to the contrary. For example, an individual's "heart disease schema" is likely to contain an element with a slot to represent the victim's weight. The default value for this is likely to be "overweight". Second, typicality can be used in a wider sense, to refer to the pattern of most commonly used elements in a schema, together with their default slot-values. This represents what a thinker expects to happen most often. For example, the most used elements in an individual's "heart disease schema" might include the victim's sex, age, and occupation. Relevant slots might have the default values "male", "52", and "stressful business", respectively. The constellation of these and other expected variables represents the thinker's heart-attack exemplar or "prototype" (Green & Coulson, 1995) and this is the meaning intended by Bishop and Converse (1986).

To test their hypothesis they presented 132 students with a list of 60 symptoms and asked them to indicate on a 7-point scale the extent to which each symptom was associated with each of 40 disease labels. On this basis, nine diseases were selected for use in the main experiment. For each, six symptoms of high mean association, designated "prototypical", were identified, and four of "low" perceived association. Next, brief descriptions of hypothetical people experiencing sets of six symptoms related to each of the nine diseases were developed. The symptom sets operationalised four levels of prototypicality. In the high prototypical condition, all six symptoms were prototypical; in the medium condition, four symptoms were prototypical and two were of low perceived association; in the low condition, two symptoms were prototypical and four were of low perceived association. Finally, random sets of symptoms were generated for the control condition.

Participants were asked to read 12 descriptions and decide whether the symptoms experienced by the stimulus person were indicative of a disease. If so, they were to name it. In the design, sex of stimulus person, the nine diseases, and three experimental levels of prototypicality were all counterbalanced.

The results showed that high prototype symptom sets were significantly more likely to be perceived as indicating a disease. Relevant percentages were 68% for "high", 45% for "medium", and 32% and 34% for "low" and "random" sets, respectively. Although the results for formally naming the disease did not reach significance, when synonyms and related conditions were both allowed, high prototype symptom sets were significantly more likely to be named correctly.

Overall, the prototype hypothesis was supported. The implication is that delays in identifying symptoms are more likely when the symptoms are not prototypical. This may well account for delay in appraising unusual combinations of symptoms as indicating an illness. However, since unusual symptom sets are also likely to be unexpected, there is some degree of mismatch between this account and Psycho-physiological Comparison Theory which suggests that unexpected symptoms are more likely to be appraised.

Interestingly, the results of this study may be interpreted in another relevant way. Overall, it shows that when six symptoms are experienced, most people do not appraise a disease at all. Even six prototypical symptoms are only evaluated as indicating a disease about two-thirds of the time. This suggests that delay in deciding that a symptom or symptoms indicate a problem might arise because most symptoms are simply not labelled as a disease.

There were a number of limitations to the study. For example, Bishop and Converse (1986) note that the prototypes were consensual and gathered for well-known diseases. It is not known whether individuals have idiosyncratic prototypes, nor what diseases they have them for. Neither is it known whether the prototypes are accurate. It is worth adding that the ecological validity of the study can also be challenged, because the experience of students earning course credits through evaluating brief descriptions of others is likely to be different to that of a person appraising his or her own symptoms with possible life-or-death consequences.

3.1.2 Schemata, inferences, and attributions

Pennebaker (1982) makes the interesting point that schema-based processing of one symptom is likely to lead to the experience of another. This means that common symptom clusters and syndromes might arise as a result of cognitive processes as opposed to some underlying clinical condition. Furthermore, relevant schema can be instantiated by external, as well as internal, stimuli. For example, an individual might notice that supper is overdue and infer that s/he is tired and hungry and so on. More paradoxically, people with high-blood pressure *developed* symptom-based strategies for monitoring their own blood pressure, even though they agreed that, in general, high blood pressure is asymptomatic (see Leventhal et al., 1984). Such studies suggest that symptom perceptions are not necessarily the building blocks of appraisals. Rather, appraisals can create symptoms.

Moss-Morris, Petrie, and Weinman (1996) explore further the role of such cognitive processes in creating the experience of chronic fatigue syndrome (CFS). They begin with a review that shows that neither organic findings nor objective tests can account for the illness. Then, in a study of 189 women and 44 men with CFS, they measured a range of variables, including "illness identity", a cognitive variable, operationalised by the number and severity of a set of 25 symptoms experienced. An interesting point was that only 13 of the set were part of the medical definition of CFS. As expected, illness identity predicted highly significant amounts of variance in participants' levels of dysfunction, psychological adjustment, and vitality *irrespective* of objective signs, which were not even measured. Furthermore, the levels of variance in a number of outcome variables predicted by illness identity were higher than those predicted by 12 coping strategies combined: the relevant figures for dysfunction, psychological adjustment, and vitality being 49%, 42%, and 50%, compared with 19%, 28%, and .07% respectively. Consistent with this picture, a recent study of 111 people with diabetes showed "personal models" to be predictive of a range of outcomes, including eating patterns, glycosylated haemoglobin, physical functioning, and mental health (Hampson et al., 2000).

Although these studies do not concern appraisal delay *per se*, they show that cognitive processes as opposed to signs can create symptoms and other aspects of illness. Moreover, these can feed back to affect signs. By inference, it is reasonable to hypothesise that similar cognitive processes can delay the appraisal that a symptom indicates an illness or, more interestingly, that they might create symptoms that do not.

In addition to symptom information and a disease label, other key elements in illness schemata are thought to hold information about cause(s), prevalence, and the typical victim. Long-term consequence(s) or timeline (duration, recurrence, and other temporal factors) and severity have also been studied (e.g., Lalljee, 1996; Lau & Hartman, 1983; Leventhal et al., 1984).

Since it is comparatively unusual for an individual directly to know why symptoms occurred, the value for the "cause" slot is likely to be inferred (Hewstone & Fincham, 1996). This is equivalent to the individual's attribution for getting sick and can be analysed using dimensions already identified by attribution theorists. For example, individuals who infer an internal, as opposed to an external, cause for a given symptom are more likely to appraise that a symptom indicates a problem that requires some further thought or action (Ingham & Miller, 1986; Lau & Hartman, 1983). Thus, individuals in a stressful situation such as an examination room are unlikely to think they are ill (see Salovey et al., 1998, for a discussion). A relevant though very different case is that of a woman who attributed her breast cancer to a punishment from God, because she had had an adulterous affair in which a central role was played by mutual pleasure in her voluptuous breasts (Fallowfield, 1991). Such attributions are likely to lead to further appraisals that indicate symptoms should simply be endured, and consistent with this interpretation, Helman (2000) argues that victims who see pain as divine punishment may be unwilling to seek relief, since they view suffering without complaint as "expiation". Overall, therefore, the inferred cause of a symptom is likely to have implications for appraisal delay (see Salovey et al., 1998, for a discussion).

3.1.3 Schemata and disease prevalence

Another element in illness schemata concerns the prevalence with which an individual believes a condition exists in the population. Its influence was observed in a study in which participants who believed they might have a fictitious disorder were more upset, and perceived it as more serious, if they believed it to be rare (Croyle & Jemmott, 1991; see Salovey et al., 1998, for a discussion). Likewise, frequently experienced symptoms can be defined as normal and are therefore tolerated, although they might be painful and treatable (Helman, 2000). Thus, differences in perceived prevalence might influence appraisal delay, irrespective of the symptoms *per se*.

3.1.4 Schemata and typicality of the victim

Lalljee, Lamb, and Carnibella (1993) hypothesised that a set of symptoms associated with a given disease is more likely to lead to the diagnosis of that disease when the sufferer is typical of its victims. To test this, students at Oxford Polytechnic read about symptoms related to mumps, typhoid, leukaemia, and heart disease together with information about a person and his or her environment. Below this was a list of eight diseases that included the four targets and the task was to indicate which of these (or any others) the person might have. Results clearly supported hypotheses. For example, 100% of respondents "diagnosed" mumps in a 6-year-old on the basis of "mump-like" symptoms, but only 17% made the diagnosis when a person from the Third World experienced the symptoms. The Action Aid advertisement depicted in Figure 3.3 provides a similar example because our schemata (as well as social reality of course) predict different prognoses of the same condition according to the supposed nature and circumstances of the victim. Although the extent to which people use these illness prototypes when appraising their own symptoms is not yet known (Lalljee et al., 1993), it might be reasoned that appraisal delay is more likely when an individual experiencing a symptom does not self-categorise as a prototypical sufferer. Much more will be said about self-categorisation both below (in Section 3.3) and more especially in later chapters.

3.1.5 Schemata, heuristics, and biases

Fiske and Taylor (1984) identify many cognitive biases that arise out of schema-based processing. These also help to account for appraisal delays. For example, a schema that has been recently or frequently used is more likely to be triggered again, and in time "personalised prototypes" are likely to develop in this way. Moreover, since most people will have experienced many minor ailments before their first major one, it follows that trivial schemata will be triggered first (Lau & Hartman,

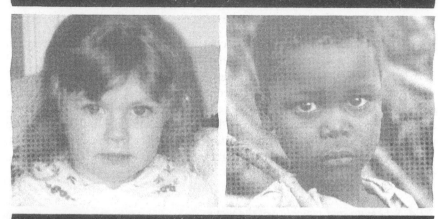

FIGURE 3.3 This advertisement for Action Aid helps us to reflect on our expectations about the typical victim of diarrhoea. Reproduced with permission from Action Aid.

1983). Once triggered, such a schema can generate its own verification by directing attention away from phenomena that are outside its frame of reference (as discussed in Chapter 2, Section 4.1.2). Thus, an inappropriate trivial schema is unlikely to be dismissed as a result of rational symptom appraisals. Rather, the appraisals are likely to be distorted to fit it, with the result that delay in rationally appraising a serious symptom occurs.

The same idea is illustrated not with a "trivial" schema, but in a cognitive approach to understanding panic attacks, in which Clark (1986) suggests that a trigger stimulus such as an internal thought, or an external event such as a theatre outing, gives rise to anxiety and associated sensations. However, instead of an exciting and pleasurable schema being triggered to appraise them, they are interpreted in terms of a catastrophic heart-attack schema, for example. The person infers they are likely to collapse and this creates further arousal and panic, which becomes self-perpetuating. The person is then likely to engage in preventive behaviour, like leaving the theatre and perhaps going home to bed. The fact that they have not collapsed does not lead them to abandon the heart-attack schema. Rather, they attribute their survival to their preventive behaviour. Sadly, such schema perseverance can ultimately result in victims simply staying home.

More generally, it follows that schema-based appraisals can be self-perpetuating and where they lead to preventive action that brings relief, the individual might delay further appraisals indefinitely or otherwise fail to understand that the selected schema is inappropriate.

3.1.6 Schemata, emotions, and motivations

In addition to "cold" cognitive processes, "hot" emotions and human motivations can influence symptom appraisals. In this section, these will not be treated as intrapersonal traits or dispositions as they were in Chapter 2 (Section 4.1.4). Rather, they will be incorporated into schema theory as part of an individual's understanding of an issue. An effective way of illustrating the importance of human emotional involvement in appraising illness is suggested by Sedgwick (1982, cited in Stainton-Rogers, 1991) who draws a parallel between events such as the invasion of a human organism by cholera germs and the souring of milk by other forms of bacteria. Objectively speaking, the two are analogous, but the response to the label "cholera" is much wider. Even a detached reader is "drawn in" and feels emotions such as curiosity, relief, or fear and much more. Clearly, if the cholera label is personally relevant, experienced emotions will be much stronger and this is why it is easier to be rational about someone else.

The concept of personal relevance raises some interesting points when thinking about pain, since the concept pain *includes* other meanings, such as fear and suffering, misfortune, or divine punishment, and the idea that it motivates action to find relief (Helman, 2000). In other words, pain is always personally relevant, and indeed, Melzack and Wall (1988) comment that experiences that resemble pain, but which do not include the notion of personal threat and negative emotions (such as those that might be practised by masochists), must be defined as something else. In effect therefore, pain is already an organised concept, consisting of appraised symptoms within a schema. These and other meanings and emotions are exactly why pain thresholds measured in a laboratory must be different from pain experienced in "real life". Thus, a term such as "hurt" might better describe them, "pain" being reserved for a more elaborated schema resulting from appraisals. An interesting speculation about self-efficacy follows. Since self-efficacy reduces laboratory-induced pain experiences (see Salovey et al., 1998, for a discussion) it might be that reduced feelings of efficacy in individuals in chronic pain serve to maintain and exacerbate pain experiences. This and other points and speculations mean that much of the previous chapter should have been included in this one, and further illustrates that there is no clear division between a symptom perception and appraisals of it. Rather, the appraisals help to create the symptom.

These ideas help to explain a number of paradoxes. One is why distraction *and* its opposite, monitoring, can both reduce pain. Many studies (some of which were reviewed in Chapter 2) have shown that distraction decreases and attention increases symptom perceptions, but Leventhal et al. (1989) found that asking women during childbirth to focus on the somatic aspects of their contractions reduced pain. The explanation was that monitoring enhanced perceptions of control. More generally, Suls and Fletcher (1985) carried out a meta-analysis of 43 studies, and concluded

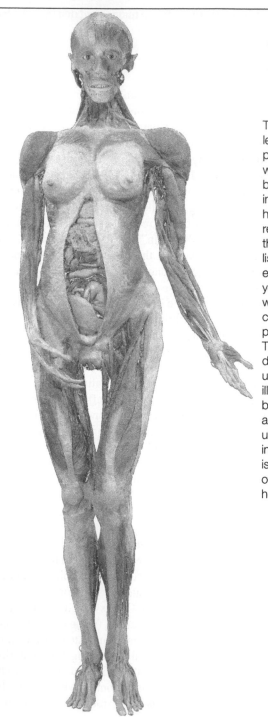

ACTIVITY 3.2 Reproduced with permission. Copyright © Prof. (RC) Dr. Gunther von Hagens, Institute for Plastination, Heidelberg, Germany.

The representation on the left is a photograph of the plastinated corpse of a woman and her unborn baby. Now you know the image is of two real humans, are you able to restrict your appraisals to the biological facts? If not, list your thoughts and experiences. Consider how your list might compare with menbers of different cultures, sexes, professions and times. These experiential dimensions of your understanding help illustrate the difference between objective disease and human illness. To understand the nature and impact of these dimensions is a fundamental purpose of social psychologists of health.

that distraction offers better strategies for coping with pain in the short term (i.e., 3 days or less) but that monitoring its sensory dimensions was better in the longer term (after 2 weeks). They suggested that distraction occurs at a lower level of processing, merely occupying cognitive capacity, whereas monitoring occurs at higher levels, effecting qualitative changes in symptom appraisals, such that a hurt is accompanied by feelings of control as opposed to fear. According to the definition given earlier, this would transform the experience into something other than pain (see also Chapter 4, Section 3.1.5).

This same principle provides an answer to the paradoxical question of whether an individual has *really* been helped if they experience the same amount of hurt but call it something other than pain (e.g. Skevington, 1995). The dilemma arises from following a scientific perspective in which the objective hurt is "the truth". From a more experiential perspective the answer is, of course they have been helped if they are freed to continue their lives—with hurt, but without fear, helplessness, and other miseries that characterise pain appraisals.

To return to the focus on delay in deciding that a symptom indicates a problem, the point is that the motivation to alleviate pain might trigger cognitive coping strategies. If successful, these might end further appraisals irrespective the presence of serious symptoms.

In fact, the first principle of Psychophysiological Comparison Theory suggests that unexplained events are aversive, (although some desired events might be happily experienced, whether they are explained or not!) and this predicts that there should be a natural tendency for psychophysiological comparison processes to be self-terminating. This is because symptoms that an individual has appraised and resolved should be less aversive than those that are unexplained. Hence an individual might be biased towards accepting an irrational appraisal, since in emotional terms, this should be preferable to not having one.

Emotions are also likely to contribute to appraisal delay through biasing choice of label information for schemata. For example, Helman (2000) suggests that avoidance of the anxiety aroused by the implications of interpreting symptoms in terms of a heart-attack schema can help explain why even people who are familiar with relevant symptoms interpret chest pain as indigestion. Similarly, the need to maintain self-esteem predicts that people will be biased against interpreting a symptom in terms of a socially undesirable illness schema. An example would be AIDS when it was seen as "a modern-day pestilence" or as a moral punishment for homosexual activity (see Temoshok et al., 1987).

Finally, "unrealistic optimism" refers to the belief that one's future holds bountiful opportunities and an absence of adverse events (Weinstein, 1987). It is conceptually similar to what Cacioppo et al. (1986) call "hedonic bias" which led patients with gynaecological cancer initially to appraise their symptoms in terms of normal events and processes like overwork or menopause. It follows that symptom appraisals are likely to be made in a way that is consistent with the idea that they are not getting worse and are transient. In other words, there is likely to be a bias towards appraisal delay (see also Section 3.2 below).

3.1.7 Conclusion

Schema theory provides a useful overall framework in which to understand how top-down cognitive processes can mean that the same "bottom-up" symptoms lead to different appraisals, which typically slow the decision that further cognitive work or action (i.e., illness) is indicated even for a serious symptom. However, schemata are defined as cognitive structures within individuals. Thus only intrapersonal influences on appraisal delay have been considered. As I argued at this juncture in the previous chapter, the choice of relevant schema as well as its content is likely to be influenced by others and hence other levels of analysis need consideration. This will be attempted next, but it is worth noting that the section also includes an attempt to incorporate more *social* social psychological influences.

3.2 Interpersonal influences on appraisal delay

"Legitimisation" refers to a social psychological process, usually in the context of informal discussions with friends and family, by means of which individuals appraise symptoms and evaluate whether they warrant further attention (Helman, 2000; Skevington, 1995). Such processes mean that symptom appraisals are not simply driven by the nature of the symptoms and intra-individual structures and processes, but also take place outside the individual, in the context of social psychological interactions. Still more complex, a recent study of 140 people with psoriasis showed that the main contributor to illness behaviours was anticipatory worry about other people's reactions, which was independent of symptom severity (Fortune et al., 2000). Thus, influential social interactions can take place within the individual's cognitive structures rather than in the real world.

3.2.1 Excitation transfer and symptom appraisals

In a famous paradigm Zillmann, Johnson, and Day (1974) demonstrated that physical symptoms, which "should" be appraised as arousal, can be attributed to the actions of another. More formally, they established that residual arousal produced by one arousing condition can be transferred to a second arousing situation. The result is that the combined physical arousal leads to an exaggerated appraisal of the second situation. A funny example occurs in the children's cartoon "Bugs Bunny", in which Bugs Bunny kisses the rabbit whom he has heroically wooed. At the same time, his rival detonates an exploding cigar between the pair. However, instead of the usual sooty faces and tattered clothing, the lovers leap into the air, hearts pounding and eyelashes fluttering. "Wow, what a kisser!" they chorus. Just as predicted in excitation transfer theory, arousal caused by the explosion was combined with arousal caused by the kiss. The pooled arousal was misattributed to the kiss, leading to an ecstatically intense experience!

Since excitation transfer depends on a misattribution of arousal from the first situation to the second, the length of time between arousing events is important because enough time has to pass for the cause of the first arousal to be "forgotten". A second crucial factor is how long the arousal lasts. If it is over before the second situation happens, there will be nothing to transfer. Thus, when arousal is created by physical exertion, a shorter time span during which transfer is possible should be the case for fit individuals because their physical parameters should return more quickly to baseline levels.

Such relationships were investigated in a complex experiment, which was ostensibly about memory and distraction (Zillmann et al., 1974). Sixty male undergraduates were assigned the role of teacher. They were told that they had been paired with a pupil who had already arrived and was well under-way with his learning task. The pupil was, in fact, a confederate of the experimenters. During pretests, participants' fitness and "unprovoked aggression" were measured, the latter being operationalised by the strength of the electric shock selected to "punish" pupils' mistakes.

The experiment consisted of a provocation phase, during which the confederate administered electric shocks to the participants, followed by an arousal phase, during which participants pedalled strenuously on an exercise bicycle for one and a half minutes. In the third phase participants were to "test" their pupils' memories, being sure to punish any mistakes. However, some time before the memory test however, came a distraction task. For half the participants, the distraction task occurred *before* the cycling. For the other half, it came after it. For the first half of participants, this meant that the memory test followed about 30 seconds after physical exertion, while arousal should still be high and its cause fresh in participants' minds. For the second half of them, it occurred about 6 minutes *after* cycling, when arousal should be relatively low and its cause most probably forgotten. During the memory test itself, the confederate made 18 prescheduled errors. The relevant dependent variable was the mean intensity of electric shock chosen by the participants as punishment. This operationalised "provoked aggression".

The results confirmed that there were no differences in levels of unprovoked aggression prior to arousal. After provocation, there was a general increase in aggression scores, but this was not of as much interest as the interaction between the two lengths of delay and three levels of fitness on aggressive behaviour. For men tested 30 seconds after exercise (when physical arousal had not had time to decay and the reasons for its presence were still salient) levels of fitness made no difference to aggressive behaviour. After 6 minutes' delay (when arousal and its cause were decaying) fit men whose arousal levels were closer to baseline were significantly less aggressive than unfit men. The interpretation was that unfit men were still experiencing higher levels of arousal which they attributed to the provocation rather than the exercise, and therefore they gave out more "punishment".

According to Hewstone, Manstead, and Stroebe (1997), different sources of arousal can be combined and it is this feature that makes excitation transfer theory relevant to interpersonal influences on symptom appraisals in general. One interesting hypothesis is that an individual experiencing symptoms may attribute them to an arousing social interaction, and delay deciding that he or she has a problem.

It is exciting is to speculate with this idea in the field of Type A behaviour. Two cardiologists who noticed that many of their patients showed cynical hostility, aggressiveness, competitiveness, impatience, and a sense of time urgency identified this famous behaviour pattern. They labelled these individuals "Type A" and those who showed a relative absence of these characteristics were labelled Type Bs (Friedman & Rosenman 1974). Subsequently, a "momentous" (Roskies, 1991) large-scale longitudinal study confirmed that the Type A behaviour pattern predicted coronary heart disease (Rosenman 1978; Rosenman, Brand, Jenkins, Friedman, Straus, & Wurm, 1975).

However, a key difficulty is that no one theory links the action–behaviour complex with the disease (e.g., Taylor, 1995). Because of this, and because of recent failures to replicate (e.g., Ragland & Brand, 1988), there have been many attempts to identify the toxic elements in the pattern together with their mode of influence (Strube, 1991). One hypothesis is that people categorised as Type A suppress or ignore physical symptoms, in order to work longer and harder. This increases appraisal delay, and therefore increases risk. Evidence for this view is that Type As push themselves closer to their limits on treadmill tests and they tend to ignore sports injuries (e.g., Carver, DeGregorio, & Gillis, 1981; Hart, 1983). Unfortunately, other studies disagree. For example, Essau and Jamieson (1987) studied 200 male students aged 19–31 who completed questionnaires that identified 28 Type As and 28 Type Bs. These two groups went on to participate in the three-phase study. First, they estimated their heart-rates, second, they did a challenging digit recall task, and third, they estimated their heart-rates again. Results showed that Type As had higher heart-rates, but also tended to *overestimate* them, which of course contradicts the idea that they suppress symptoms.

More recently, Toates (1996) has suggested that the toxic element in the Type A complex is a "cynical heart" or an expectation of hostility from others. The previous discussion of excitation transfer theory suggests that he might be right. Perhaps rather than suppressing symptoms, a hostile heart predisposes Type A individuals to transfer excitation onto social interactions, with the net result that cardiac symptoms are attributed (say) to the insulting behaviour of others. Not only is this likely to be self-perpetuating, because the enhanced experience of these insults should lead to further arousal, but also this misattribution should lead to increased delay in recognising that a symptom needs attention. This idea can reconcile the opposing results concerning symptom repression that were described above, since sporting situations are more likely to afford an opportunity to make such misattributions than situations in which challenging mental arithmetic is being carried out. However, these possibilities must await further research, because the social characteristics of testing situations do not seem to have received much attention.

Before leaving the subject of excitation theory, it is worth reviving issues of accuracy laid to rest in the last chapter. Excitation transfer occurs when an individual is tricked into making a misattribution, which assumes that calibration between level of aggression and objective physical arousal is the normal state of affairs. Thus, under normal circumstances an individual can accurately partition arousal into that caused by (say) running upstairs and a subsequent rude remark, using the latter to generate exactly the right degree of sarcasm in retaliation. Such accuracy in perception and discrimination of symptoms seems extremely unlikely.

3.2.2 Social comparisons, unrealistic optimism, and appraisal delay

Another way in which interpersonal interactions can delay symptom appraisals occurs in the context of unrealistic optimism (which was briefly introduced in Section 3.1.6). Harris and Middleton (1994) argue that there are least three intrapersonal and one interpersonal underpinnings for this concept: it could be a trait; it could arise out of an illusion of control; or it might simply be "unrealistic" in the sense of statistically inaccurate. Fourth, it might depend on interpersonal comparisons. To explore these possibilities, 192 undergraduates were asked about the risk of developing 15 medical conditions. In a between-subjects design, risks were rated for self, an acquaintance, a friend's friend, and a student, using an 8-point scale in which 0 denoted no risk and 7 denoted that a disease would certainly occur. To focus on the results for AIDS, students rated their own risk lowest at .71. For an acquaintance, risk was higher at 1.47, rising to 1.97 for a friend's friend, and 2.75 for a student.

The interpretation was that unrealistic optimism arises out of downward comparisons with negative views of others from whom people distance themselves. The role of social comparisons will be more fully explored in the context of subjective health status in Chapter 6. The important point for present purposes is that unrealistic optimism, and hence the delay in deciding a symptom indicates a problem, might vary according to changes in person's social context.

3.3 Group-level influences on appraisal delay: An important transition to more social social psychological influences

Helman (2000) argues that ordinariness is central to making sense of health and illness. However, what is ordinary depends on common sense knowledge of everyday life, including the social norms of reference groups (see Stainton-Rogers, 1991). From this point of view, a symptom indicates illness if it interferes with ordinary activities and since many symptoms do not, it is easy to see that appraisal delay might occur.

However, it might be argued that most of the studies so far reviewed do not describe "truly" social psychological influences. This is because intra-personal structures and processes have typically mediated the social influences so far described. Like the Russian doll analogy that was described in Chapter 1, the assumption is that cognitive structures are nested within the individual and the individual is nested within dyads and groups and so on. Nested dolls usefully enable us to picture the systems of an individual's social ecology, but the idea of each individual at the centre of his or her own little universe is misleading because it affords no way to picture the shared sense of belonging that humans can experience. In other words, the analogy cannot accommodate the changes that occur when the little doll at the centre transforms from "I" to "we".

To understand such phenomena is exactly what Tajfel and subsequently his many colleagues set out to do. In 1978 Tajfel (1978a) suggested an interpersonal–intergroup behaviour continuum (Tajfel & Turner, 1979, p.34):

> at one extreme . . . is the interaction between two or more individuals which is fully determined by their interpersonal relationships and individual characteristics and not at all affected by various social groups . . . The other extreme consists of interactions between two or more individuals (or groups of individuals) which are fully determined by their respective memberships of various social groups

In terms of this continuum, the examples so far reviewed all locate the individual at the interpersonal extreme, because during symptom appraisals the focus has been on personal characteristics and cognitive processes. Some might have been "reset" by social influences, but they still pertain to individuals. In order to find truly social psychological influences on symptom appraisals and delay, it is necessary to find examples in which the appraiser is functioning at other loci along the continuum. Such an example is to be found in a seminal study (Levine & Reicher, 1996) in which appraisal of a given symptom was a function of the currently salient social identification. The study was grounded in Social Identification Theory (e.g., Tajfel, 1978a) and because of its importance, some background to the theory will be given before the study is described.

The relevant aspect of the theory begins with Tajfel's realisation that, para-doxically, the self-concept was the only common factor to underpin examples of intergroup conflict. More specifically, he realised that the individual's knowledge that he or she belongs to a social group was not only necessary, but also sufficient for intergroup behaviour.

In 1972, Tajfel defined social identity as: "the individual's knowledge that he [sic] belongs to certain social groups together with some emotional and value significance to him of the group membership." Clearly, social identity is an aspect of self-concept. Turner (1981) took this as a starting point, using the term "social identification" to refer to any social categorisation used by the individual in self-definition and the individual's social identity to refer to the repertoire of such social identifications. Personal identity, on the other hand, refers to idiosyncratic traits, characteristics, and preferences. As an aside, it is worth noting that social and personal identifications cannot be distinguished by linguistic means alone (i.e., social identity is not necessarily flagged by use of group names and personal identification is not necessarily flagged by use of personal traits). What counts is whether the functioning aspect of an individual's self concept is rooted in a group membership or in his or her individuality.

ACTIVITY 3.3 Give 10 answers to the question " Who are you?"

- The self concept may be operationalised as the answer to the question "Who am I?" (see Kuhn & McPartland, 1954).
- Typically, Western respondents generate a number of personal descriptions such as "I am 5 feet 6 inches tall"; "I sing"; "my favourite colour is . . ."; my name is . . ." etc. together with a number of self-descriptions are grounded in group memberships, such as "I am a psychologist"; "I am a mother"; "I am British" etc. The theoretical importance of this distinction was extensively discussed and developed by Taifel (e.g., 1972) and later by Turner (e.g., 1981).
- Observe whether you have made these distinctions.

Next, Turner (e.g., 1981) focused on the function of the self concept which, like that of other cognitive structures, is to enable a perceiver to make better sense of the environment, including his or her own role in it, in order to behave more adaptively. In more familiar terms, the self-concept is a schema. Thus, incoming experiences are either symbolised, perceived, and organised in some relationship to self-knowledge, ignored because they have no perceived relevance to the self, or perhaps they are distorted to become more consistent with it (e.g., Fiske & Taylor, 1984; Markus, 1977). According to circumstances, individuals define themselves in terms of a particular social identification. At such times, the salient self-schema, which guides cognitions and behaviour, may be entirely based on beliefs about a single group, whereas at other times other social identifications or personal identity will be salient. Indeed, just such a switch from personal to social identity is likely to underpin the switch from interpersonal to intergroup behaviour. Moreover, since individuals possess numerous social identifications, they "switch" between them in order to behave adaptively between, or even within, situations.

It is the consequences of such "switches" that have fundamental *social* psychological implications for symptom appraisals. Tajfel (e.g., Tajfel & Wilkes, 1963) had argued that social categorisation has both inductive and deductive aspects. Induction concerns the process by which information about a social category is built up, whereas deduction refers to the process by which a person is assigned an attribution on the basis of category membership. Turner (1981, 1987) extended this process to the self. He argued that self-categorisation as a member of a given social group results in self-assignment of the characteristics associated with that group. Furthermore, individuals who share a given social identification will assign themselves essentially the same set of characteristics in a situation that enhances its salience. This results in cognitive and behavioural conformity to the relevant group norms whenever that identification becomes salient. Turner (1981, 1987) named this process "referent informational influence".

The stage is now set on which to describe the study of 68 men and women PE students (Levine & Reicher, 1996) mentioned earlier. A pilot study had suggested that the symptoms of most importance to women were those that threatened physical attractiveness. More important to PE students were symptoms that would prevent them from taking part in physical activity and those of most importance to males concerned physicality and therefore tended to overlap with the PE ones. Experimental materials were built on these distinctions. The dependent variable was an inventory, which included three types of symptoms. One type was designed to be relevant to a female gender identity and concerned such issues as scarring. A second was designed to be relevant to a PE/masculine identity and concerned such issues as knee damage, while the third type was a control that concerned the symptoms of a virus.

Participants completed the inventory under one of two experimental conditions. One was designed to promote the psychological salience of gender and the other that of a PE student social identification. A number of interactions were predicted and found, but those concerning symptoms that threatened physical attractiveness are sufficient to give the overall flavour. Female participants rated these symptoms as more serious when their female gender identification was salient, as opposed to their PE student identification. Male participants' ratings of these, on the other hand, were not affected by the identity manipulation.

More recently, Levine (1999) part-replicated and extended the study with reference to self-categorisation theory (Turner, Hogg, Oakes, Reicher & Wetherell, 1987). Self-categorisation theory will be discussed in more depth in Chapter 6. It is sufficient for present purposes to say that it extends referent informational influence to incorporate the idea that the social identification that becomes salient in a given situation does not necessarily pre-exist in the individual's self concept, but can be actively constructed with reference to the current social context in order to maximise the ratio of intergroup to intragroup differences. Consistent with this extension, Levine (1999) predicted and found that 40 men from a rugby club appraised symptoms differently according to whether "new men" or "women" provided the social context in the form of an imaginary contrast group.

These studies have far-reaching implications. They show that the way in which people make sense of symptoms *can change* according to the social identification that is currently salient. However, in both Levine and Reicher's (1996) and Levine's (1999) study participants were evaluating hypothetical situations as opposed to their own symptoms. However, at least two other studies suggest that the principle applies to individuals' own symptom appraisals. In the first, Buss and Portnoy (1967) famously found that strength of group identification predicted the amount of pain participants were willing to tolerate, when they were told their group had a lower pain tolerance than a salient, relevant comparison outgroup. More recently, St. Claire and Clift (2003) predicted and found an interaction between the presence of a cold and the self-definition as a cold sufferer on the experience of cold-relevant symptoms. In this study, participants were randomly assigned to one of three identity conditions. In Condition 1 they received a manipulation designed to make their social identification as a current cold-sufferer or non-sufferer salient. Condition 2 controlled for the salience of colds *per se*, by repeating the focus on them, but

TABLE 3.1 *Symptoms of a cold: Having a cold and self-categorising as a cold-sufferer are both important.*

	Cold present	Cold absent
Cold identification salient	17.29	3.85
Colds central, but cold identification not salient	12.63	5.25
Exercise identification salient	11.38	4.63

omitting the encouragement to self-categorise, and Condition 3 was designed to make salient participants' social identification as an exerciser or non-exerciser. A second independent variable was whether or not participants currently had a cold. The dependent variables were (i) a scale that reflected the perceived number (0–11) and severity (1–4) of cold-relevant symptoms, and (ii) a scale that concerned other physical symptoms. Results on the cold-relevant scale are given in Table 3.1.

As expected, participants who had a cold endorsed more cold-relevant symptoms. Of more interest was a significant interaction which showed that the number and severity of symptoms endorsed by individuals who had a cold was greater in the condition in which their social identification as a cold-sufferer was salient. Furthermore, these relationships were not found for other symptoms.

Taken together, these studies suggest that the social psychological act of self-definition leads to differences in symptom perceptions and appraisals, and by inference to variation in the nature and duration of appraisal delay.

3.4 Summary

Referent informational influence and self-categorisation theory provide a means to explain how top-down social psychological influences can lead to symptom appraisals that reflect group memberships as well as, or perhaps even instead of, the symptoms themselves. In this way, the social identity approach provides a powerful and truly social psychological way to understand why delay might characterise appraising a painful, dangerous, or bothersome symptom as indicating a problem or why delay might impede the understanding of such a problem. Furthermore, the approach suggests that variation in the appraisals of a given symptom set might occur not only between, but also within, individuals according to changes in salient social identifications. Thus, the individual who perceives no illness as, say, a dancer on a Saturday night, might perceive they are too ill to work on Monday. In spite of appearances, this difference might reflect normal cognitive processes, not malingering. Moreover, the framework provides an alternative to explanations, based on learning and modelling, for positive correlations between symptoms such as headache and menstrual pain and the number of pain sufferers reported to be in the family, the crucial factor being identification with other sufferers rather than exposure to them

4. Towards a More Social Social Psychological Model of Symptom Appraisals

Symptom appraisals do not always follow the predictions of common sense. In a more social social psychological model, symptom perceptions are not necessarily the building blocks of later rationally constructed illness representations. Rather schema-based processing can lead to biases, especially those that delay recognising and understanding an illness. Although common sense has it that contact with objective reality is a good thing, in the wider context of the social world, positive biases might be adaptive (Taylor & Brown, 1988). Furthermore, it is likely that these social cognitive influences contribute to the creation of the symptoms themselves (as discussed in the previous chapter). Thus, a social psychological rival to a common sense explanation of the relationship between symptom perceptions and appraisals needs to accommodate bi-directional influences.

A social psychological model differs even more from common sense in allowing for many potential relationships between a given symptom set and appraisals for a given individual. This is because s/he might use a range of different schemata according to changes in salient self-image. Thus, whereas there is one true diagnosis from a common sense perspective, there are many rival truths from a social psychological viewpoint.

5. Summary and Conclusions

This chapter was about the ways in which people think about their symptoms. In the first section a common sense model was suggested in which people appraise painful, debilitating, or bothersome symptoms as requiring further cognitive work.

- Appraisals were assumed to be rational and therefore to reflect the nature and severity of the symptoms.
- When individuals cannot reach an understanding of their symptoms, it was assumed that they would recognise this and seek help.

In the second section this common sense model was challenged by empirical and case studies which showed that:

- irrational delays occur when appraising that symptoms indicate illness;
- irrational delays and misunderstanding occur when appraising illness.

In the third section, social psychological explanations for the relationship between symptom perceptions and appraisals were suggested as rivals to common sense explanations.

- The bulk of the section was pitched at the intrapersonal level and used schema theory in order to explain many ways in which delays could occur.

- At the interpersonal level of analysis, excitation transfer theory showed that interpersonal encounters could influence symptom appraisals.
- At group levels of analysis, referent informational influence showed that symptom appraisals could depend on the salient self-image of the appraiser.

In the fourth section it was concluded that the common sense model of illness reflects a scientific perspective in which symptom perceptions are elaborated in a rational manner, the nature of rationality being defined by the fit between the symptoms and the appraisals. In a more social psychological approach, the appraisals might construct the symptom perceptions. Furthermore, the appraisals are shaped by social influenced from all levels of analysis and the entire relationship between symptoms and appraisals might be recalibrated by a change in salient self-image.

So far, the focus has been on delay in deciding that a symptom indicates illness, and on delay and misunderstanding in illness appraisals. However, once the individual has understood that s/he is ill, s/he needs to plan how to remedy the situation. More specifically, s/he decides whether or not to seek professional medical help, and this is the focus of the next chapter.

4

I'm Ill! Shall I See my Doctor?

Chauntecleer the cockerel has had a nightmare. His wife, Pertelote the hen, advises:

> For Goddes love, as taak som laxatyf!
> Upon peril of my soule and of my lyf,
> I conseille yow the beste, I wol nat lye,
> That bothe of colere and of malencolye
> Ye purge yow; and for ye shal nat tarie,
> Though in this toun is noon apothecarie,
> I shal myself to herbes techen yow
> That shul been for youre hele and for youre prow;
> > From Chaucer's *Nun's Priest's Tale*

The attainment of fitness is the duty of each one of us as far as lies in our power, and no woman has any right by neglecting her health to bring unnecessary trouble and suffering upon herself and other people.
> Barbara Crawford, MBE MB ChB, former Senior Resident Medical Officer
> at the Borough Isolation Hospital and Sanatorium, Leicester, undated.

This chapter begins where the last chapter ended, that is, when the individual has appraised serious, painful, debilitating, or bothersome symptoms and understands s/he is ill. The previous chapters dealt with the antecedents to this understanding. This chapter is about what happens next. In particular, the focus is on whether the person decides to seek professional medical help in the form of a visit to a GP.

In Section 1 key concepts are discussed, and a common sense model of illness behaviour simply predicts that people will decide to seek professional medical advice when they have appraised themselves as ill with painful, debilitating, or bothersome symptoms. Again, the level of analysis is weighted heavily at the intrapersonal level because this decision is a result of intra-individual cognitions.

In Section 2 this model will be challenged by empirical studies and a case study, which demonstrate that delay characterises the progression to professional help.

In Section 3 different stages of delay are outlined and social psychological explanations for delay in deciding to seek professional help are reviewed, in order to suggest alternatives to common sense. The lion's share of the discussion is in Section 3.1 which overviews the role of many intrapersonal influences in the form of social cognition models of health behaviour, and personality and relational models of stress and emotion. In Sections 3.2 and 3.3 interpersonal and group-level influences on delay in seeking professional medical help are briefly sketched.

In Section 4 some suggestions for a more social social psychological model of seeking help are suggested as a rival to the common sense idea that people will decide to seek professional medical advice when they have appraised themselves as ill with painful, debilitating, or bothersome symptoms. The social psychological model also attempts to integrate conclusions from Chapters 2 and 3 about symptom perceptions and appraisals.

It is concluded that illness behaviours in response to a given set of symptoms can fly in the face of common sense because the seriousness of the symptoms does not necessarily determine whether or not medical help is sought. Moreover, the appraised seriousness of the symptoms does not necessarily depend on their nature, and still more surprising, there is not necessarily a reliable relationship between underlying signs and perceived symptoms. Rather, social psychological variables at all four levels of analysis both influence and create cognitions, symptoms, and sometimes even signs. This means that responses to symptoms depend on salient meanings in the context of individuals' social ecologies, as opposed to the nature of objective signs. Furthermore, the relationship between symptoms and illness might be entirely recalibrated according to changes in the way the individual self-categorises.

1. Introduction and a Common Sense Model of Seeking Professional Help for Illness

The previous chapter focused on predicting what an individual would think about perceived symptoms. This chapter is still about illness, but focuses on predicting what the individual will do. Of the various steps taken to remedy the situation it focuses on the decision to seek medical help. Since this is an observable action taken with respect to an illness, it may be defined as an "illness behaviour" (Helman, 2000; Turpin & Slade, 1998).

Visiting a GP represents the gateway through which the individual in Britain must pass, if he or she is to become formally ill. This is because medicine is elevated above other forms of healthcare and upheld by law. In addition, the individual's illness needs to be legitimated by a GP if s/he is to have access to publicly funded treatment and social support (Helman, 2000). In this sense, the general practitioner is the professional gatekeeper to illness.

According to Helman (1994), modern medicine is a profession because it is based on specialised knowledge, which is designed to meet the needs of clients and which is not easily acquired. In addition, it is organised and controlled by peers, who amongst other functions also protect their own interests. Within the profession, hospital medicine enjoys higher status than general practice (Helman, 2000), probably because hospital medicine has a longer and more illustrious history. Its precursor, the Royal College of Physicians, was founded in 1518 and is described as a "traditional domain of the educated elite" (Crossley, 2000). The precursors of GPs, on the other hand, were apothecaries, or specialised tradesmen who were only licensed to sell drugs prescribed by physicians during the 17th century. Whatever its source however, this difference in status further fits the characterisation of the general practitioner as gatekeeper, since he or she also permits access to hospital consultants if expert opinion is needed. Interestingly, Cornwell (1984) found this difference reflected in lay beliefs, which construed GPs as competent to deal with "normal illness", and serious cases as needing to be tackled in hospital.

Figure 4.1 depicts a common sense model of deciding to seek professional help. The model begins with the individual's understanding that she/he is ill with non-trivial symptoms, that is, with symptoms that have been appraised as painful, debilitating, or otherwise bothersome (antecedents to this understanding were the topic of Chapter 3). The fast track is intended to represent the situation when the individual seeks professional help without further deliberation. Common sense suggests this route will be taken when the individual "feels really bad" (Telles &

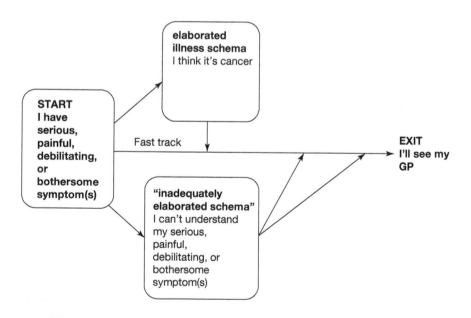

FIGURE 4.1 A common sense model of illness behaviour: seeking professional help for symptoms appraised as serious.

Pollack, 1981) or appraises his or her symptoms as extremely serious. Where symptoms are not so overwhelming, the model predicts that the individual will carry out further cognitive work to plan how to remedy them.

Again the model is based on an information-processing perspective and its major assumption is that the decision to seek professional medical help is a rational outcome of processing symptom-related information. Its second assumption is that humans are motivated to preserve themselves and this determines what is rational. Thus the goal of the decision (and subsequent action), is to remedy the symptoms because they cause current distress and discomfort and/or threaten long-term consequences. Since the symptoms have already been appraised as serious, the common sense model simply predicts that the individual will decide to seek medical help, which means seeing his or her GP. Where the schema includes identity information this decision is assumed to be a direct schema-based inference (see Chapter 3, Section 3.1). Where the schema is not organised enough to allow such understanding, the decision to seek help is assumed to follow for two main reasons. These are to obtain symptomatic relief and to gain understanding or help in elaborating an "inadequate" schema.

Although the model is not drawn to any scale and no detailed predictions about time are made, the distance to the exit decision could be scaled to represent time, and the underlying assumption is that a rational decision is also a prompt one. Two subsidiary predictions follow. First, there should be a correlation between appraised seriousness and the speed with which the decision to seek help is made. In the model, this could be represented by the angles of ascent or descent onto the fast track. The quickest is perpendicular, which as depicted in Figure 4.1 is the rational outcome when the individual understands that his or her symptoms indicate cancer. When the individual cannot decide what the symptoms indicate, more painful or bother-some symptoms should predict a steeper gradient and therefore a faster decision to seek help (as indicated by the steeper pathway). The second subsidiary prediction is that mistakes in deciding to visit the GP will be characterised by Type 1 errors (false alarms) since individuals should err on the side of safety.

People who are rapidly overcome by incapacitating symptoms might not be able rationally to process information and seek help, and the model is not strictly relevant in these cases, nor in cases where people do not make their own decisions. The model also assumes that medical help is believed to be available. However, empirical and case studies show that the common sense model of deciding to seek professional help is inadequate.

2. Challenges to the Common Sense Model of Seeking Professional Help for Illness

---

ACTIVITY 4.1 Insights into seeking help for medical symptoms

Have you, or anyone you know, visited a GP for something trivial? How do you explain this?
    Reconsider Activity 2.1 (p. 23)

● Are you experiencing any symptoms? If so, what actions have you taken to gain relief from them?
    If you have taken no actions, why not?
● Have you consulted your GP? If so, how much time elapsed between noticing symptoms and visiting him or her?

2.1 Empirical studies

In a seminal study, three quarters of a sample of 1344 people who were registered with a GP, but not currently in treatment, were experiencing symptoms. Because they had not sought help, common sense would predict that they had appraised their symptoms as trivial. On the contrary, however, one quarter of the sample had pain, a disability, or worries, or were suffering inconvenience (Hannay, 1979). Thus, they had appraised themselves as ill with serious symptoms but had not sought medical help. Similarly, Taylor (1995) estimates that 60% of people who have appraised themselves as ill and who feel ill do not seek professional help in the USA. Second, although common sense suggested a negative correlation between the perceived seriousness of a symptom and the time taken to seek help, even alarming and potentially life-threatening symptoms, such as rectal bleeding, often go untreated (Bishop & Converse, 1986).

Consistent with this picture, survival rates and quality of life following treatment of cancer are typically inversely proportional to the extent of disease at diagnosis and many lives are lost because of patients' delay in seeking help (Andersen & Cacioppo, 1995). For example, Hackett, Gassem, and Raker (1973) studied 563 cancer patients. Only a third had consulted within 4 weeks of perceiving the first symptom and 8% waited until they could no longer function independently. This untreated majority was famously labelled the "illness iceberg" (Hannay, 1979). It challenges the common sense model of deciding to seek professional help.

The common sense model also predicted that mistakes should be characterised by Type 1 errors, because people should err on the side of safety. However, unnecessary visits to the GP are estimated to occur about half as often as untreated symptoms (Hannay, 1979). Thus, help seeking seems more to be slowed by Type 2 errors than accelerated in the interest of self-preservation. Again, this challenges common sense.

2.2 Case study

> *Mike Pugh had a large, deep melanoma removed from his nose. It began as a crater-like spot, which would weep, then form a scab. However, when the scab dropped off, the cycle would begin again instead of healing. It was bothersome, because it would bleed profusely, staining towels whenever he washed his face. He became worried when friends repeatedly told him he had a teardrop on his nose. However, he endured it for several years, until he visited his GP about an eye complaint and while he was there, he asked for it to be examined. He was immediately referred to a consultant. On more than one occasion, he arrived at the clinic, but turned away because it shared an entrance with the Special Clinic.*

This case study shows that people do not necessarily visit a health professional even when they know they have a prominent, inconvenient, and serious symptom.

2.3 Summary

Empirical and case studies show that contrary to common sense, rational decisions to visit a doctor do not necessarily follow the appraisal of serious symptoms. Social psychological explanations of the "long-standing socio-medical habits, attitudes and practices collectively labelled chronic patient delay" (Goldsen, Gerhard, & Handy, 1957) will form the focus of the next section in an attempt to find rival explanations to common sense.

3. Do I Need to See my Doctor? Social Psychological Influences on Delay in Seeking Professional Help for Illness

Safer et al. (1979) systematically identified qualitatively different stages of delay in seeking medical help (see also Andersen & Cacioppo, 1995; Cacioppo, 1995; Sarafino, 1998; Suls et al., 1997). Four such stages are shown in Table 4.1.

First, there might be a delay between detecting an unexplained symptom and inferring a problem or illness. This stage is labelled "appraisal delay" and it formed the focus of the previous chapter. Subsequently, a further delay (labelled "illness

TABLE 4.1 *Stages in delaying seeking professional medical help (after Safer et al., 1979)*

Appraisal delay	Time between detecting an unexplained symptom and inferring illness
Illness delay	Time between deciding one is ill and deciding to seek professional help
Behavioural delay (also known as schedule delay)	Time between deciding to seek professional help and doing so
Treatment delay (also known as utilisation delay)	Time between seeing the professional and taking his or her advice

delay") might elapse between deciding one is ill and deciding to seek professional help. Third, "behavioural delay" (also known as "schedule delay") refers to the time between making the decision and actively seeking professional help, for example, by making an appointment. Finally, "treatment delay" (also known as "utilisation delay") is the time between seeing the professional, and acting on his or her advice. There is some conflict between these labels and the definition of illness quoted at the beginning of Section 1 of the previous chapter. This is because "illness delay", "behavioural delay", and "treatment delay" are all responses to symptoms and therefore would all be defined as illness (see Helman, 2000). For consistency, the descriptions of stages in delay rather than the labels will be preferred in the rest of this chapter.

To give some idea of the relative duration of these stages, a study of 39 women with gynaecological cancer found a mean total patient delay of 97 days (Andersen & Cacioppo, 1995). It took 77 days to infer that a problem existed. On average, 10 more days passed before the women decided to seek medical help followed by a further 5 days before they saw a doctor. Finally, another 5 days elapsed before they began treatment.

In practice, it is often not possible to distinguish between the last three stages of delay, because the only evidence is that the person is not undergoing treatment. This chapter attempts to do so where possible by focusing on the period between appraising that a symptom indicates a problem and deciding to seek medical help. The attempt is justified because compared with making a decision, implementing it and carrying it through in the real world are increasingly subject to non-psychological factors.

3.1 Intrapersonal influences on delay in seeking professional help for illness

The prediction of behaviours from intrapersonal structures and processes is a core topic of social psychology. In fact, so many studies have extended what has been learned into the health field that there is simply not space to do justice to them here and only a few major approaches will be considered. Recent and comprehensive reviews are to be found in Stroebe and Jonas (2001) and Conner and Norman (1996), respectively. In order to narrow the focus further, selected approaches will not be reviewed in depth. Rather, those features will be highlighted that offer rivals to the common sense view that individuals will decide to visit a doctor when they appraise themselves as ill with serious symptoms. In addition, I will focus on a single example throughout. It is a recent case in which a man who had a serious pain in his testicles, which he feared might be a symptom of cancer, delayed a week before deciding to visit his GP. This example fits with current attempts to raise awareness of prostate cancer as depicted in Figure 4.2 and a male-oriented example is also appropriate because Chapter 7 will focus on women.

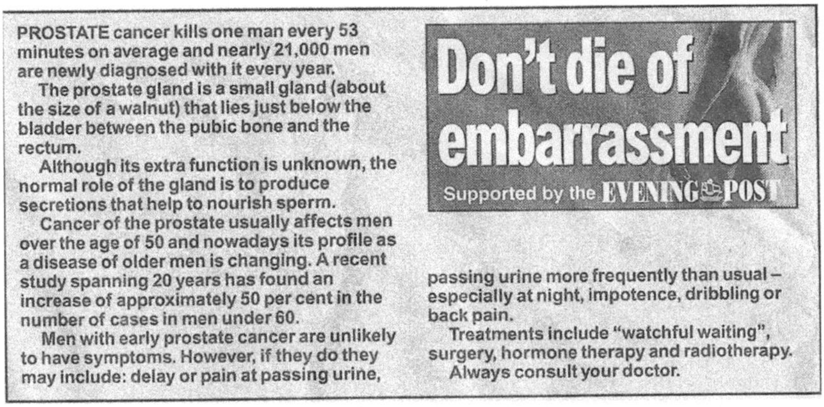

PROSTATE cancer kills one man every 53 minutes on average and nearly 21,000 men are newly diagnosed with it every year.

The prostate gland is a small gland (about the size of a walnut) that lies just below the bladder between the pubic bone and the rectum.

Although its extra function is unknown, the normal role of the gland is to produce secretions that help to nourish sperm.

Cancer of the prostate usually affects men over the age of 50 and nowadays its profile as a disease of older men is changing. A recent study spanning 20 years has found an increase of approximately 50 per cent in the number of cases in men under 60.

Men with early prostate cancer are unlikely to have symptoms. However, if they do they may include: delay or pain at passing urine,

passing urine more frequently than usual – especially at night, impotence, dribbling or back pain.

Treatments include "watchful waiting", surgery, hormone therapy and radiotherapy. Always consult your doctor.

Don't die of embarrassment

Supported by the EVENING POST

FIGURE 4.2 Don't die of embarrassment. Reproduced with permission from the *Bristol Evening Post*.

3.1.1 The Health Belief Model

In order to try to understand why people failed to make use of screening tests to detect and prevent disease, Hochbaum (1958) developed the Health Belief Model. This was underpinned by the assumption that health decisions and behaviours are best understood with reference an individual's perceptions of the social environment, which are rationally processed. Whether a person will carry out a given health behaviour is predicted by two major variables. The first is perceived vulnerability to the relevant threat, which in turn depends on perceived susceptibility to the threat and the perceived severity of its consequences. The second variable is an evaluation of the act, which is based on perceived benefits weighed against perceived barriers to performing it. The Health Belief Model is credited with inspiring more research than any other (Sheeran & Abraham, 1996) and it has met with "moderate success" in predicting a wide range of health-related behaviours (e.g., Calnan, 1984; Conner & Norman, 1996; see Sheeran & Abraham, 1996, for a review).

The Health Belief Model offers a number of explanations to rival the common sense idea that a man who appraises serious testicular pain, which he fears indicates prostate cancer, will seek prompt professional help. It is annotated with respect to this example in Figure 4.3. The first explanation is that the man believes his susceptibility to prostate cancer is low. He might also believe that its long-term consequences are mild even though its symptoms are currently appraised as serious, although this begs the question as to the meaning of "serious" (by splitting it into independent constituents and conveniently redefining some as not serious after all). Better rivals to common sense are therefore likely to revolve around the second explanation, which concerns evaluations of the act. For example, the man might delay visiting his GP in spite of serious symptoms if he has little faith in doctors,

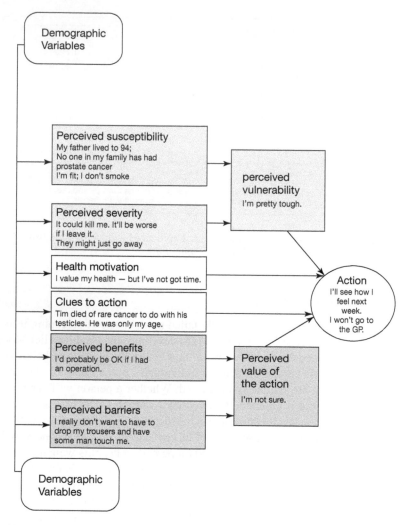

FIGURE 4.3 The Health Belief Model: The example of a man who has pain in his
testicles, which he fears indicates cancer.

or sees barriers, such as embarrassment, to the visit. Taylor (1995) notes that women
who fear they have breast cancer delay seeking help because they believe they
will have to undergo mastectomy and other cures, which they perceive to be worse
than the disease. Similarly, 33% of women who had not consulted for distressing
menstrual symptoms were described as "alienated" (Scambler & Scambler, 1985)
and did not believe the medical profession could help them. Similar influences
might be relevant in the field of prostate cancer, since once diagnosed some men
never return for treatment (Key, 2001).

Clearly, such evaluations are not based on symptom or illness information *per se*, but include beliefs about treatment and other factors, which were missing from the common sense model. Curiously however, how symptoms make the individual feel does not play any role (see Telles & Pollack, 1981).

In some versions of the Health Belief Model, the action of the two key variables is moderated by other factors such as cues to action, and how symptoms feel might be incorporated here as an additional cue. Demographic variables and the individual's motivation to care for his or her health are included as other moderators (Sheeran & Abraham, 1996). In the first instance, Taylor (1995) cites a number of large-scale surveys, which show that poor and uneducated people are less likely to visit doctors, because they have less means to do so. Similarly, in a study of cardiac rehabilitation patients in a UK hospital, we found that patients were less likely to attend if they had problems with public transport or parking (St. Claire & Turner, 1995). Thus, although it is grounded in the individual's cognitive structures and processes, the model includes other, not necessarily social psychological, variables and further highlights that symptom-relevant information is not the only source of influence on the decision to seek help.

It is also worth noting that the model predicts that perceived vulnerability is likely to be relatively low when the man has little understanding of his symptoms. This is because vulnerability results from appraisals, which presuppose that there should be some knowledge of the threat to appraise. This fits with the finding that individuals with strong illness identity (and cure components) are more likely to seek professional help (Lau, Bernard, & Hartman, 1989) and offers a successful rival to the common sense idea that individuals will seek help when they are unable to understand.

The Health Belief Model has been criticised because each variable can be operationalised in many ways (Stainton Rogers, 1991). It is easy to understand this point when observing Figure 4.3, which includes a few example beliefs, since many other beliefs to represent the key variables immediately spring to mind. The problem most likely indicates inadequate construct definition (Sheeran & Abraham, 1996) and support for this interpretation has already been illustrated earlier where it was not clear whether serious symptoms could be defined in ways that did not entail serious consequences.

Another criticism is that the model is too static. In research, once questionnaires are printed, new items cannot be added, and less important items cannot disappear. Likewise, once completed, questionnaires are analysed without revision. A moment's reflection, however, reveals that real-life decisions are often of the "to be or not to be" variety—that is, they are characterised by twists, turns, and changes. The model is also too static in the sense that there is no indication of the psychological processes that link variables and no indication of how variables should be combined (Stainton Rogers, 1991). Indeed, there is some doubt as to whether some of them should be combined at all. For example, a single index is unlikely to be appropriate to represent the qualitative differences between costs and benefits, to say nothing of the multiple components that contribute to each (Sheeran

& Abraham, 1996). Notwithstanding, most researchers seem to add susceptibility to severity, to give personal vulnerability. To this total they add benefits and then they subtract costs. Rather than this additive combination, Stroebe and Stroebe, (1995) and Stroebe and Jonas (2001) argue that an interactive model is necessary since perceived vulnerability will be very low if either susceptibility or severity has the value zero, no matter how high the other. For example, a man discovering a lump in his breast might (mistakenly) believe that men do not develop breast cancer and decide not to seek help even if he thinks breast cancer has very serious consequences. However, although it makes sense, the suggestion has not received empirical support and further research is needed to resolve the issue (Sheeran & Abraham, 1996).

A final criticism is that although perceived susceptibility, severity, benefits, and costs are individually significant in a majority of studies, the amount of variance they explain in behaviour is limited (Sheeran & Abraham, 1996). On average it is only between 0.5 and 4% (Harrison, Mullen, & Green, 1992).

Overall therefore, the Health Belief Model usefully identifies many variables that were overlooked in the common sense model of seeking help for serious symptoms, especially those relating to evaluation of the act. However, because it has a number of weaknesses and accounts for little variance in behaviour, it does not provide a convincing rival.

3.1.2 The Theory of Reasoned Action and the Theory of Planned Behaviour

The common sense model of seeking help for serious symptoms is assumed to be schema-based. However, a general weakness of schema theory is that it does not specify the ways in which knowledge-based inferences can be turned into procedures and actions in the real world (Kahney, 1993). Unlike schema theory, however, a major goal of attitude research and theory has been to predict behaviour (Bohner, 2001). Of course attitudes and schemata are different concepts because (for example) attitudes specifically concern evaluation (Ajzen, 1988) whereas schemata do not. Notwithstanding, there are convenient overlaps between them since both are higher-order cognitive structures that organise thinking and experience (Eagly & Chaiken, 1993). These overlaps mean that research into attitude–behaviour links offers a paradigm that might yield a rival to the common sense idea that an individual who has appraised him or herself as ill with serious symptoms will seek medical help.

In the Theory of Reasoned Action (Fishbein & Ajzen, 1975) the relationship between attitudes and behaviours was reformulated. A reformulation was badly needed because early studies had attempted to predict behaviour directly from attitudes. Unlike the common sense model, these would have predicted whether a man who had a pain in his testicles would visit his doctor on the basis of his attitude to doctors, visits, medicine, health, or even "life" and not on the basis of symptom severity. Like those of the common sense model, however, predictions were unsuccessful (e.g., Ajzen & Fishbein, 1977; Ajzen & Timko, 1986; LaPierre, 1934).

TABLE 4.2 *Target, action, context, and time elements relevant to a visit to the GP for a man with pain in his testicles*

Target at which attitude is directed
Relieve pain; understand what is wrong; gain reassurance; cure any underlying problems

Action at which attitude is directed
Visit Dr Smith

Context in which actions occur
University Health Centre

Time
1st December 2001

In building their theory, Fishbein and Ajzen (1975) first argued that target behaviours and intrapersonal measures needed to be compatible. In the present case, this means that attitude measures gathered to predict whether the man will visit his doctor should not be pitched at general levels (e.g., to doctors) but must concern the relevant visit, specifying its time, date, and purpose. A few relevant examples are illustrated in Table 4.2 and it can be appreciated that compatibility means that the visit to be predicted is likely to be more closely tied to the man's understanding of his symptoms (see Salovey et al., 1998 for a recent review).

Second, Fishbein and Ajzen (1975) argued that a given behaviour is a direct result of a compatible behavioural intention, rather than of the attitude to it. However, the attitude to the behaviour still figures prominently because, barring unforeseen events, behavioural intention "flows reasonably" (Ajzen, 1988) from a linear combination of the relevant attitude and another variable, known as the subjective norm.

The model also specifies how to predict the relevant attitude and subjective norm. The attitude flows reasonably from salient beliefs about outcomes and attributes of the behaviour. These are called behavioural beliefs and three examples are included in Figure 4.4. More formally, an expectancy-value equation defines the attitude as directly proportional to a sum calculated over salient beliefs about the outcomes of an act. For each salient belief, the subtotal contributed consists of the subjective probability that performing the act will lead to the given outcome, multiplied by the subjective value of that outcome (Ajzen, 1988). Illustrative (verbal) probabilities and values are included in Figure 4.4 and suggest that our example man's attitude is likely to be neutral or negative.

Subjective norms, also called normative beliefs, represent the thinker's perceived social support for his or her behavioural intention and are therefore social psychological in nature. They can be calculated by identifying a range of salient people for an individual, such as friends, family members, and experts. For each of these, the extent to which the individual believes that person would approve of the behaviour, and the individual's motivation to comply with him or her are measured, then multiplied together. The summed total over all salient people gives the individual's subjective norm for that behaviour. Three examples are included in Figure 4.4 and also suggest that the man's subjective norm is likely to be neutral or negative.

The Theory of Reasoned Action offers many ways of understanding why a man with pain in his testicles might not intend to seek medical help, even if he has appraised his symptoms as serious. First, and unlike the common sense model, the visit as opposed to the symptoms takes centre stage and symptom appraisals might play a relatively small role in the attitude to this, which might be negative if he believes it will not do much good and will be excruciatingly embarrassing. However, the attitude to the visit is only one predictor of the intention to visit. The other is a relevant subjective norm. Again, symptom severity might play a relatively small role here and normative beliefs might be negative if the visit falls in working hours and the man's work-mates have told him they cannot manage to complete a crucial project without him.

The Theory of Reasoned Action is especially useful because it distinguishes between intention and actual behaviour. In the case when the man does intend to visit his doctor, he might simply miss the bus or find he has lost the requisite telephone number and cannot make an appointment. Alternatively, he might lack the resolve to carry his intention through and find himself distracted by the opportunity of an unexpected night out.

The current interest is on the decision or intention to seek help rather than the ways in which implementing it might be disrupted by unforeseen contingencies. However, it can easily be appreciated that the man might not bother to form the intention to visit his doctor if he is not permitted to take the time off work, knows he will be standing on the bus stop while his appointment time comes and goes, or knows that he has a lousy record of keeping appointments. The Theory of Reasoned Action was formulated to deal with situations under volitional control in which beliefs about control are not an issue. The model was extended by the addition of perceived behavioural control in order to accommodate behaviours over which individuals have incomplete control (Ajzen, 1985, 1988). The extended model is called the Theory of Planned Behaviour and it is shown in Figure 4.4, annotated with respect to our example. Perceived behavioural control is a complex concept which represents a wide range of beliefs relevant to the act, the person, and the circumstances, including the person's expectancy of the ease with which s/he can perform a behaviour. It includes knowledge of relevant skills, experience, emotions, and past track record as well as knowledge of external circumstances such as the inhibitory role of others and opportunity (Ajzen, 1988; Povey, Conner, Sparks, James, & Shepherd, 2000; Salovey et al., 1998).

Perceived behaviour control was also missing from the common sense model and it suggests that, irrespective of symptom severity, anticipated obstacles to visiting a GP might mean an individual decides not to bother. Although it is not so relevant to the present interest in understanding delay in making the decision to seek help, it is also worth noting that perceived behaviour control can sometimes accurately reflect actual control. Under these circumstances it can be used as a

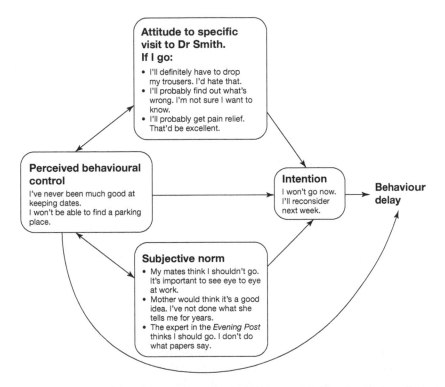

FIGURE 4.4 The Theory of Planned Behaviour: The example of a man who has pain in his testicles, which he fears indicates cancer.

partial substitute for a measure of actual control, and therefore it can help predict behaviour independent of its contribution to behavioural intention (Ajzen, 1988; Schifter & Ajzen, 1985; Sutton, 1998). This pathway is indicated by the curved arrow in Figure 4.4.

The Theory of Planned Behaviour has been extensively applied and tested in the field of health and it performs well, with correlations between behaviour and behaviour intention averaging about .70 (Norman & Conner, 1996; see Conner & Sparks, 1996, for a review). A more recent review found that multiple correlations, which predicted intention from the variables of the model, ranged between .63 and .71, whereas correlations between intention and behaviour ranged between .48 and .58 (Sutton, 1998). A recent example was a postal questionnaire study of 1215 women who had never had breast screening. The predictor variables of the model were used to categorise them on a 5-point intention scale into those who definitely intended to attend for X-ray mammography and those who definitely did not. As predicted, the former group was least likely to attend (Rutter, 2000).

In spite of its good performance, the Theory of Planned Behaviour has been criticised because of its mathematical complexity and because the prediction of behaviour is dependent on such proximate measures that the researcher might as well wait to see what happens (see Stainton Rogers, 1991). This is because the demands of compatibility mean that a researcher who wants to predict whether someone will visit a health professional cannot simply refer to global measures, such as the person's attitude towards doctors, that might even have been collected previously. Rather s/he needs to measure a range of predictors to discover what the person feels about that visit, at a given time and place, and with respect to the appraised symptoms (see Table 4.2 above). Thus, to discover how the predictor variables interact for the behaviour of interest is likely to involve a great deal of meticulous work for each individual, which contrasts with the immediate appeal of common sense (Richard et al., 1995).

Overall, the Theory of Planned Behaviour offers a useful approach to rival the common sense idea that an individual who has appraised that s/he is ill with serious symptoms will promptly seek professional medical help. The main reason is that it changes the focus from the symptoms to the visit, and the symptoms and their seriousness might not play the central role in evaluating this. In addition, the theory includes more social social psychological influences in the form of the subjective norm and perceived behavioural control.

3.1.3 Personality and health locus of control

An early attempt to predict health behaviours from personality variables was based on the work of Rotter (1966) who had suggested that people could be categorised into "externals" or "internals". Externals believe that what happens to them is largely a matter of chance, whereas internals see themselves as having control over their own lives. From this perspective, individuals with an external locus of control should take a *laissez faire* approach, and hence they should be more likely than internals to delay seeking medical help. Thus a man who has a pain in his testicles might decide not to seek help from a medical doctor even though he has appraised himself as seriously ill, because he believes fate, or perhaps his genetic constitution, has already decreed whether he will get better or succumb to cancer.

Early use of the scale was criticised because externality might have nothing to do with a weak personal disposition. Rather it might reflect an accurate assessment of control by others (Levenson, 1981; Stainton Rogers, 1991). Thus, a third dimension, Powerful Others, was added and the Multidimensional Health Locus of Control Scale was born (Wallston, Wallston, & De Vellis, 1978). On this, any individual could be classified according to his or her position on three subscales. As before, the main prediction was that individuals endorsing internal items would take active responsibility for their health. However, a lack of faith in Powerful Others offers an additional rival to the common sense idea that a man who has appraised serious symptoms that he fears indicate prostate cancer will decide to visit his GP. A few items from the scale are given in Table 4.3.

The Multidimensional Health Locus of Control Scale has been applied to a wide range of health behaviours including preventive behaviour, exercise, and alcohol

TABLE 4.3 *Typical items from the Multidimensional Health Locus of Control Scale*

Internal dimension
The main thing that affects my health is what I myself do

Powerful Others
Whenever I don't feel well, I should consult a medically trained professional

External
No matter what I do, if I'm going to get ill, I'll get ill

---

use but the results have been mixed (see Norman & Bennett, 1996, for a review). One problem noted by Stainton Rogers (1991) is that the addition of Powerful Others was at odds with the rationale that demanded it, because they were not operationalised as negative political forces that controlled or constrained individuals' health. Rather, they were operationalised as medical professionals with positive influences. Furthermore, after reviewing the literature, Stainton Rogers concludes that the scale is inadequate, and her own by-person factor analysis of responses on a Multidimensional Health Locus of Control scale yielded sixteen, not three factors. Although two did resemble internal and external dimensions, the remainder, which accounted for 50% of variance, bore no resemblance to them or to Powerful Others.

Another serious omission from the scale is a measure of the value the individual places on his or her health, since theoretically, internally oriented individuals should only take active control of their health if they value it (Norman & Bennett, 1996).

Overall therefore, the scale is not likely to offer a successful rival to the common sense idea that an individual who understands him or herself to be ill with serious symptoms will seek professional medical help.

Many studies have examined the relationship between other personality factors and the decision to seek medical help for symptoms. For example, individuals who seek professional (as opposed to lay) consultations are more likely to have high self-esteem and less likely to be self-disclosing, submissive, and trusting (Sanders, 1982). Individuals with so called "hardy personalities" are also less likely to consult professionals, whereas high self-monitors, who seek information in anxiety-provoking situations, are more likely to do so (Skevington 1995). From such studies extensive lists of individual traits that are associated with delay in approaching the professional healthcare system may be drawn up. However, criticisms of this approach have already been made in the context of predicting symptom perceptions from personality traits (see Chapter 2, Section 4.1.4). For example, the direction of causality cannot be settled and links between personality and delay might have been caused by previous experiences with health professionals. As previously argued therefore, such variables *per se* are unlikely successfully to offer a rival to the common sense idea that an individual who understands him or herself to be ill with serious symptoms will seek professional medical help. Notwithstanding, personality variables play important roles in wider models as we have seen, and shall see.

3.1.4 Fear and Protection Motivation Theory

The approaches so far reviewed concern "cold cognitions" which fail to capture the human experience of illness. In the example used throughout this section, the man is described as *fearing* that his pains might indicate cancer, and a moment's reflection reveals that this is likely to be a very different experience from making an actuarial calculation of susceptibility and seriousness. The common sense model assumed that health-relevant information is rationally processed. However, the impact of fear might disrupt rational processing, and therefore it might offer a rival explanation to the common sense idea that an individual who appraises serious symptoms will seek prompt medical help.

Early social psychologists believed that fear was a drive state that, like other drives, motivates instrumental responding (Eagly & Chaiken, 1993). Since drive reduction was inherently reinforcing, cognitive or behavioural responses that reduced fear would be reinforced and therefore would become more likely. Early researchers applied this principle in the health field. They hypothesised that persuasive messages that contained frightening depictions of what would happen if respondents did not take the recommended course of action should be more successful than less frightening messages. This was because deciding to take the action would reduce fear, and hence be reinforced. However, the drive-reduction model was "subtly complex" (Eagly & Chaiken, 1993) because people might use a range of idiosyncratic strategies to reduce their fear as opposed to the danger (see Salovey et al., 1998 for a discussion). For example, they might deny the message altogether. Researchers also discovered that fear was more likely to have the desired effect when their recommendations were presented immediately afterwards and were portrayed as effective and easy to carry out.

Early experimental manipulations of persuasive communications are a world away from the present focus. Notwithstanding, the drive-reduction approach usefully suggests that the common sense correlation between the seriousness of appraised symptoms and speed of help seeking might not accrue because people are frightened by serious symptoms and find non-rational ways of reducing their fear. The approach, annotated with respect to our example, is depicted in Figure 4.5.

In Protection Motivation Theory, Rogers (1975, 1983) set out more systematically to understand the impact of fear appeals on attitude change (Milne, Sheeran, & Orbell, 2000). The theory has been described as a hybrid because it incorporates key variables from the Health Belief Model and the field of stress, and because it has been revised and extended (Conner & Norman, 1996; Milne et al., 2000).

In the theory, an adaptive behaviour is predefined as the one that reduces a health threat, and is conceptualised as a function of "protection motivation" which is the intention to carry it out. Whether an individual forms a protection motivation is predicted by two major variables. The first is an appraisal of the threat constituted by continuing with maladaptive behaviour and the second is an appraisal of the recommended behaviour as a means to cope with the threat (Floyd, Prentice-Dunn, & Rogers, 2000).

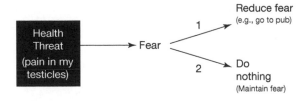

Fear reduction is inherently reinforcing. Response 1 reduces fear and so becomes more likely. It shows there are many ways to reduce fear besides visiting a GP.

FIGURE 4.5 Drive Reduction Model of fear.

Threat was originally predicted by perceived severity and vulnerability, essentially as it was in the Health Belief Model, plus fear. In the revised version of the model, perceived rewards associated with the maladaptive behaviour were also included and hypothesised to reduce perceived threat (Rogers, 1983). However, it is worth noting that the relationship between threat and maladaptive behaviours is complex because, as noted above, threat can sometimes initiate maladaptive behaviours such as denial.

Coping appraisal was initially predicted by perceived efficacy of the behaviour. In the revised model however, the person's self-efficacy in performing it was added. Costs and other barriers, such as embarrassment, were also added and hypothesised to reduce coping appraisal (Boer & Seydel, 1996; Eagley & Chaiken, 1993; Milne et al., 2000; Rogers, 1975, 1983).

In the model, exposure to a fear-arousing communication is thought to arouse three cognitive processes relevant to susceptibility, vulnerability, and efficacy. Higher levels of fearfulness are thought to increase perceived severity and vulnerability, and therefore to increase the likelihood of performing the adaptive behaviour (Boer & Seydel, 1996). This means that a threatening message accompanying a health recommendation is more likely to lead to the acceptance of the recommendation than a non-threatening message (Eagley & Chaiken, 1993).

The model suggests two new reasons to rival common sense. First, instead of increasing the likelihood that help will be sought, high levels of threat might trigger denial and so sabotage help seeking. Paradoxically therefore, attempts to reassure an individual might have the undesired effect of reducing the likelihood that s/he will seek help. Second, advantages to *not* seeking help might also reduce feelings of threat, with the result that the individual chooses not to go to the GP. Thus, a need to conceal symptoms at work to protect one's job might mean delay in seeking help. The model annotated with respect to our example is depicted in Figure 4.6.

The model has been successfully applied in a number of health-related areas including reducing alcohol use, enhancing healthy lifestyles, and preventing disease (see Boer & Seydel, 1996, and Eagly & Chaiken, 1993, for reviews). For example,

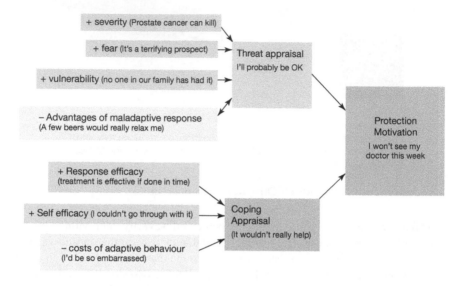

FIGURE 4.6 Protection Motivation Theory.

a study of the intention to participate in breast cancer screening found that severity and vulnerability accounted for negligible amounts of variance in protection motivation, whereas response efficacy accounted for 22% and self-efficacy, for an additional 14% (Boer & Seydel, 1996). A recent meta-analysis of 27 studies in the context of health threats supported this picture (Milne et al., 2000) because although all variables of the model were significantly correlated with protection motivation, the association with severity was small while that with response efficacy was most robust. This led the authors to conclude that coping variables are more important than threat.

However, precisely how the variables should be combined has been subject to doubts and revision. For example, there is no agreed formula to accommodate the idea that perceptions of higher threat will only increase protection motivation if they are supported by response and self-efficacy (Rogers, 1983; Stroebe & Jonas, 1996). Another problem is that the effects of fear are more marked on protection motivation than on adaptive behaviours (Boer & Seydel, 1996; Eagly & Chaiken, 1993).

Overall, protection motivation is more relevant to experimental variations of scare tactics in public health campaigns than to the present interest in finding social psychological rivals to the common sense idea that an individual will seek help when s/he appraises that s/he is ill with serious symptoms. Notwithstanding, it usefully suggests variables that were missing from the common sense model, the novel one being the attractiveness of maladaptive acts. Furthermore, because threat variables are poor predictors of help seeking compared with coping appraisals, it can be seen that the appraised seriousness of symptoms, which is the driving force of the common sense model, might not determine whether a man will seek help for serious symptoms. His views about the treatment and his own abilities to cope might carry more weight. Interestingly, a second recent meta-analysis suggests that this suggestion might prove premature with respect to our example of a man who fears he might have prostate cancer. To explain, Floyd et al. (2000) reviewed 65 studies, which represented 29,650 participants. Not all of the studies were in the health field, but separate analyses of studies related to different health problems were carried out. Compared with smoking cessation, adherence to medical regimens, AIDS prevention, health, diet, and exercise, variables behaved differently in the field of cancer. In this field, it was threat, as opposed to coping, that was more closely associated with protection motivation. Clearly, further research is needed to clarify this issue, but it might be resolved by a consideration of the function of the behaviour in question. This is because beliefs about the severity of a threat are more relevant than beliefs about vulnerability when predicting screening behaviour, but when predicting preventive behaviour, vulnerability is the more important (Salovey et al. 1998).

3.1.4 Stress and emotion

From fear and protection motivation, it is a small step to the field of stress, which offers a wider paradigm from which to draw rivals to the common sense idea that an individual who appraises him or herself as ill with serious symptoms will seek professional help. A consideration of stress also raises interesting issues about the ways in which social psychological influences can cross physical boundaries.

The term "stress" was first used in the 14th century to mean hardship or affliction (Cooper, Cooper, & Eaker, 1988). In the 17th century, the developing science of engineering introduced a view of stress as the ratio between a load and the area over which it was applied. Stress in this sense was thought to cause strain in its recipient (Lazarus & Folkman, 1984). However, such approaches proved inadequate to understand human stress because individual differences in responses meant it was impossible to say what stimulus characteristics made something stressful (Lazarus, 1999).

The term did not enter the psychological literature until 1944 when the Second World War generated concern that fighting men might be less effective under the stress of battle (Lazarus, 1999; Lazarus & Folkman, 1984). Lazarus (1966) was the first to emphasise the role of thinking and appraisal in understanding human stress, which he famously defined as: "A particular relationship between the person and the environment that is appraised by the person as taxing or exceeding his or her resources and endangering his or her well-being."

Appraisal means more than passive perception. It means evaluating events with respect to personal goals and values. There are two broad categories of appraisal. The first is primary appraisal, which is an evaluation of the extent to which circumstances are relevant to the person's well-being, and Lazarus (1966) distinguished three types of stress based on three types of primary appraisal. Harm or loss refers to damage that has already taken place; threat refers to damage that might happen; and challenge is the sensibility that, although difficulties stand in the way of gain, they can be overcome with verve, persistence, and self-confidence.

Primary appraisal is relevant here because, as in the models already reviewed, serious symptoms can pose a threat, intimately related to loss of control and esteem (e.g., Baron, 1985; Wood, Taylor, & Lichtman, 1985). However, of fundamental importance, primary appraisal does not necessarily depend on rational evaluations of stimuli, such as symptoms and associated probabilities and prognoses. Rather, stimuli are evaluated in relation to the individual's own goals, values, and well-being. Thus, contrary to common sense, it might be that a man welcomes the possibility of prostate cancer and wants to succumb to it as quickly as possible. This might be because he has religious convictions, which lead him to appraise it as an opportunity to demonstrate the strength of his faith and as a means to an early union with his god.

The second sort of appraisal is called secondary appraisal and this is the person's evaluation of the coping resources they can marshal to deal with stress. It entails choosing what to do and when and how to do it. It also entails evaluating the ability to act together with advantages and disadvantages of the action (e.g., Lazarus, 1999; Lazarus & Folkman, 1984). Because the assessment of coping resources is likely to underpin the ensuing behaviours, coping is an integral part of stress. Indeed actual coping and secondary appraisal cannot always be distinguished because finding out what is to be done, for example, can fall into both categories.

Secondary appraisal is relevant here because seeking help from a GP can be seen as a coping strategy. However, of fundamental importance, secondary appraisal entails evaluating ways of reducing stress, not ways of reducing the stressor *per se*. To explain, coping behaviours are often categorised into those that are active (also known as problem-oriented) and those that are passive (also known as avoidant). The former are attempts to solve external problems identified as causing stress, whereas the latter are aimed at managing internal emotions and accommodating to the situation (Lazarus, 1999; Lazarus & Folkman, 1984; Stroebe & Stroebe, 1996). In the case of a threatening symptom, a problem-oriented coping strategy would entail actions aimed at removing it, including seeking instrumental professional help. An emotion-focused strategy would entail reducing stress by other means, including denial, joining a support group, or perhaps just talking it through. Although it is often assumed that active coping is more likely successfully to remove the appraisal of stress, the best strategy depends on the situation. For example, emotion-focused coping might be more effective in the short term, and it is all that is available if the stressful situation is uncontrollable (Sutherland & Cooper, 1992; Suls & Fletcher, 1985; Taylor & Clark, 1986). Interestingly, Broadstock and Borland (1998) found use of a cancer helpline had both active and passive functions depending on the use made of the information. They also found that it was particularly valuable because patients frequently failed to elicit the information they required from their GPs.

The appraisal approach to stress usefully accommodates the role of many personality traits because, for example, an optimist may be reconceptualised as an individual who appraises coping potential positively (Spencer, 1998a). Even dimensions relevant to health locus of control such as attributions of controllability and accountability parallel some components of secondary appraisal and there is evidence that the latter are the stronger predictors of (stress and) emotion (Frijda, Kuijpers, & ter Schure, 1989).

In spite of this promise, however, Lazarus's approach can be criticised because its cognitive emphasis fails to capture the emotional and biological turmoil that characterises human stress. In addition, it is inconsistent about its evaluative status, which is positive when described in the context of challenge, but exclusively negative when described in the context of emotions (Lazarus, 1999). A useful second definition of stress therefore, is that of Baum (1990) who defines it as: "a negative emotional experience accompanied by predictable biochemical, physiological, cognitive and behavioural changes that are directed either toward altering the stressful event or accommodating to its effects."

Of course, the question "What is stress, really?" is nonsense because stress is a "fuzzy" concept constructed by humans to refer to a wide range of chosen phenomena (see Mercer, 1973; Rosch, 1975). Thus, it makes pragmatic sense to build a working model of stress, in which Lazarus's contribution represents the cognitive components and Baum's contribution represents physiological arousal, feeling states, and action tendencies. The model is depicted in Figure 4.7, annotated with respect to our example, but to accommodate feedback and reappraisals it is best viewed as cyclic and dynamic (see Chapter 3, Section 3.1.5, for an example in which a full-blown panic attack began with appraisals of normal physical events).

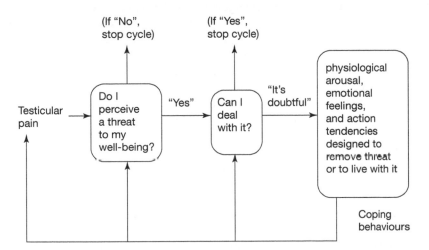

FIGURE 4.7 A working model of stress (annotated with respect to a man who has perceived pain in his testicles which he fears indicates cancer).

This working model preserves the advantages of appraisal theory but because it does not specify harm, loss, or challenge, it neatly avoids confusion over the evaluative status of stress, which is always a negative experience. The model is close to Scherer's (2001) view of emotion, but the important difference is that it is inherently unstable, since it is characterised by doubt and uncertainty and so represents a state of emotional turmoil that does not resolve into one (or more) specific emotions.

Thus, contrary to common sense, whether a man who appraises a serious pain in his testicles, which he fears might indicate cancer, seeks prompt professional help is not so much a function of the appraised seriousness of the symptoms, but of his ways of coping with stress. Likewise, the effectiveness of seeking professional medical help is not evaluated with respect to the efficacy of the act in removing the threat to health, but with respect to its efficacy in removing stress. The model predicts that delay in seeking professional help is likely, because many actions are likely to achieve the latter end.

A further advantage of the approach is that it prompts speculations about the ways in which stress and symptoms might interact. To explain, Selye (1956, 1974) had observed what appeared to be a core pattern beneath traumas such as burns, ingestion of toxins, infections, and other diseases in medical patients. In general they lost their appetite, weight, strength, ambition, and motivation. Selye suspected that this pattern might reflect biological laws governing the body's attempt to return to normal and that weight loss associated with cancer, for example, might be due to this effort rather than the disease. In order to investigate his idea he studied the physical aspects of (dis)stress in rats that he repeatedly exposed to different severe stressors. The General Adaptation syndrome was the resulting discovery. In its first stage, adrenal activity and hormone levels, particularly corticosteroid secretions, were raised and they caused enlargement of the adrenal cortex, suppressed immunity, and gastrointestinal ulcers. Resistance to the stressor was low and death occurred if the stressor was too intense. In the second stage of the syndrome, the signs of alarm disappeared, as the animals adapted by channelling energy into the organ system best equipped to resist the repeated exposures. The cost of this resistance was paid in the third stage, in terms of increased vulnerability of other systems. Alarm signs reappeared but were irreversible and specific symptoms arose, depending on specific effects of the stressor and individual differences. Ultimately, the systems would break down and the animal would die (e.g., Selye, 1974).

Although it is unwise to generalise from animal studies to humans, and flaws in Selye's interpretations have been identified (e.g., Lazarus, 1999), people can and do adapt to chronic stress and many recent studies suggest that it leads to disease via immune system down-regulation. For example, Cohen, Tyrrell, and Smith (1991, 1993) exposed subjects to common cold viruses under controlled conditions and found that those who reported more stress were more likely to develop a cold and that the severity of their symptoms was correlated with their stress levels. Similarly, the prognosis of breast cancer, HIV, and AIDS, together with autoimmune diseases such as rheumatoid arthritis, is worse for stressed individuals (Evans, Clow, & Hucklebridge, 1997; Levy, 1986; Levy et al., 1990).

Chronic stress can also contribute directly to the risk of heart disease because chronic sympathetic arousal means chronically raised heart-rate, tendency of the blood to clot, and raised levels of serum lipids (Evans et al., 1997; Girdano & Everly, 1986; Stroebe & Jonas, 2001; Stroebe & Stroebe, 1996). Third, in rest periods after stress, rebound overactivity of the parasympathetic system might contribute to the development of ulcers or even heart failure (Kalat, 2001).

These studies show that the boundaries between stress, disease, symptoms, and wider social psychological factors are permeable. Since adaptation to stress can lead to disease, an illness that has no signs might develop them through the action of psychological stress. Thus, a man who has appraised pains that alarm him might be in physical danger because of the alarm as well as, or even instead of, the symptoms. Furthermore, emotion-focused coping, if successful, will ameliorate hormonal and chemical changes associated with stress and hence might improve immune function and ameliorate underlying disease processes (Pennebaker, Kiecott-Glaser, & Glaser, 1988). Thus, not seeking professional help might paradoxically mediate a "cure" if alternative behaviours, including simply doing nothing, reduce stress.

Overall, an appraisal model of stress offers a complex rival to the common sense idea that an individual who has appraised himself ill with serious symptoms will seek prompt professional help. The important difference is that the meaning of the symptoms in relation to personal well-being is more important than their severity and the efficacy of the visit in removing stress is more important than its efficacy in removing the symptoms.

3.1.5 Some conclusions and a note on stage models

Although a wide range of intrapersonal variables help to explain why a man who has serious pain which he thinks indicates prostate cancer does not behave as common sense predicts and seek medical help, the models reviewed draw upon the same core variables, and consequently share a family resemblance. The possible exception is the Multidimensional Health Locus of Control Scale, which alone does not include an appraisal of threat or of outcomes. In fact, the models might be closer than at first appears, because differences in the labelling of variables often mask theoretical similarity between underlying constructs, and Norman and Conner (1996) conclude that there is probably little to choose between them. Indeed, performance of the models is likely to converge and improve (i) if the most powerful variables, such as self-efficacy, are added to those that do not already include them; (ii) if moderator variables, such as the value an individual places on his or her health, are used to identify subpopulations in which approaches such as the Multidimensional Health Locus of Control Scale might perform as hoped; and (iii) and if new variables that capture sufficient variance, such as moral norms and affective beliefs, are added (Conner & Armitage, 1998; Salovey et al., 1998; Sparks & Guthrie, 1998).

However, Norman and Conner (1996) also point out that current interest is moving away from reformulating variables in order to fine tune and compare models. Rather, interest is more focused on qualitative changes at the different stages of making a decision, carrying it out, and maintaining it (Salovey et al., 1998). The distinction is of relevance here, because it maps neatly on to the stages of delay identified at the beginning of the chapter and facilitates a focus on the decision to seek help. In the Precaution Adoption Process there are seven stages (Weinstein & Sandman, 1992) and in the Transtheoretical Model of behaviour change (Prochaska, DiClemente, & Norcross, 1992) there are five stages of change. Although the model was designed to be relevant to the treatment of addictive behaviour, it suggests useful pointers for present purposes. In the first, precontemplation, stage, an individual is unaware of relevant health risks associated with a maladaptive behaviour and has no plans to change. This would be analogous to the situation when an individual has no symptoms and no plans to visit a GP. In the second, contemplation, stage the individual begins to think about risk and possible change and this is analogous to symptom perceptions and appraisals. It is not until the third, preparation, stage that the individual forms an intention to change and begins to make relevant plans. Clearly, this is the stage of most relevance here as it involves making the decision to seek professional help. In the fourth and fifth stages, the individual implements change and if change is successful, s/he moves into the maintenance stage. A transtheoretical approach provides a formal framework in which to examine the weakening relationship between predictor variables, intention, behaviour, and subsequent behaviours. It also provides a fresh strategy to help answer the criticism made above that models are too static. For example, state-space analysis of transitions as opposed to cross-sectional analysis of individual differences might usefully be pursued by future researchers since variables relevant to risk and the efficacy of visiting a GP might be heavily weighted in early symptom appraisals while those relevant to self-efficacy and behavioural control might play a greater role when making the decision to seek help (see Stroebe & Jonas, 1996).

With the exception of the Multidimensional Health Locus of Control Scale, the approaches are grounded in rational information processing. Even behaviours that appeared irrational with respect to removing symptoms make sense after all if the individual's goals are discovered. Likewise, emotional feelings follow cognitive appraisals. However, people are not always motivated or do not have the opportunity to expend energy and effort to carry out rational information processing (Bohner, 2001; Eagly & Chaiken, 1993) and one possibility is that behaviour is based on habit. Thus, the man in our example might decide not to visit his GP simply because he never does so. In this case, his behaviour would be guided by automatic processes, as opposed to beliefs about past behaviours. Hence, rational social cognition models would be inapplicable (Aarrts, Verplanken, & van Knippenberg, 1998; Salovey et al., 1998). Alternatively, behaviour might simply be guided by the most accessible compatible attitude (Bohner, 2001; Stahlberg & Frey, 1996). The reality of this possibility is illustrated in Figure 4.8, which suggests that a man

Beating macho barrier

BIRAL Patel is nearing the end of the 12-year training that it takes to be a surgeon.

His job at the moment is research-based and he has undertaken the task of trying to find out why the incidence of prostate cancer is so much higher in black people than in white Europeans, Asian and white Americans.

His research is called the Process study – standing for Prostate Cancer Study of Ethnic Subgroups.

Hardly any studies have been carried out into black men and Mr Patel says there are many more aspects to the condition in this race than purely medical.

He said: "In this community, there is some amount of machoism that means many of the men who come to us are in the very latest stages of cancer.

"In fact, we've had patients who have never come back to us once they have found out they have it, and unfortunately it's something that is passed on through the generations," he said.

"We simply don't know why there is such a high rate of prostate cancer in black men and we desperately need to find out.

"It's great that we're carrying out the research because it quite literally is the first of its kind."

FIGURE 4.8 Beating the macho barrier. Reproduced with permission from the *Bristol Evening Post*.

who had appraised a serious and possibly life-threatening symptom might not seek professional help because his attitude to machismo was more salient than any other.

Similarly, the Heuristic–Systematic Model of attitudes assumes that people are motivated to attain accurate attitudes that square with relevant facts. However, it acknowledges that cognition can occur in an heuristic mode, in which simple decision rules as opposed to rational processing predominate (Eagly & Chaiken, 1993). Thus, a flaw in, or a hidden goal of, rational processing might not be the reason why a man does not seek medical help for serious symptoms. Rather, he might be influenced by a salient negative attitude to medical help formed as a result of absent-mindedly watching a television drama (see also Bohner, 2001).

The level of analysis relevant to the reviewed models is intrapersonal and the ongoing reality of living with active others plays little if any role in them. In the next sections, influences at interpersonal and group levels of analysis will be considered but because "health psychology is dominated by social cognition models" (Lowe, 2001, personal communication) the sections will be short.

3.2 Shall I see my doctor? Interpersonal influences on delay in seeking professional help for illness

In the previous chapter it was suggested that early caregiver reactions to children's symptoms are internalised and later influence adult symptom perceptions. It is likely that caregivers similarly provide schemata, which influence decisions about when to seek professional help. Consistent with this view, Quadrel and Lau (1990) found that teenagers' decisions to consult were very similar to those of their parents. However, although this influence comes from others, it is not necessarily truly interpersonal because it might not involve meanings created between individuals. For example, the perceiver might simply have internalised another's schema, which has therefore become an intrapersonal structure of his or her own.

Delay in deciding to seek professional help does not mean that a person is doing nothing other than cognitive processing. On the contrary, an early study of 1000 patients in a GP's surgery revealed that 96% had received advice or treatment *before* coming (Elliot-Binns, 1973; 1986, cited in Helman, 1994). Excluding self-advice and treatment, patients averaged 1.8 sources of help, although 35 had received advice from more than 5 sources. The most popular sources were friends, spouses, and relatives. More recently, Suls et al. (1997) have found similar results in a sample of young adults and argue that these lay consultations are likely to provide opportunities for interpersonal comparisons that the perceiver can use to evaluate whether symptoms indicate a visit to a professional. Beyond these close relationships, homoeopaths and acupuncturists, for example, offer an alternative to the "official" health system and an informal health-care sector comprises people who are perceived to have relevant experience, such as doctors' spouses or receptionists and those who are regularly in contact with the public, such as hairdressers (Helman, 2000). To give some idea of the prevalence of such consultations, a study of 79 women who kept health diaries for 6 weeks found an average of 11 lay consultations for each professional visit (Scambler, Scambler, & Craig, 1981). It is worth adding that a potentially serious effect of "over-the-fence" consultations is hoarding and sharing of drugs. This was demonstrated in two early studies which showed an average hoard of 26 tablets per person and that 68% of young adults admitted to receiving psychotropic drugs from friends or relatives (Hindmarch 1981; Warburton, 1978; both cited in Helman, 1994).

For present purposes, however, the important point is that an individual might delay seeking professional help because she is busy consulting family and friends. Again, these examples are not necessarily truly interpersonal since the other individuals might simply provide additional information to be processed by the perceiver.

As well as exerting influence because their views have been internalised, members of an individual's social network can influence them by virtue of sharing their social world. A study of the effects of changes in partners' smoking behaviour on the smoking behaviour of 662 women during pregnancy illustrates the point (Appleton & Pharoah, 1998). Effects were assessed independent of a range of psychosocial variables and results for early pregnancy showed that partner continuing or increasing smoking was associated with failure to quit, whereas partner stopping smoking was associated with success. Similarly, the odds of continuing smoking at the same level were higher if the partner continued at the same level and were decreased if he reduced. Results for later pregnancy showed that cessation of partners' smoking was associated with maintaining quitting, whereas women whose partners had not changed were more likely to fail to stay off cigarettes. In three out of the four analyses described, partner's behaviour was the only significant proximal social variable associated with women's smoking. By extrapolation therefore, a partner's behaviour might contribute an interpersonal influence on a man's decision not to seek medical help for serious symptoms, which is independent of the partner's cognitive structures and processes.

It is frequently the individual's spouse who first notices a symptom and has to decide what to do. A spouse literally "shares the burden" (Key, 2001), because a threat to a partner constitutes a threat to the relationship. Furthermore, it is also the case that members of an individual's social network can influence them without being consulted, both proactively and intentionally. They are likely to interrogate him or her if they suspect s/he is unwell and as caricatured in the first quotation at the start of this chapter, a bossy spouse might even take over cognitive processing for an individual. Delay might result as the individual follows the spouse's home remedies. However, empirical studies suggest the opposite also occurs. For example, a large, active kinship network predisposed towards consulting a professional (Scambler & Scambler, 1985). Moreover, relatives' advice led to more appropriate visits (see Suls, Martin, & Leventhal, 1997). Following their review, Suls et al. (1997) concluded that interpersonal consultations can increase or decrease delay.

More interestingly, common sense is oriented towards maximising individual, medically defined health. However, maximising interpersonal well-being might be the goal, and behaviours directed towards this might work against preserving the self. Furthermore, relevant appraisals might be negotiated between partners as opposed to processed within the individual. This idea was illustrated in an interpretative phenomenological analysis of interviews with 25 gay men about sex and relationships (Flowers, Smith, Sheeran, & Beail, 1997). In the context of loving relationships, new meanings of unprotected anal intercourse emerged. For example, it was an expression of commitment and "becoming one". These meanings were magnified by the threat of HIV, because consenting partners literally entrusted their lives to each other. One man even described how unsafe sex allowed a relationship to be put before the self, since "really loving somebody" entailed wanting semen exchange, even knowing that the other is HIV positive, so that a couple could die together. Thus the individual's decision to delay seeking medical help for serious symptoms might have little to do with intra-individual cognition, but might reflect interpersonal meanings.

In summary, a range of social psychological variables at the interpersonal level of analysis influence the decision to seek medical help for symptoms, and therefore offer rivals to the common sense idea that an individual will seek professional medical help on appraising serious symptoms.

3.3 I'm ill! Shall I see my doctor? Group-level influences on delay in seeking professional help for illness

In addition to having personal consequences, illness has consequences for others, especially family members who might have to care for the sick person or work-mates who might have to take on extra tasks to cover for him or her. In fact, Telles and Pollack (1981) note that individuals frequently visit their doctors in order to legitimise their symptoms in the eyes of others. It might be reasoned that the opposite is also the case and an individual might choose not to seek help of the sake of others, or perhaps in order to maintain a social function. For example, s/he might wish to conceal symptoms in order to protect his or her employment.

Telles and Pollack (1981) also point out that individuals are less likely to consult when "there is something going round" in their group since their symptoms are less likely to need legitimising by a doctor. Likewise, group norms might prescribe that high levels of symptoms should be tolerated, and in a study of 2700 individuals living in just under 800 families, Osterweis, Bush, and Zuckerman (1979) found that family context variables were better predictors than individual variables of individuals' use of medicine. Thus, contrary to common sense, whether an individual consults might depend on a comparison between personal symptoms and those of other group members and not on the severity of the symptoms.

A frequent reason why wives and mothers seek professional help is to stop being unfair to family members. However, some also give exactly the same reason for not seeking help (Cornwell, 1984). The reason for the apparent contradiction is that the former believe that delay now will cause future inability to care for their families, whereas the latter feel they cannot take time off from caring at the moment. Clearly, these women are not evaluating illness with reference to their individuality. Rather they are evaluating it with reference to their family roles, which is the position caricatured in the second quotation at the beginning of this chapter.

Many studies indicate that men are less inclined to seek professional help for symptoms than women (e.g., Pennebaker, 1982). While this might reflect social pressures on men, Helman (1994) argues that the mediating processes can only be understood with reference to the cultural lens through which individuals interpret their social world. Quite simply, help seeking is incompatible with ordinary male roles (see also Meininger, 1986, and Helman, 2000, also Figure 4.8 which can be interpreted in this way). A few minutes' reflection highlights that intergroup differences have been a recurrent, if implicit, theme throughout this chapter. The psychological validity and stability of researcher-defined social categories has simply been accepted. Thus, a final issue concerns changes in the decision to seek help for serious symptoms according to changes in salient self-categorisations within individuals. The role of Referent Informational Influence and Self-categorisation Theory on symptom appraisals was outlined in the previous chapter (Chapter 3, Section 3.3) and this may be extended to provide an explanation of how top-down social psychological influences can lead to decisions that reflect group memberships as well as, or perhaps even instead of, symptom severity. In this way, a social identity approach provides a powerful and truly social psychological way to understand why delay might characterise appraising a painful, dangerous, or bothersome symptom one day, but not another. Thus, the individual who perceives they are too ill to work on Monday and who decides to visit a GP might delay making such a decision as, say, a dancer on a Saturday. In spite of appearances, this difference reflects normal cognitive processes, not malingering.

To sum up, different gender, cultural, and other social identifications can translate into conformity to different patterns of help seeking and delay in spite of similar signs and symptoms. These help to explain why seeking professional help may not be predicted in a common sense manner from symptom severity.

3.4 Conclusions

Social psychological influences at all levels of analysis influence the decision to seek medical help for symptoms appraised as serious and help offer rivals to the common sense idea that people make the decision based on the seriousness of their symptoms. Influences were heavily weighted towards intrapersonal analyses and it was difficult to escape from the gravity of social cognition models because most if not all influences at other levels could potentially be incorporated into them. For example, in the Theory of Planned Behaviour, interpersonal meanings of unprotected sex could be represented in attitudes towards condom use or in subjective norms. However, it seems paradoxical to represent social psychological influences in the form of relatively stable intra-individual cognitive structures, which serve as proxies for direct influences. Second, it does not seem practicable for a researcher to discover and incorporate a range of private meanings created by participants and their social networks. Neither in a social cognition approach would such a strategy be desirable. Rather such shifts and changes are likely to be interpreted as "noise" and their influence masked by aggregation. In the next section, some alternative suggestions are tentatively made.

4. Towards a More Social Social Psychological Model of Illness

Illness does not follow a common sense pathway from objective sign to symptom perception, from symptom perception to rational symptom appraisal and from symptom appraisal, to rational decision to seek professional help. It is worth commenting that what is common sense is often judged retrospectively, in the light of a secure medical diagnosis confirmed by a fulfilled prognosis. By definition, the knowledge necessary to make such appraisals is not available to lay people in advance, or indeed at all, and it is likely that people simply cannot decide whether their symptoms are serious or not. Thus common sense reflects the influence of biomedical expertise, against which the lay person is found wanting.

Notwithstanding, many social psychological influences on help seeking have been reviewed. Most of these were grounded at an intrapersonal level and many focused on appraisals of threat and seriousness in the form of anticipated consequences. A strength of the common sense model is that it began with the idea that symptoms might be serious because they are appraised as painful, debilitating, or otherwise bothersome, and how symptoms make people feel physically seems to have been lost in the emphasis on information processing and cognition. For example, Telles and Pollack (1981) describe the case of a woman who could touch lumps that were tumours from her advanced cancer, but who had never felt ill until she was treated, and it can be imagined that cognitive appraisal might be sometimes less motivating than feelings.

For this reason, feelings as opposed to appraisals of threat *per se* remain central in the preliminary attempt to draft a social psychological model of professional help seeking that is shown in Figure 4.9. The model is intended to help explain why people who appraise themselves as ill with serious symptoms might delay seeking professional medical help and it is intended to represent just one active social identification as opposed to one individual. This important feature is represented in its title.

Perhaps the most obvious feature of the model is that (signs, and subsequently) symptoms are no longer its building blocks, except where symptoms are overwhelming, in which case a fast track to professional help is envisaged. In fact, the model has no obvious beginning because although it starts with an early representation, it is not possible to distinguish the extent to which bodily signs, environmental cues, existing knowledge structures, or other social perceptions contribute to it. This feature allows for the transfer of excitation, or for top-down influences to create or interact with symptom perceptions as discussed in Chapter 2.

In the model, appraisals are based on this early representation, but the heavier arrow is intended to represent the idea that appraisals are biased towards positive outcomes. Thus, appraisal delay is likely to occur as the individual repeats Circuit

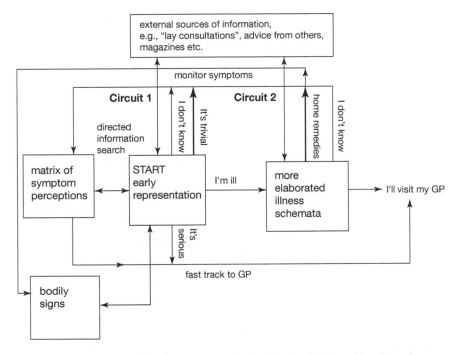

FIGURE 4.9 A social psychological model of professional help seeking for a given salient identification.

1 until symptoms can no longer be dismissed as trivial or set aside without being understood. Because the early representation is likely to direct the search for confirmatory symptoms, delay might be extensive and perhaps permanent. Alternatively, the symptoms might disappear. In the event of an exacerbation or an appraisal that something is seriously amiss, the fast track to professional help might be joined.

Symptoms that are appraised as serious, painful, debilitating, or otherwise bothersome are hypothesised to trigger a more elaborate illness schema, which is sufficiently developed to generate an illness, that is, a response to the symptoms. Based on an assumption that to be ill is less positive than to be well, the process in the model is biased such that schemata with identities that lead to positive outcomes are tried first. Thus, individuals are more likely to believe they have indigestion or flu as opposed to heart disease or cancer. This suggests that the individual in doubt does not err on the side of safety and simply visit a GP because s/he is attempting to find explanations that do not entail self-categorising as seriously ill. Moreover, within a currently active schema, appraisals and inferences are also hypothesised to be positively biased, so even when an individual believes s/he has a serious disease, s/he believes s/he will be one of the lucky ones who will escape its consequences. Thus, delay in seeking help is likely to occur as the individual repeats Circuit 2 and self-medicates or consults friends and otherwise copes. The model shows that these actions can feed back to have effects on symptom perceptions through interventions directed at bodily events (i.e., medicines and other remedies) and through changes in beliefs, since the individual might feel better due to reduction of stress. In other words, successful coping does not necessarily mean that symptoms disappear, but that they are no longer appraised as serious, painful, debilitating, or otherwise bothersome. However, feedback (from the early representation) to bodily cues is intended to represent the ways in which psychosocial stress can have a physiological effect.

The dynamic of Circuit 2 may be characterised as a snowball accelerating down a hill. Thus, the circle of advisors and actions might grow larger if earlier coping fails. The process terminates with activation of a schema-based inference that indicates a visit to the health professional. This coping strategy marks the exit from the model. For some identities, however, this might be late or never. Notwithstanding, it might be that the schema upon which this decision is made is comparatively undeveloped, because the perceiver has exhausted his or her repertoire without finding an identity that fits his or her experiences.

As in Figure 3.2, the separate "boxes" are intended to represent different moments, not different cognitive structures (this is why feedback is shown only from the early representation to bodily signs). Thus, an ongoing process of elaboration is envisaged as the individual develops strategies to deal with perceived symptoms.

An important feature of the model is that under different circumstances, a given individual might self-categorise in terms of another identification, with the result that the valence of biases, the selection and order of schemata, and other features of the model are reset. An interesting possibility is that individuals sharing a salient social identification might follow essentially the same pathway through the model, perhaps evincing similar patterns of delay, and this might account better for similarities in their behaviour than symptom severity.

An interesting final point is that the model suggests that an individual might be in "two minds" about the seriousness of a symptom and what to do, because of switches between self-categories as a function of changes in social context—as illustrated in the struggle to decide whether a symptom that one has decided merits a day off work, is serious enough to stay in bed, when one remembers it is Saturday!

5. Summary and Conclusions

This chapter was about the ways in which people act when they have appraised a symptom as serious, debilitating, painful, or otherwise bothersome. More especially, it focused on why people delay seeking professional medical help.

In the first section the key concepts of signs, symptoms, disease, and illness were distinguished and a common sense model was suggested, in which people are assumed to seek professional medical advice when they appraise a symptom as serious, painful, debilitating, or otherwise bothersome.

- This decision was assumed to be a rational one and therefore to reflect symptom severity.
- The goal of help seeking was assumed to be self-preservation.

In the second section this common sense model was challenged by empirical studies and a case study which showed that irrational delays characterise the progression to professional help.

- Stages in "patient" delay were described.
- Delay in deciding to visit a GP was identified as the focus for the remaining sections.

In the third section social psychological explanations for delay in deciding that symptom requires medical help were suggested.

- The bulk of the section was pitched at the intrapersonal level. Social cognition models, health locus of control and personality factors, protection motivation and stress approaches were reviewed in order to offer rival explanations to the common sense idea that people will seek prompt medical help if they appraise themselves as ill with serious symptoms.
- At interpersonal and group levels the influence of lay referral systems together with family and cultural influences mediated by self-categorisations were highlighted.

It was concluded that social psychological factors at all levels of analysis influence seeking professional help as well as, and sometimes in spite of, the severity of symptoms.

In the fourth section it was concluded that common sense reflects a medical perspective in which objective signs are paramount, and that self-preservation and rationality are defined in relation to medical outcomes.

- A more social psychological approach to delaying seeking medical help was suggested in which meanings, as opposed to symptom severity, play the key role, and in which appraisals are biased towards positive outcomes and stress relief.

Once the individual has decided to seek professional help, he or she has to communicate with a doctor to request and receive it. The next chapter begins in the doctor's surgery and considers how the patient is likely to fare.

5

I've Seen my Doctor, but I'm Still Not Sure: Doctor–Patient Communication

Psychologist: Do you think it matters how doctors communicate with patients?
Medical student: [After some thought] No, I don't really think so because the facts about disease are the facts however you talk about them.

Doctor: Oh no . . . I'm not one of those doctors who play God. In fact, I can't stand doctors like that . . . I always ask my patients if they want me to let them die.

This chapter begins where the last chapter ended, that is, at "the gateway to illness" or the visit to a doctor. Its focus is on the mutual understandings that develop between doctor and patient, and therefore it is pitched predominantly at an interpersonal level of analysis.

In Section 1 a common sense model of doctor–patient communication is suggested. The model predicts that the patient tells the doctor about the symptom(s) and appraisals that triggered his or her visit, and that the doctor uses this information to build a schema of the problem. Next, the doctor gives relevant information to the patient who as a result acquires an expertly grounded coping plan or remedy, which s/he subsequently follows.

In Section 2 each of these assumptions is challenged with empirical evidence or case studies.

In Section 3 key concepts are discussed, a working definition of communication is developed, and differences between interactions and relationships are highlighted, together with their implications for communication.

In Section 4 these considerations are used in reviewing social psychological influences that help to offer rival explanations to the common sense model of doctor–patient communication.

Finally, in Section 5 a social psychological model of doctor–patient communication is suggested, followed by some suggestions for improvement.

1. Introduction and a Common Sense Model of Doctor–Patient Communication

1.1 The importance of doctor–patient communication as "the gateway to illness"

Doctor–patient communication is essential for effective health care (Pendleton & Hasler, 1983). It is of fundamental importance in getting appropriate help because in spite of a range of objective tests, health professionals are often unable to identify what will be a source of suffering for their patients (Skevington, 1995). Communication is also the means whereby patients receive the expert advice they need.

1.2 A common sense model of doctor–patient communication

Figure 5.1 depicts a common sense model of doctor–patient communication, set in the context of a first consultation about an illness. The major assumption of the model is that information about the patient's problem passes efficiently between him or her and the doctor.

The model begins with the illness schema upon which the patient decided to seek professional help. It is labelled "inadequate" because it failed to provide the patient with relief, which of course is why the visit to the doctor resulted. On its basis, the patient encodes symptom information to communicate to the doctor, most probably

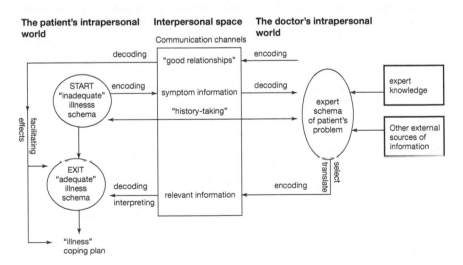

FIGURE 5.1 A common sense model of doctor–patient communication.

using language for the purpose, although other communication channels are also likely to be involved. For example, the patient might show a sign to the doctor or gesture the whereabouts and nature of a pain.

In stage two of the common sense model, the doctor decodes the patient's communications and uses them as variables in an expert schema of the problem. In addition to information offered by the patient, the doctor might ask questions, take a history, look at case-notes, and carry out a physical examination in order to build and fine-tune the schema. The common sense assumption is that s/he backtracks through patient communications of symptoms to real signs and the underlying disease.

In stage three, the doctor selects, encodes, and communicates relevant information to the patient, to help him or her to understand and treat the problem. Ong, de Haes, Hoos, and Lammes (1995) use the term "bilingual" to capture neatly the idea that doctors "speak" both medical language and the everyday language needed to achieve this task.

In the fourth stage of the common sense model, the patient receives the information, which in effect is his or her original illness schema appropriately transformed by the medical expert so that it now provides the remedy that the patient was unable to work out alone. At the end of the common sense model, it is assumed that relevant corrective action follows, with the result that the patient becomes formally ill and in so doing, begins the road to recovery.

A second function of doctor–patient communication in the model is to build "good relationships". It is common sense that these can contribute significantly to the patient's well being *independently* of the clinical aspects of his or her case. This is because information and reassurance from the doctor can reduce uncertainty and stress (see Chapter 4, Section 3.1.4). Knock-on benefits include improvements in recall, understanding, emotions, and other psychological states (e.g., Buckman, 1993; Cohen & Herbert, 1996; DiMatteo & Friedman, 1982; Levy, 1986; Ong et al., 1995; Smits, Meyboom, Mokkink, Van Son, & Van Eijk, 1991). Where patients are anxious, it follows that good relationships are especially important (Fallowfield, 1988). One such example is likely to be when cancer is diagnosed, and one study found that perceived social support from physician (and husband) were the most significant of five variables which together explained 39% of variance in the immune system activity of patients with breast cancer (Levy et al., 1990).

"Good relationships" are usually operationalised in terms of three characteristics of doctors: good manners, psychotherapeutic qualities, (chiefly empathy), and due emphasis on the patient's concerns (Ong et al., 1995). Thus, in the common sense model they are depicted as flowing from the doctor to facilitate the patient's understanding and coping skills.

Many empirical and case studies challenge the common sense model. A few will be reviewed in the next section.

2. Challenges to the Common Sense Model of Doctor–Patient Communication

2.1 Empirical studies

In the first stage of the common sense model, the patient begins by telling the doctor about his or her symptoms. Interviews with several hundred patients in a psychiatric walk-in clinic, however, showed that 99% came intending to request help with symptoms, but only 37% did so (Lazare, Eisenthal, Frank, & Stoeckle, 1978 cited in Murphy, 1996). These surprising figures do not seem to be unique to psychiatric patients, since Stimson and Webb (1975) concluded that virtually all patients visit their doctor with at least one specific request or question, but less than half spontaneously express it. Similarly, 60% of a sample of general practice patients who reported symptoms on a questionnaire did not mention some of them in their consultation with the doctor (Tuckett, Boulton, & Olsen, 1985). The figures are not low because they focus on spontaneity, perhaps overlooking requests coaxed into the open by doctors. On the contrary, in over two-thirds of a sample of consultations, physicians intruded on patients' statements and redirected talk, on average taking only 18 seconds for the first interruption (Beckman & Frankel, 1984). Moreover, a study of two standardised cases presented by trained patient simulators to 43 primary care practitioners found that the doctors elicited only slightly more than 50% of the scripted information (Roter & Hall, 1987). Similarly, a famous meta-analysis revealed that the chief concerns of patients were not even mentioned in more than 25% of interviews (Beckman & Frankel, 1984).

These data suggest that between a quarter and half of patients do not tell the doctor about their symptoms. This might be because patients lack the knowledge necessary to encode symptom information correctly (e.g., Burnett & Thompson, 1986), and a number of studies that support this possibility have already been mentioned in the context of schema-based appraisals of symptoms (Chapter 2, Section 4.1.2). In another, 59% of 234 patients thought the stomach occupied the entire abdomen from waist to groin, and 14% of a sample of 81 hospital patients awaiting surgery thought that humans possess two livers (see Helman, 1994). Whatever the cause, however, the first stage of the common sense model is challenged.

In the second stage of the common sense model, doctors decode information from their patients. Few studies focus on difficulties at this stage, but Herz et al. (1996) studied 100 physicians' and 418 patients' understanding of the term "constipation". Only 46% of the doctors agreed on the medical definition (of defecation every 4 days or less often) and taking variation in patients' definitions into account, the authors concluded that more than half of patients presenting with constipation are talking about something other than the entity the doctor understands.

Having built a schema of the patient's problem, the third stage of the common sense model predicts that the doctor selects information relevant to the patient's needs, translates it to fit his or her social world, and encodes the results into everyday language that s/he can understand. Many studies challenge this part of the model.

A global challenge is that lack of communication causes more complaints than any other aspect of the doctor–patient relationship (Burnett & Thompson, 1986). For example, patients with incurable cancer want to know as much information as possible about their case, and seem to benefit from it (Centeno-Cortes & Nunez-Olarte, 1994; Maguire & Faulkner, 1988). However, reviewers agree that physicians currently convey more information than was common in the past, but doubt that current levels have yet reached adequacy (e.g., Siminoff, 1992). In one study, 68% of terminal cancer patients had not been informed of their diagnosis (Centeno-Cortes & Nunez-Olarte, 1994) and in another, 40% of a sample of cancer specialists agreed that patients preferred not to know too much about their condition, *even if the patients said otherwise* (Greenwald & Nevitt, 1982). Other studies have shown that the physician's attitude and attributions about the patient, or their feelings about communicating disturbing news, can determine whether information is given (De Monchy, 1992; Skevington, 1995). Lack of information is not exclusive to cancer patients. In a study of 347 drugs prescribed for 153 patients, how long to take the drug and how regularly to take it was explained in only 10% and 17% of cases, respectively. In 29% of cases the drug was not named, nor was its purpose mentioned (Svarstad, 1976, cited in Skevington, 1995).

Where information *is* given, a complaint is that it does not match patients' needs. In particular, doctors in cancer wards frequently give facts that are precise and relevant from a biomedical point of view, but not relevant to the patients' bio-psychosocial concerns (see Ong et al., 1995). Still more bizarre, Byrne and Long (1976) famously analysed some 2500 consultations only to find very little flexibility in the doctors' behaviour. In fact, differences between consultations reflected consistent differences between doctors' interests and purposes, rather than differences between patients and their problems. Further studies showed such inflexibility increases rather than decreases with experience (Burnett & Thompson, 1986) even though older doctors perceive themselves as less dominant and more effective (McManus, Kidd, & Aldus, 1997). Studies in the fields of prescribing and cancer have come to similar conclusions. For example, heavy use of "favourite" drugs in five European countries could not be explained by variation in patients' problems (O'Brien, 1984, cited in Helman, 1994). Similarly, Siminoff (1992) describes a study in which the communications of breast cancer surgeons were patterned according to their routines rather than the needs of patients.

Doctors' translations from medical into everyday language also attract criticism. One complaint is that hedging or euphemisms are used when breaking bad news (West & Frankel, 1991). Another complaint is that medical jargon is not translated at all. This occurred in a study of 800 paediatric visits, in more than half of which physicians used specialised terms that patients and their parents could not understand (Korsch & Negrete, 1972, cited in West & Frankel, 1991). Still more challenging is the finding that doctors frequently use such words without *expecting* their patients to understand them (Burnett & Thompson 1986).

The fourth stage of the common sense model assumes that the patient decodes the information received from the doctor. At this stage, it is difficult to distinguish between jargon that doctors should translate, and everyday language that patients should be able to decode for themselves. This difficulty is illustrated in an early study, in which 60 medical terms were presented to a sample of patients. Virtually the whole sample did not understand "metastasis" and "prognosis"; almost 80% did not understand "lesion" but 10% did not know what "cancer" meant; and 4% did not understand relatively common terms such as "infection" (Redlich, 1949, reported in Ley, 1990). Clearly it is impossible to say whether four or ten or some other percentage of patients should have been able to understand their doctors. However, even where there is no difficulty in decoding terms, the ways in which patients interpret phrases to fit their social world might not match the doctor's intentions. For example, one patient questioned about family history of cardiac arrest, replied that he "never had no trouble" with the police (West & Frankel, 1991)!

The exit point of the model is an adequate illness schema, which provides the patient with understanding, including how to remedy the situation. The assumption is that s/he follows this coping plan. Probably the oldest challenge to the common sense model is that patients often do not follow medical advice. This problem was identified by Hippocrates around 200 BC, and currently up to 25% of medical in-patient beds are estimated to be occupied because of it (Ley, 1990). Numerous ways to operationalise it include: taking incorrect doses of medicine; not taking medicine at all; taking medicine at the wrong time; and a host of other variants. Thus, it is not surprising that rates vary tremendously, between 6% and 95% according to Pendleton, Schofield, Tate, and Havelock (1984).

Traditionally, patient compliance was conceptualised in terms of patient control, mediated by the persuasiveness of doctors' communications. From this perspective, studies identify poorer compliance rates when patients are not given understandable instructions or when other aspects of the doctors' communication is poor (see Ley, 1990, for a review). More recently, the term "adherence" has been suggested because "compliance" casts the patient in too passive a role. From this perspective, studies identify patients' characteristics such as their memory or unrealistic expectations as reasons for poor levels of adherence (see Skevington, 1995, for a review). However, whether compliance or adherence is the preferred term is immaterial from the point of view of the challenge to the common sense model.

Throughout the common sense model of doctor–patient communication, exchange of clinical information and other positive effects are facilitated by good relationships, which are mediated by good manners and empathy flowing from the doctor. In a meta-analysis however, fewer than 5% of doctors' comments were friendly or sociable (Beckman & Frankel, 1984). Furthermore, studies of closing strategies routinely employed by physicians included high incidences of clock watching; making a rapid "getaway" rather than giving a farewell; or even just walking from the room with no other indication to the patient that the consultation is over (Roter & Frankel, 1992). Thus, the assumption that good relationships flow from the doctor is also challenged.

2.2 Case study

ACTIVITY 5.1 Opportunity survey of experiences of communication with doctors

Ask four or five people about their experiences of medical consultations. Consider the same question for yourself. Reflect on these experiences. Can you gain an overall impression? What defined experiences as positive or negative? What were the consequences of people's experiences? How generalisable do you think your results are?

The literature is replete with case studies that further challenge the common sense model of communication in vivid and often distressing ways. Fallowfield (1991) gives the following example:

> *I felt terrible; I was scared stiff and shaky and really embarrassed lying there on the examination couch with just this flimsy gown that didn't cover me right up. He came in with a couple of young doctors, and oh I was so ashamed, the way he examined me—I've got such big breasts you see. He just didn't seem to act as though I was there and kept talking to the others about the difficulty in knowing what to do with big breasts. I asked him what was wrong with me. He said 'You must realise it's cancer; we'll have you in next week sometime' and walked out.*

2.3 Summary

Jarvinen (1955) noted that sudden deaths often followed ward rounds, and suspected they might be triggered by stressful doctor–patient communications. Over the half century since then, the common sense idea that information is freely and accurately exchanged, and good relationships flow during doctor–patient communication has been extensively challenged. At the dawn of the third millennium, doctors' communication still attracts more complaints than any other aspect of medical care (Neubauer, 2000, personal communication).

It is important to build more successful rival explanations to common sense for doctor–patient communication, because according to Wiemann and Giles (1996) a negative spiral of unsatisfactory communication contributes to poor health and can accelerate both ageing and death. Because this task is complex, it is first necessary to discuss some key concepts and issues. These will be introduced in the next section before social psychological influences will be reviewed in order to offer some rivals to common sense.

3. Thinking About Doctor–Patient Communication

Progress in improving doctor–patient communication has been hampered because researchers mean different things by communication and often do not define it at all (Epstein et al., 1993). Furthermore, doctor–patient communication occurs during interactions between doctors and patients, but a given social interaction might exist in the context of a relationship or it might not. Because of these complexities, it is useful to develop a working definition of communication and to discuss differences between interactions and relationships and their implications for communication. These tasks will be attempted in the coming section in order to provide a consistent basis for the remainder of the chapter.

3.1 Conceptualising doctor–patient communication

In the *Compact Oxford English Dictionary*, the word "communicate" is given 10 meanings. All derive from the Latin *"communicare"* which means to make common to many, to share, impart, or divide. Leaving aside two meanings (which concern Holy Communion and connecting rooms!) the following remain: to give to another as a partaker; to impart by way of information to the readers of a journal etc.; to give or bestow; to share in, partake of, to use in common with, either by receiving or bestowing; to have a common part; to hold conversation; to impart, transmit, or exchange thought or information.

The emphasis of the definitions is on active sending and sharing of information. In keeping with this, and following Kaye (1984), communication will be defined as "the intentional sharing of meaning(s)". Thus, to qualify as "communication", the sender must intend to share a meaning with the recipient and it must be made common, that is, it must coincide with the meaning understood by the receiver.

Clearly, this is a more complex concept than the idea of information exchange. An advantage of this complexity is that two types of miscommunication follow directly from the definition. First, a sender may not intend to share a particular meaning with its recipient. For example, information from case notes or physical signs is only communication if the patient *intends* to share and use it with his or her doctor. Similarly, a doctor's yawns or smiles are not communication unless the doctor intends them as gestures. If s/he does not, they are "leaks" (see Ong et al., 1995) even though the meaning grasped by the patient might be correct. The second way in which miscommunication occurs is when the meaning intended by the sender does not coincide with the meaning understood by the receiver.

Although language is the dominant channel of communication in human affairs, many other channels include: physical appearance, which may be manipulated in order to communicate impressions; and physical movements, which can function as the components of formal sign languages, or less formally as gestures (Spencer, 1998b). For example, people who like or agree with each other often mirror each other's movements, and more generally, liking can be communicated by an open posture. Accent and intonation might also be used but more often the face is the primary vehicle. For example, eye contact typically communicates liking, and it is also used in the regulation of turn taking when conversationalists characteristically look away from each other on beginning an utterance and then look back as they near its end. Since the face can also betray information about internal states, Spencer (1998b) suggests a continuum with universal innate facial expressions at one end and learned, culture-specific expressions at the other. Both extremes convey information, but by definition the former are not communication channels, unless intentionally used for that purpose. Interestingly, it will be remembered that both extremes have been incorporated into measures of pain, the former perhaps appealing to those seeking objective measures, while the latter perhaps appeal to those more interested in measuring the experience of pain (see Chapter 2, Section 3.3).

Finally, Spencer (1998b) lists physical context, proxemics, and touch as additional communication channels. An interesting further addition to his list is music, which is increasingly used in therapeutic settings as a means of communicating with those who are unable or unwilling to use other channels (Malone, 1996; Robb, Nichols, Rutan, Bishop, & Parker, 1995).

3.2 Differences between doctor–patient interactions and relationships: Some implications for communication

A doctor and patient might interact only once, because the patient simply requires a signature from a locum on a repeat prescription. On the other hand, an interaction might be in the context of a relationship that spans from cradle to grave. Such differences have implications for communication.

To explain, an interaction can be defined as the joint engagement of two or more individuals in an activity, the elements of which may be observed (Miell & Dallos, 1996). Although the elements can be observed, however, their meaning depends on the social setting and the purpose of the interaction (Radley, 1996). For example, the phrase "I've got trouble with my plumbing" is likely to mean different things in a builder's yard and a consulting room. Doctor–patient interactions are different from everyday interactions because they occur by appointment and exist because the patient has need of the doctor's professional expertise. They fit well the criteria of professional interactions that (i) take place at restricted, appointed times in specific places, (ii) take place for specific reasons, and (iii) include a competence gap between the advice giver and seeker (Stimson & Webb, 1975).

Unlike interactions, relationships cannot be observed because they are charac-terised by three features that are only apparent to the participants. The first of these is meaning. Meanings are constructed and shared by participants in a relationship, who have come to understand the other's perspective. These mutual understandings are used to shape and interpret elements of interactions (Radley, 1996). For an example, an observer might evaluate a doctor as cold if s/he fails to touch a weeping child. However, in a previous consultation a sympathetic touch might have distressed the child further, and the doctor and child might have agreed that the next time, the child would be allowed to compose itself in a grown-up manner. Similarly, a pat on the shoulder and use of a first name might be observed in two identical interactions, in which a woman receives the good news that a biopsy result is clear. In the context of one relationship this might communicate comforting reassurance, but in another it might communicate a patronising affirmation of differences in status. The difference depends on past events invisible to the observer, but known and understood by participants.

Because it takes time and effort to develop mutual understandings, a second feature of relationships is that they are characterised by developmental histories. Periods of conflict and changes in affiliation levels and the distribution of power are likely to have happened in the past. Third, relationships have many functions, which implies some "fit" between mutual needs and the idea that, in order to continue, a relationship must be rewarding somehow (Miell & Dallos, 1996).

For a doctor–patient relationship to exist, it follows that joint meanings need to be constructed and used to shape and interpret interactions. This is likely to involve an investment in terms of time and effort, and perhaps more than one meeting. However, the development of doctor–patient relationships is likely to be constrained in at least three ways, which extend the special characteristics of professional interactions identified by Stimson and Webb (1975) which were outlined above.

First, the purpose of the relationship is to access professional expertise. This means that doctor–patient relationships are likely to be intergroup in nature. Thus, participants are likely to communicate with each other as undifferentiated representatives of social groups such as "doctor" and "patient" (Wiemann & Giles, 1996) irrespective of the fact that only two people are involved and the consultation might be of an extremely private nature. In terms of Tajfel's (1978a) interpersonal–intergroup continuum (see Chapter 3, Section 3.3) doctor–patient relationships are towards the intergroup end. This means there is likely to be relatively little scope for initial attraction and later change, since the doctor should always have the power of expertise and is not expected to reciprocate self-disclosure, so the patient is unlikely to develop much understanding of the doctor's personal world. Other interpersonal norms are also suspended during doctor–patient relationships and increase the likelihood that they will remain intergroup. For example, the patient can expect stress relief, symptom relief, and emotional support, but is unlikely to have an opportunity to reciprocate the help (see Bierhoff, 2001, for a discussion of aid relationships). These constraints and theoretical distinctions have important implications for language and communication.

First, the role of language is likely to be more central during intergroup communication because in it, less can be taken for granted. Constraints on the development of intergroup relationships are likely to maintain an intergroup emphasis. Moreover, differentiation between social groups is likely to increase the semantic distance between the social worlds of the patient and the doctor, so that sharing meaning and hence communication becomes more difficult (e.g., Burnett & Thompson, 1986). Notwithstanding, the doctor is expected to communicate "good relationships" through good manners, empathy, and due emphasis on patients' concerns. The latter in particular implies a movement towards interpersonal communication. Thus, a tension seems inherent in doctor–patient communications. In order to fulfil clinical and relational functions, the doctor is simultaneously expected to interact at intergroup *and* interpersonal loci, which is not possible in terms of Tajfel's (1978a) interpersonal–intergroup continuum. Alternative possibilities are that multiple continua exist within single situations, or that rapid switches between relevant identities can be made. More recently, Worchel, Iuzzini, Coutant, and Ivaldi (2000) have argued that several identity concerns might act simultaneously. It follows that characteristics of personal identity such as empathy might after all affect a professional doctor–patient relationship.

A second, important implication is that the meaning communicated by a given element of an interaction cannot be determined by observation alone. For example, clock watching as a closing strategy employed by doctors might leak that it is time the patient left, together with a rather negative attitude towards him or her. In the context of a relationship however, it might communicate good relationships since the doctor might know about the patient's regular choir practice and the difficulty s/he has with promptness! In other words, the success of communications might be underestimated by researchers where an interaction occurs in the context of a relationship. Under such circumstances, the fact that the patient's chief concerns were not mentioned, is no guarantee that they were not communicated.

Having discussed some of the complexities inherent in doctor–patient commu nication, it is time to review some ways in which social psychological influences offer rival explanations to the common sense model depicted in Figure 5.1. The model predicts that the patient tells the doctor about his or her symptoms of concern; that the doctor uses this information to build an expert schema of the problem; that the doctor selects and translates information that is relevant to the patient; and that the patient assimilates the information.

4. Social Psychological Influences on Doctor–Patient Communication

4.1 Intrapersonal influences

It is common sense that a reticent patient might fail to describe embarrassing symptoms, and that a doctor who is uncaring, or whose native language differs from that of the patient, might fail to translate medical jargon so that patients can understand it. In this section, the task is not to review such barriers but to focus on the personal worlds of the doctor and patient, and how these might "sabotage" communication between them.

4.1.1 Why didn't the patient tell the doctor about his or her main symptoms? Why didn't the patient follow the doctor's advice?

Much research in cognitive psychology concerns the knowledge structures individuals must possess in order to communicate by using language. In addition to lexical meanings, syntactic structures, semantics, and general knowledge, the individual possesses knowledge of inference and discourse rules (Greene & Coulson, 1995). From consideration of the latter, a paradox arises. According to the principle of "audience design" (Clark & Murphy, 1982) communicators intend their messages to be understood and therefore give their audience all necessary cues and background. However, the patient is unlikely to know what cues and background the doctor needs. Indeed, if he or she *did* know, the professional's services might be redundant! In other words, patients might have difficulty spontaneously telling the doctor about their problems, because they do not know where to start the presentation.

Another interesting way in which information flow from the patient might be inhibited arises from a consideration of the ways in which multiple channels are used during communication. A good example is personal distance, which is

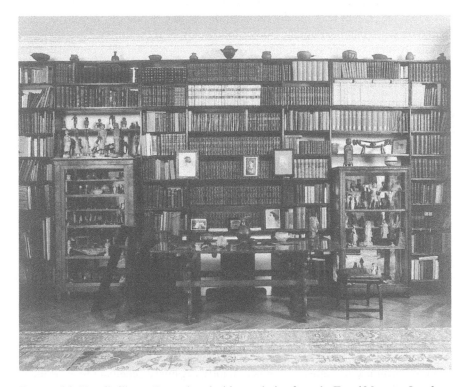

FIGURE 5.2 Freud's library. Reproduced with permission from the Freud Museum, London.

normally 0.5–1.5 metres in British society (see Spencer, 1998b). Distances are shorter in more intimate situations and longer in more formal ones, and people adjust not only distance, but also eye-contact, touch, facial expressions, and other channels as the topic changes, in order to negotiate a mutually comfortable level of intimacy (Argyle & Dean, 1965). In a consulting room, the doctor controls most channels. Usually the patient's chair is ready-positioned, it is the doctor who initiates handshakes or touch, and s/he can choose to look at notes or a computer screen rather than at the patient. Even the surroundings might be chosen by him or her to communicate a chosen image and level of formality. Unable to effect changes in these communication channels, the patient's ability to adjust to a change in intimacy as the topic shifts from opening gambits to his or her personal problems might be inhibited. As a result, s/he might simply talk about something else.

In Chapters 2 and 3, much was said about the ways in which schema-based processing influences symptom perceptions and appraisals. The recall of symptom information and the way in which it is presented is also subject to prototypicality effects (Bishop & Converse, 1986) and this means that information given by patients is likely to regress to a prototypic mean, perhaps glossing over key personal symptoms.

Thus, there are at least three social psychological rivals to the common sense idea that the patient tells the doctor about his or her symptoms. Moreover, it is common sense that the patient will not follow advice if the advice does not offer a remedy for his or her symptoms of concern.

4.1.2 Why didn't the doctor listen to the patient? Why did s/he keep interrupting?

To turn the focus onto the personal world of the doctor, an assumption underpinning the common sense model of doctor–patient communication is that the doctor is an impartial, scientific expert, able to backtrack to the cause of the patient's symptoms without human distractions. This means that doctors might sometimes listen for the signs of disease and not to their patients' descriptions of symptoms. Baron (1985) describes just such an example. He was carefully auscultating a patient's chest when the patient began to ask a question. He interrupted him with, "Quiet, I can't hear you while I'm listening."

Much has already been said about schema-based heuristics and biases and these are relevant to doctors as well as to patients. Consistent with this idea, Reiss and Szysko (1983) found that information that a patient had learning difficulties "overshadowed" diagnoses and guided questions in a confirmatory direction, so that the other problems, with which the patient had more difficulties, were not raised. Information that is consistent with the central and most used aspects of schemata is processed more efficiently. In fact, experts derive their superior decision making from frequent use of highly elaborated, tightly organised schemata (e.g., Roth & Bruce, 1996).

A prediction that runs counter to common sense is that these biases might be more pronounced in medical experts. This is because these should be especially vulnerable to prototypicality effects. They might be relatively slower than novices in deciding a case is *not* an instance of their speciality, because they have more material to search. They should also have more difficulty in generating unconventional therapies because they have more information to re-organise and stronger links to break.

4.1.3 A note on framing effects

Also within the personal world of the doctor, how he or she typically frames therapeutic options is likely to affect patient adherence (Wilson et al., 1987). For example, McNeil, Parker, Sox, and Tversky (1982) asked participants to imagine they had lung cancer and to choose between surgery or radiation therapy under one of two conditions. In Condition 1, the "frame" for surgery was: "if adopted you will have a 32% chance of dying after 12 months". In Condition 2, its frame was: "if adopted you will have a 68% chance of surviving after 12 months". Results showed that 58% chose surgery in the first condition and 75% in the second, although rationally the outcomes were identical. The underlying theory derives from studies of cognitive heuristics and biases (Tversky & Kahneman, 1981) which revealed that perceivers seemed more swayed by possibilities framed in terms of gaining a benefit than making an equivalent loss (see Salovey et al., 1998 for a discussion). Thus, advice framed in terms of possible losses might paradoxically undermine decisions to follow treatment recommendations (Siminoff & Fetting, 1991).

4.1.4 Summary

Intrapersonal characteristics of both patient and doctor, including knowledge of discourse rules, the ability to control communication channels, schema-based heuristics and biases, and framing might all sometimes sabotage doctor–patient communication. As such they offer social psychological explanations to rival the common sense idea that the patient tells the doctor about his or her symptoms and the doctor listens.

4.2 Interpersonal influences on doctor–patient communication

Although this chapter began with an assertion that the level of analysis for a discussion of doctor–patient communication is interpersonal, the common sense model in Figure 5.1 depicts the work of communication as intrapersonal. It takes place in the encoding and decoding of messages that criss-cross between participants as they take turns at sending and receiving, like players in a game of tennis. Messages are communications or hits if the pattern of meaning in the recipient's working memory matches the pattern intended by the sender, and individuals are good communicators if they can encode and fire messages that efficiently trigger relevant meanings in others, scoring more hits in less time.

Interpersonal analyses, however, focus on properties that emerge between individuals. At this level it is acknowledged that the patient might not encode a prepared meaning at all, because his or her meaning might be incomplete. Indeed, in the previous chapter it was hypothesised that inadequate understanding was the key trigger of the visit. This means that the patient's meaning might only emerge as a result of the doctor's response (Radley, 1996). Thus, his or her schema can be constructed in, and belong to, the consultation as opposed to being prepared by him or herself. For example, "I'm worried about lung cancer" will have different meaning for the patient according to whether the response is "With your history, I am confident you have nothing to worry about" as opposed to "I'll arrange an emergency referral".

ACTIVITY 5.2 Insights into communication

Consider, or better still, observe the following:

(i)   yourself having some conversations on an answering machine;
(ii)   an international phone call (or TV interview where there is a time delay between people's comments);
(iii) an email correspondence;
(iv)   a purchase made in the presence of a convincing salesperson which, when examined at home, seem less attractive.

What do such experiences suggest about the ways in which communication differs from an exchange of thought-out messages?
What is striking about everyday use of language? What differences can you notice between language in personal and social relationships?

4.2.1 Why didn't the patient tell the doctor about his or her main symptoms? Why didn't the patient follow the doctor's advice?

Much recent progress in understanding interpersonal communication has been made by considering multiple meanings and purposes that are shared between participants (Wiemann & Giles, 1996). In particular, language is not only used to convey the information represented in its words, but also to achieve other goals, which emerge as the interaction progresses. The result is that the lexical meaning of an expression can be different from its intended function. Moreover, the meaning of the same expression might vary with each repetition, if the goals of the person change (Potter, 1996).

To focus first on the patient, an important goal during communication is the construction of a self-image (Wetherell, 1996a). Pursuit of this goal might sabotage the communication of symptom information. For example, a patient might assert that presenting physical symptoms are "not too bad", in order to construct a stoical self-image. Following this lead, the doctor might cease asking about them, perhaps pursuing another line of questioning about emotional problems. Next, the patient might attempt to redirect conversation towards the seriousness of his or her physical symptoms, because seeking relief has become the salient goal. However, from the doctor's point of view, this might be contradictory. It might even confirm a diagnosis of emotional problems. Consequently, the patient's chief concerns might not be aired! Moreover, it is common sense that the patient will not follow advice if the advice does not offer a remedy for his or her symptoms of concern.

Although little if any research seems to have investigated the idea, it seems that such miscommunication will be less likely in the context of relationships, because the doctor is more likely to share knowledge of the patient's preferred self-image and symptom history.

4.2.2 Why didn't the doctor listen to the patient? Why did s/he keep interrupting?

To focus now on the doctor, another important goal of language use is to construct the social context in which an interaction occurs. Wiemann and Giles (1996) identify control and affiliation as the two major dimensions of social context constructed in this way, although these are rarely addressed directly but are more usually constructed through discursive strategies such as silence, talking more, interrupting, rate of speech or choice of pronouns, vocabulary, or accent. It will be remembered that doctors frequently interrupt their patients. In Section 2.1 this served as a challenge to the common sense model of doctor–patient communication, because to stem the flow of information upon which the consultation depends seemed irrational. However, an interpersonal analysis raises the possibility that interruptions might not be not failed attempts to illicit clinical information, but successful attempts to assert control.

It is important to pursue this possibility because use of controlling styles has detrimental implications for patients' health. To illustrate, 98 diabetics were randomly assigned to experimental and control groups (Greenfield, Kaplan, & Ware, 1988). Those in the experimental group were trained in assertiveness skills, how to negotiate with their doctors, and how to ask questions of him or her. About 12 weeks later at the next scheduled visit, the latter were doing significantly better on a range of measures such as blood sugar levels, disease severity, and quality of life. To take just one example, perceived health status scores could range from 1 (good) to 4 (bad), and at the start of the study the experimental group had scored 2.38 compared with 2.17 for controls. At follow up, their scores were 2.04, whereas scores for controls had deteriorated to 2.82. More generally, six out of eight studies showed a direct relationship between doctors' communication styles and patients' health status, the overall pattern being for patients with doctors who were less controlling to show better outcomes (see Kaplan, Greenfield, & Ware, 1989, for a review). The authors reasoned that reduction in the extent to which doctors controlled communication triggers a sense of active control in patients, which better motivates them to look after themselves. This leads to important benefits in the context of chronic disease, because it is the patient who has to manage treatment.

There are at least four problems with this interpretation. First, although it ostensibly casts the patient in a less passive role than the idea that his or her behaviour is determined by the persuasive communications of the doctor, the assumption seems to be that the patient's locus of control has been reset from external to internal by the doctor. This means that the patient's behaviour is still ultimately determined by his or her communications. Second, the failure of an internal locus of control reliably to predict compliance with health-related behaviours is well known (see Chapter 4, Section 3.1.3). Third, just why doctors seem so often to use a controlling style is left open. Fourth, in circumstances where social norms already establish the expectancy of control, such as might be expected in a professional consultation with a doctor, little if any negotiation should occur (Wiemann & Giles, 1996).

4.2.3 Summary

At an interpersonal level, the ways in which information is encoded to serve social psychological purposes might be at odds with its literal meaning and this might serve to sabotage communication between doctor and patient. This offers a rival explanation to the common sense view that doctor–patient communication is about the patient's problem. In particular, interruptions and the like by doctors might be better understood as an interpersonal strategy designed to establish control, rather than a failure to elicit information. However, the fact that doctors seem to use controlling styles, in circumstances where social norms already cede control to them, suggests that a group-level analysis might be needed to explore the issue more fully. In the next section, the issue will be pursued at this level.

4.3 Group-level influences on doctor–patient communication

Because they are based on a professional relationship, doctor–patient interactions are likely to occur at an intergroup level of analysis. Referent Informational Influence (e.g., Turner, 1987, as described in Chapter 3, Section 3.3) predicts that self-categorisation as a patient or as a doctor will lead to conformity with the norms associated with those groups. This has far-reaching implications for doctor–patient communication in general, but specifically offers a social psychological explanation for the use of controlling styles of communications by doctors.

A study in the field of mental retardation supported the idea that doctors' self-categorisations can shape their perceptions of patients (St. Claire, 1993). Three findings provided the impetus for the study. First was the robust finding that most people evaluate "the mentally retarded" more negatively than other social categories.

Second was the finding that professionals evaluate them more negatively than lay people do, and (although evidence is sparse) the third finding was that medical professionals evaluate them most negatively of all (e.g., Bogdan & Taylor, 1976; Butt & Signori, 1976; Gottlieb & Gottlieb, 1977; St. Claire, 1986; Valpey, 1982). The question that the study investigated was why medical professionals seem to hold such negative attitudes towards people with learning difficulties. Common sense explanations included the idea that medical professionals have a better grasp of the truth about them; that admission criteria for medical schools focus too narrowly on academic as opposed to caring skills; or even that traditional medical teaching "dehumanises" students (Ewan, 1987; Zeldow & Daugherty, 1987, respectively).

The alternative hypothesis tested in the study is that medical professionals' beliefs reflect conformity to professional norms, mediated by a shared "medical professional" social identification (St. Claire, 1993). Since mental retardation is an anathema within the medical model (Mercer, 1973) because it cannot be objectively observed, measured, or cured, and since the medical model encourages a focus on pathology (Booth, 1978; Helman, 1994), such conformity might entail self-assignment of negative attitudes towards mental retardation.

An opportunity sample of 45 medics aged 18 to 33 was recruited. There were 19 males and 26 females; 23 were first-years, 15 were second-years, and 7 were qualified as doctors. Participants were randomly assigned to one of two conditions. Condition 1 was designed to enhance the salience of a professional medical social identification and Condition 2 was designed to enhance the salience of personal identities. If a shared social identification mediates doctors' especially negative beliefs about mentally retarded people, participants in Condition 1 should express more negative beliefs than those in Condition 2.

A second hypothesis concerned the effects of this evaluative gradient on diagnoses. Tajfel (1972, 1978a, 1981) had argued that evaluation biases the mistakes that people make when judging the group membership of others. Misclassifying a member of a negatively valued group into a valued group is more serious than misclassifying a member of a positively valued group into a negative one. This is because the first mistake contaminates the positive group and so threatens the values it represents. The second mistake might be unfortunate for the misclassified individual, but it keeps the valued group pure and therefore its underlying values safe. Consequently, the second error is less likely. On this basis, doctors and medical students whose shared "medical social identification" is salient, were predicted to class more people as "mentally retarded" when in doubt.

There were two experimental tasks. The first was to complete a 46-item semantic differential questionnaire designed to measure attitudes about mentally retarded people. The second was to view slides of 20 children and judge who was "retarded" and "normal", giving associated confidence ratings. Ten of the children had received medical diagnoses that included severe learning difficulties and the other ten were so-called normal.

Results for the first task showed that doctors and medical students whose medical social identification was salient, gave the more negative opinion on 40/46 scales

($p < .0001$, Sign Test). For the second task, a signal-detection approach was used to calculate how accurately participants could discriminate between the two groups of children, and the preferred direction of guesses (McNicol, 1972). Results indicated no difference between conditions of subjects' ability to discriminate, (Mann Whitney's $U = .209$, $p = .317$, two-tailed). However, participants whose medical social identification was salient were significantly more biased towards responding "retarded" when in doubt ($U = 161$, $p = .018$, one-tailed).

Thus salience of a medical social identification as opposed to personal characteristics or experience that medics might share mediated the negative evaluations of mentally retarded people typically evinced by medical professionals. Thus the study was consistent with a view of medical education as an enculturation of the student with medical concepts and values (Helman, 1994; Murphy, 1996).

4.3.1 Why didn't the patient tell the doctor about his or her main symptoms? Why didn't the patient follow the doctor's advice?

If a consultation occurs at an intergroup level then a patient social identification will be salient as well as a doctor social identification. Some feel for what this identification might entail can be inferred from the *Oxford English Dictionary*, which defines a patient as a person who shows patience and as a person receiving, or registered to receive, medical treatment. It defines "patience" as calm endurance of hardship, provocation, pain, or delay. Conformity to a patient identification is likely to involve passive behaviours and speaking when spoken to, as opposed to a spontaneous presentation of symptoms. In other words, a person is less likely to voice his or her concerns as a patient than as an individual.

A number of studies are at least consistent with these possibilities. For example, families often establish their own rules for using medication, and patients often follow these and community norms rather than medical advice (Osterweis et al., 1979; Suchman, 1972, cited in West & Frankel, 1991). Even stronger anecdotal support may be found in a rich and deservedly well-known study of meanings relevant to health and illness expressed by an opportunity sample of 24 people living in London's East End (Cornwell, 1984). An ethnographic approach, in which respondents were repeatedly interviewed, allowed for the discovery of two sorts of health beliefs. The first, labelled "public accounts" were expressed more frequently and were characterised by deference to medical authority. These were used in response to direct questions and were especially noticeable in interviews when the interviewer seemed cast in the role of formal "expert", for example asking impersonal, authoritative-sounding research questions. In these accounts, respondents seemed to "put on a good face", reflecting and recreating their version of scientific medical opinion and positive images of doctors, which over-rode any negative experiences with them. Similarly, an idealised presentation of respondents' own social worlds was given, depicting family members as fulfilling expected and valued norms. This picture was frequently at odds with medical case histories and

Expectations about the roles of doctors and patients can be gleaned from current media, including hospital dramas on television, such as "Casualty". Actors and actresses preparing to play these roles can offer useful insights. Here are the comments of professional who recently played a surgeon in "Casualty".

> . . . *there were so few lines. Most of my preparation was learning medical terms. I had a position of power compared with other doctors and nurses in the scene . . . It was terrific! I'd say "Get some medicine" or something, and they'd have to sort it out. If they were agitated, I'd be the one to calm them down. The good thing about the situation was, you're the one in control. You're the one who looks calm while everyone does your bidding. Some of the authority of the character rubs off on you. It's like playing The King on stage . . . some of it rubs off you afterwards and you are more authoritative.*

Do you think the professional was an actor or an actress? Why? Reflect on your last experience as a patient. How did you feel about your doctor? Did you feel s/he was in control? Were you aware of putting on a "best face"?

FIGURE 5.3 Interview with a thespian.

personal life events and is close to the picture that might be expected from people interacting in terms of a salient patient identity.

The second kind of health beliefs were labelled "private accounts". These were far less frequent, and emerged in interviews where social distance between respondent and researcher was small, perhaps as a result of increased familiarity and trust, or when shared experiences as women were salient. In private accounts, the goal was no longer to maintain appearances. Unlike public accounts, these reflected complex networks of causes, effects, circumstances, and hypothetical alternatives arising from respondents' personal worlds. Private accounts revealed a less "rosy" view of doctors, and frequently referred to social distance arising out of doctors' power, and a feeling of being in an unequal contest. These could be contradictory, reflecting the vicissitudes of real life and are close to the accounts that might be expected from people interacting in terms of salient roles or their personal identities. Consistent with this view, Stimson and Webb (1975) note that lay accounts of consultations can be best interpreted as reactions to relationships in which people feel inferior.

When a patient leaves a consultation s/he will switch to a personal identification or another social identification, such as an ill student for example. A treatment plan that made perfect sense from the perspective of a patient identification might not survive the ecological transition from the consultation to home, work, or some other setting because it might not be relevant to identities that are salient in those places. Consistent with this view, Morgan (1997) notes that patients frequently attend surgeries for repeat prescriptions in order to keep up appearances, and do not take the medicine prescribed. From an intrapersonal perspective the Jekyll and Hyde quality of patient adherence is irrational, but from a group-level perspective it can be seen as an appropriate response to a change in social context. Clearly, the impact of such changes in salient identifications on adherence and other outcomes offers a rich, new seam for future research. They also offer a group-level rival to the common sense expectation that patients tell doctors about their symptoms and follow their advice.

4.3.2 Why didn't the doctor listen to the patient? Why did s/he keep interrupting?

The social identity approach might be generalised to speculate that doctors' use of controlling styles represents conformity to a salient "doctor" social identification and not some interpersonal jockeying for control. This speculation still leaves open the question as to why control as opposed to something more positive seems to be a criterial behaviour of that identification. An explanation can be found in the minimal group paradigm, which was devised some 30 years ago (e.g. Tajfel, 1970). To establish a baseline for the study of intergroup conflict, Tajfel and his colleagues wanted to identify an intergroup situation in which no conflict characteristically appeared. They attempted to isolate social categorisation *per se*, by devising a paradigm in which there was no face-to-face interaction, no rational link between criteria for categorisation and responses, no instrumental value to responses, and anonymity of group membership. In a series of experiments schoolboys were assigned to one of two such minimal groups, (Tajfel, Flament, Billig, & Bundy, 1971). Their task was to allocate points to various recipients, identified only by group membership. Allocations were to be made using specially prepared booklets of matrices, which forced them to choose between various decision strategies. The major finding was that participants persistently showed outgroup discrimination, even when it entailed a cost to their ingroup.

It was Turner (1975) who realised the theoretical significance of social identity theory for understanding this discrimination. First, he accepted the axiom that humans generally desire positive self-esteem. Second, he argued that in an intergroup situation the only way an individual can derive positive self-esteem is by means of social comparisons between ingroup and relevant outgroups. In the minimal group paradigm, the only available evaluative dimension is money. Hence, the desire for positive self-esteem motivated the establishment of positive distinctiveness between the boys' own and other groups, such that they preferred to win rather than to maximise profits or be fair. In this way, the apparent irrationality of their behaviour is explained: gratuitous discrimination improved self-esteem at an objective cost. Turner (1975) called this phenomenon "social competition" to distinguish it from objective competition for scarce resources.

The next task is to speculate with this theory to explain the triggering of controlling styles in the realm of doctor–patient communication. Social competition not only predicts that members of high-status groups should act to maintain positive distinctiveness, but also that they are likely to construct an intergroup context that affords them the opportunity to do so (Oakes & Turner, 1980). From this point of view, doctors might use controlling styles of communications as a cause as well as a consequence of conformity to doctor and patient roles in order to maintain self-esteem. From this perspective, the construction of an intergroup context may be seen as a manifestation of this universal human need, as opposed to a gratuitous assertion of interpersonal control over an individual who has come to ask for help.

Further interesting questions concern the interaction between salient medical and other identifications during consultations and these lead to yet another, more critical explanation of the use of controlling styles by doctors. For example, another assumption underlying the common sense model of doctor–patient communication is that doctors are somehow genderless or "objective and emotionally detached" (Morgan, 1997), so that patients can talk to them about sexual matters or undress in front of them. Similarly, they are assumed to talk neutrally and equally to men and women patients during consultations. Outside consultations, many gender differences in communication styles have been identified. For example, men tend to act as experts and give advice when asked for help, whereas women tend to share experience and offer reassurance. Men are also more likely to initiate new topics (see Radley, 1996). Other studies have shown that women are likely to use powerless language, to interrupt less, and to be better at decoding non-verbal messages (Knapp & Hall, 1992; Lakoff, 1975). Rather than being fixed properties of the sexes, such differences reflect the social reality that men more often occupy powerful roles (Cameron, McAlinden, & O'Leary, 1988; Noller, 1980).

Interestingly, masculine speech characteristics resemble those that give cause for complaint in doctors. To some extent this is not surprising, because as the dominant system of healthcare, medicine reflects and maintains the ideology of the society from which it arises (Helman, 1994). Thus, medical hierarchies in the UK reflect those of society itself, such that white males occupy the most prestigious, powerful, and well-paid posts, with the proportion of women and ethic minorities increasing with decreasing status. Amongst consultants, women are also under-represented in prestigious "higher risk" specialities. To illustrate, in 1989 they made up 11% of accident and emergency staff, 12% in obstetrics and gynaecology, and only 3% in surgery, compared with 21%, 23%, and 26% in radiology, pathology, and psychiatry, respectively (Scambler & Scambler, 1993). Elaborating on this theme, Scambler and Scambler (1993), argue that one reason why women physicians are under-represented among medicine's elite is a belief that medicine needs to be decisive and "masculine" in order to be effective. As illustration, they cite Shelvin (1981) who warns of the dangers inherent in "feminine medicine". These include unnecessary visits and sick notes, which make doctors popular and caring, but ineffective. He further points out that errors in treatment or impending inquests make him practise like "a little old lady", afraid of decision-making, treatment side-effects, upsetting people, and complaints.

Based on these ideas, a critical hypothesis is that the controlling style of doctors' language has no direct "technical" function, but serves to maintain social order. In particular, the "scientific knowledge" of doctors can be social messages about the proper behaviour of women, wrapped up in technical language (Helman, 1994; Stainton Rogers, 1991). At a more mundane level, control can be exerted through use of patronising terms, and Wallen, Waitzkin, and Stroeckle (1979) showed that male doctors underestimate patients' medical knowledge in general, but particularly underestimate that of women. Notwithstanding, male doctors perceive themselves as more effective communicators (McManus, Kidd, Aldus, 1997).

A pressing question therefore concerns "criss-crossing" (Brown, 1996) of medical and female categories. Young (1981) for example, argues that "doctor" is a masculine concept and that women doctors are seen as "honorary men". As an aside, it is worth pointing out that the history of women in medicine suggests that this status, if it has been won at all, has been hard-won. For example, a parliamentary edict was passed in 1421 in response to a petition from male physicians. It included the clause that "no women use the practice of Fisyk on pain of long imprisonment" (Brierley & Reid, 2000). Women were excluded from the Royal College of Physicians and the Royal College of Surgeons, although in 1815, the Society of Apothecaries stated that it would examine any person who fulfilled its requirements. The first woman to attempt to do so was Elizabeth Garrett. Even so, the Society at first refused and only gave way when her father threatened legal action. She became a Licentiate in 1865. Quickly, however, women were effectively excluded because a new resolution required all candidates to have studied at medical school at a time when no British medical school would accept women! For present purposes however, the question is whether power associated with being a doctor cancels out powerlessness associated with being female. This is an empirical question, although the answer is not easily available, because the majority of research has been carried out on male doctors (Murphy, 1996) and in some cases there are simply no female consultants in post (Motsiou, 1999). One relevant study, however, found that the usual pattern for the doctor to interrupt the patient is reversed when the doctor is female and the patient is male (West & Frankel, 1991). Similarly, a "creeping specialisation" has been identified (Williams, Whitfield, Bucks, & St. Claire, 1991), caused by women patients choosing to consult women doctors and there is evidence that female physicians are more attentive and give more information than their male counterparts, who are more presumptuous and imposing (Meeuwesen, Schaap, & van der Staak, 1991).

Taken together, this evidence is more consistent with the critical idea that male rather than female doctors use controlling (masculine) communication styles that reflect and reinforce normative power differentials. Perhaps inequality in the distribution of men and women doctors lies behind an overgeneralisation. Clearly, however, the issue merits future research. Of particular interest is whether some women doctors conform to masculine speech characteristics and effectively act against their own interests as women. Research could be extended to include identifications relevant to other categories identified as experiencing similar problems when communicating with doctors, such as "elderly", "working class", and "ethnic minority" patients (Morgan, 1997).

4.3.3 Summary

At the group level, conformity to doctor and patient roles is likely to impede doctor–patient communication. In particular, the high status of doctors and positive self-esteem gained therefrom is likely to trigger controlling styles that lead to negative outcomes for patients. Alternatively, controlling styles might reconstruct normative social structures. In addition, switches between patient and other identities might have implications for the survival of coping plans agreed in the context of consultations

4.6 Conclusion

Social psychological influences at all levels offer more successful rivals to the common sense expectation that clinical and relational meanings are freely exchanged in order to help the patient. In the next section, a preliminary attempt is made to build a social psychological model of doctor–patient communication, which will be used in order to suggest strategies for improvement.

5. Towards a More Social Social Psychological Approach to Doctor–Patient Communication

5.1 A draft social psychological model of doctor–patient communication

A draft social psychological model of doctor–patient communication is depicted in Figure 5.4. The model begins with the "inadequate" illness schema, which failed to resolve the patient's symptoms and suggest a remedy. As discussed in the previous chapters this schema is likely to include a great deal more than symptom information and might have little to do with medical facts. On its basis, the patient selects, translates, and encodes information to impart to the doctor. These processes might be inhibited by sketchy knowledge of what the doctor needs to know. In addition, they might be effected in a manner that conveys a particular self-image, or expectations about the doctor and how to behave in his or her presence. Much variation between patients presenting with the same symptom is therefore expected. At one extreme, the patient's initial contribution might simply entail showing a sign to the doctor. At another, it might be a much-rehearsed, lengthy narrative.

Next in the model, the doctor decodes the patient's information, combining it with expert knowledge, in order to build a working schema of the patient's problem. Information from other sources such as case notes, the patient's appearance, or a medical examination might be incorporated, and a history might also be taken.

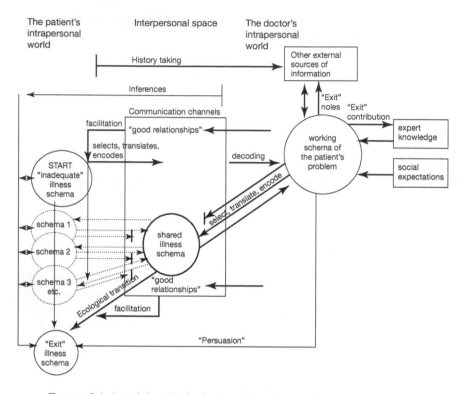

FIGURE 5.4 A social psychological model of doctor–patient communication.

So far, however, communication *per se* has not occurred. Rather, a volley of meanings has been sent by the patient and processed by the doctor. Indeed, it might be that something like this *is* what happens in some consultations, but during communication *per se*, both doctor and patient actively elaborate a mutual illness schema. Therefore, a key feature of the model is that the communicated schema of the patient's problem belongs to interpersonal space as opposed to the cognitive structures and processes of either participant. Fully, elaborated, the shared illness schema might include a diagnosis (identity information), a timeline, a coping plan, and other slots, each with a value tailored to the patient. For example, some patients might not wish to know values for prototypical slots, such as diagnosis or prognosis, yet may wish to know something unusual, such as the ways in which a proposed treatment might affect pursuit of their favourite hobby, hang-gliding. In the model therefore, the doctor selects and translates what information to contribute, on the basis of feedback from the developing shared schema.

In the common sense model, the doctor's contribution is grounded in medical facts of direct relevance to the patient's problems. In contrast, a feature of the social psychological model is that social expectations contribute to his or her working schema. It might be speculated that these include expectations about prototypical victims of diseases, the respective roles of doctors and patients, and other non-medical beliefs that will subsequently colour his or her contribution. Relevant selections and translations are unlikely to be consciously deliberate or, indeed, verbal. Rather, nuances in vocabulary, posture, and discursive strategies are likely subtly to introduce social constructions into the mutual understanding of the patient's problem(s) developed during a consultation. In some consultations, such non-medical influences might even predominate in the doctor's contribution.

In the model, contributions from the patient to the shared schema are represented by dotted arrows, flowing from dotted schemata which represent updated versions of his or her original illness schema. Dotted arrows also flow from the shared schema to these updates. These mutual influences are important: the active contributions of the patient allow for his or her needs to be more fully explored and assimilated into the shared schema. Simultaneously, communications transform the original inadequate schema, which not only shapes but also converges towards the shared one. When the contribution of the patient to the shared schema is small, the original inadequate illness schema might be relatively unchanged and the shared schema might contain more of relevance to the doctor's world.

The exit point of the model is the patient's illness schema after the ecological transition from the medical consultation to another social world. Since this is likely to be affected by a switch of identity, it really requires a different name to acknowledge that the individual is probably no longer formally "the" patient. Rather s/he is likely to self-categorise in terms of a different social identification or to return to self-categorising as an individual who has appraised him or herself as ill. The model suggests that communication results in a closer match between this and the shared illness schema constructed during the consultation. As a result, patient understanding, adherence to coping plans, and other positive outcomes seem more likely. Where there is little correspondence between the shared schema and the schema taken away by the patient, a number of possibilities may be tentatively suggested on the basis of the model. Although the shared illness schema might have made perfect sense in the social context of the consultation and associated salient patient identification, the more it was constructed by the doctor, the less likely it is to be relevant to the patient in his or her other social worlds. Perhaps it will only survive the transition to these other contexts if crucial aspects of the consultation are maintained, such as a salient patient social identification. In addition, common sense suggests that the individual's memory and the doctor's persuasiveness might influence its longevity.

In the model the outcomes for the doctor are simply a contribution to his or her expert knowledge, and perhaps a written contribution to the patient's notes.

Although the importance of the patient's contribution has been stressed, the fact that doctor is consulted as the professional means that the main responsibility for success (or failure) falls upon his or her shoulders (Brickman et al., 1982). For this reason, "good relationships" flow from the doctor in the model. They are depicted as having a facilitating effect on the patient's initial encoding of information, on the active contribution he or she makes to the shared illness schema, and on the likelihood that the shared schema survives the ecological transition from the consultation. Since "good relationships" include due emphasis on the patient's concerns, the model houses an implicit vector towards relationships as opposed to interactions. However, because its reason for existence is based on the doctor's professional expertise, the model is also pitched towards intergroup relationships. Thus, the model is inherently dynamic, with a tension between these two pulls.

In Section 3.1, two types of miscommunication were identified. In the first, the sender did not intend to share a message with its recipient. The inference and history-taking pathways in the model represent this type of miscommunication. Inferences drawn from the doctor by the patient are likely to be made on the basis of the original inadequate illness schema. For example, hypertensive patients often infer representations at odds with the biomedical model of the disease from physicians' courteous enquiries concerning how they feel (Leventhal et al., 1984). A patient who infers, as opposed to communicates, is likely to leave the consultation with his or her original inadequate illness schema relatively intact, perhaps feeling that the consultation was a waste of time, and s/he still does not know what to do. Similarly, a history that is taken from the patient by the doctor is equivalent to information taken from other external sources. A doctor who takes histories, as opposed to communicates, is likely to save time by interrupting with quick closed questions to confirm what s/he "knew" as soon as the patient entered the room.

In the second type of miscommunication, the meaning intended by the sender did not coincide with the meaning understood by the receiver. This type is represented by encoded meanings that do not contribute to the shared schema, but which end in interpersonal space, because they are blocked by interruptions, heard but not shared, or simply not picked up. Such miscommunications might be more frequent when goals vary or interactions are not supported by relationships. Thus, the model not only accommodates the common sense idea that communication will be sparse when participants impart little, but also accommodates the idea that sending large quantities of information does not guarantee good communication. An interesting point is that many such miscommunications need not matter, because they might become irrelevant as the shared schema develops, or because later attempts are more successful. Furthermore, some meanings might be incomplete when first uttered, but might be taken up and completed later during the interaction. A *preponderance* of such miscommunications, however, will impoverish the construction of the shared schema. Finally, there might be rare attempts at persuasion without communication, in that a doctor might directly intend to influence a patient's schema, without intending to participate in a mutual under-standing of his or her case. The persuasion route in the model represents this. This route embodies the bleak view of Friedson (1986, cited in Stainton Rogers, 1991) in whose eyes "lower-class" patients in particular hold such irrational and mis-conceived beliefs that doctors give up attempts to communicate with them, keeping them in ignorance "for their own good".

5.2 Using the model to suggest improvements

Because the doctor shoulders the responsibility for the success of a consultation, the focus will be on improving his or her communication skills. In fact, roughly half a million consultations take place every working day in Britain and the average physician will perform at least 200,000 medical interviews during a 40-year career, yet receives little training for this "most common procedure" (Epstein et al., 1993; Morgan, 1997). Common sense suggestions to improve outcomes include the tape-recording of bad news consultations so that patients can listen as often as they need, in order to take in all the information (e.g., Fallowfield, 1991). According to the social psychological model, however, this strategy is unlikely to affect doctors' communication skills *per se*. It paradoxically suggests that communication might sometimes happen after the event, when the patient catches up with the meaning intended by the doctor. General social skills training can also lead to improvements. For example, doctors might be taught not to interrupt patients, especially female ones (Pendleton et al., 1984). According to the social psychological model, this strategy is likely to work by reducing the number of lost attempts at communication.

Other common sense strategies include teaching medical students a little about the lifestyles of their patient populations, in order to reduce the semantic differences between them (Burnett & Thompson, 1986). Although this might help the doctor with selecting and translating information that is relevant to the patient, the social psychological model warns that this is unlikely to affect doctors' communication skills and might even sabotage them, because learning about patient populations carries with it a danger of increased stereotyping. This is because communication involves constructing shared meanings, rather than feeling more confident about selecting meanings on the other's behalf.

According to Maguire, Fairbairn, and Fletcher (1986), and McGuire, Roe, and Goldberg (1978), the most successful method to improve doctors' communication skills is to videotape interactions with simulator patients. Afterwards, doctors receive feedback in the form of discussion and evaluation of their performance. The social psychological model suggests that the success of this method might lie in its potential to reveal meanings. In this way, it tackles one of the most problematic aspects of communication, namely the fact that it cannot be seen and therefore that there is no objective check that it has occurred. In the context of a close relationship, for example, participants just know that the intended meaning of an eyebrow flash has been shared. Indeed, if they are not sure, they can use other gestures to communicate that! This is because participants in a relationship have an "insider's view" of emergent meanings (Radley, 1996). Doctor–patient relationships seem unlikely to be so close. Like outsiders (and researchers) participants are unlikely to have had enough experience of each other to have a mutual history on which to create understandings. Thus, the opportunity to ask simulator patients what they intended to impart, what they understood from the doctor, and what they thought of him or her is likely to prove invaluable to the doctor, who gains the sort of feedback that might normally take years to discover.

TABLE 5.1 *Seven communication skills*

Greeting the patient
Beginning the interview
Eliciting a full account of the patient's problem
Receiving the patient's communications
Offering a full account of the patient's problems
Sending the patient communications
Ending the interview

It follows that communication *per se* cannot be measured by observation, and this is likely to prove a handicap to evaluating attempts to improve it. However, St. Claire (2000) has identified seven open-ended measurable communication skills and they are listed in Table 5.1. An important theoretical point is that the skills are hypothesised to emerge during interactions and do not necessarily reflect the characteristics of doctors. In this respect, the approach differs from others, such as McManus et al. (1997) who assume doctors possess "true communicative ability". Although these skills were developed as a basis on which to assess the videotaped performance of final-year medical students talking about cancer with simulator patients, they follow directly from the social psychological model and offer some general guidelines for improvement.

The first two skills pertain to good relationships. "Greeting the patient" is designed to assess whether the doctor attempts to establish the basis for a positive new relationship (or sets the interaction in the context of a continuing one). This is operationalised in terms of behaviours that adjust to match the patient, rather than in terms general social skills. For example, standing to meet the patient and offering a handshake might not be relevant for a patient with whom a doctor is already on first-name terms. Thus, what is *not* done is sometimes the preferred option. Second, when the doctor as opposed to the patient has requested the consultation, a supplementary skill, "Orienting the patient", is relevant. Under such circumstances, good relationships and indeed successful understanding are likely to be promoted if the doctor prepares the patient for what is to come. The skill is assessed by observing whether the doctor reminds him or her of relevant information and reassures them about available time. In terms of the social psychological model, this skill not only promotes good relationships but might also facilitate the patient's retrieval of a relevant schema to guide the current interaction.

A third skill is the doctor's success in *eliciting* a full and active contribution from the patient. Thus, the breadth of information from the patient, and not the number of questions the doctor asks, assesses it or the amount of history he or she takes. In particular, whether the patient discusses social and emotional issues relevant to presenting symptoms is noted. In terms of the social psychological model, this skill promotes the likelihood with which the patient's meanings and concerns are accommodated in the shared schema. Such meanings may update the original inadequate illness schema and extend its relevance to a constellation of social worlds. A second dimension of the skill is assessed in terms of behaviours likely to promote good relationships, specifically those that are likely to create an atmosphere in which the patient can contribute.

The fourth skill acknowledges that a good communicator is not the same thing as a good listener. It is assessed by observing whether the doctor checks that his or her interpretations concur with the patient's intended meanings. In terms of the social psychological model, this promotes the likelihood that the initial information from the patient was correctly decoded and that his or her subsequent contributions are harvested in the shared schema as opposed to miscommunicated. Additionally, these checks indirectly reduce the likelihood that the doctor's own contribution is based on inferences as opposed to communications.

The next skill directly concerns the doctor's contribution. Fallowfield (1991) has criticised the "modern day clinical glasnost assumption" that patients must always be given the choice of treatment and full information. She argues that old-fashioned paternalism and reassurance may suit some better. In this spirit, the fifth skill is assessed in terms of the doctor's efforts to find out and comply with the patient's wishes. In particular, whether the doctor *offers* information on physical, mental, and social aspects of the patient's problem(s) is observed *and* whether s/he complies with the patient's response to the offer. Again, it is the match between doctor and patient as opposed to quantity of information that is the basis of high evaluations. Indeed, instances where the doctor gives information in spite of the patient's wishes are scored negatively. In terms of the social psychological model, the emphasis on offering and complying ensures that the selection and translation from the expert working schema to the shared schema is tailored to the patient's needs. It also allows for incompleteness, since offers might be harvested later, as their relevance to the patient emerges. A second aspect of the skill is assessed in terms of good relationships flowing when advice is given. Particularly if breaking bad news, it is important that the doctor communicates humane confidence, openness, and optimism.

In order for communication to have occurred, the doctor must ensure that s/he is not vainly talking at the patient, but that the meanings he or she intends to convey are being shared. Hence, the sixth skill is assessed by observing whether the doctor avoids or clarifies technical jargon and monitors what the patient has understood. In terms of the social psychological model, therefore, this skill promotes the likelihood that joint meanings are indeed being constructed.

Finally, the seventh skill concerns ending the interview. It is assessed by checking whether the doctor has given a clear resumé of clinical information and what to do next, together with an impression of good relationships. In terms of the social psychological model, this skill enhances the fitness of the shared schema to survive the ecological transition from the consultation.

In addition to suggesting skills that might be targeted in order to improve doctor–patient communication, the social psychological model suggests that deprofessionalisation of doctor–patient interactions offers a group-level strategy that will launch many improvements, including the reduction of doctor-centred styles. However, the worrying prediction of social competition theory is that this strategy is likely to be handicapped by motivational biases. Because the doctors' role is of high status, doctors should derive self-esteem from their positive distinctiveness compared with patients. This means that a universal human need for positive self-esteem is likely to encourage them to construct an intergroup social context. Indeed, this helps to explain the finding that doctors are "negatively affected" by more active patients (Tuckett et al., 1985). One successful strategy to reduce intergroup conflict in general is to encourage members of two or more groups to redefine themselves in terms of a single group (Gaertner, Dovidio, Anastasio, Bachman, & Rust, 1993, Gaertner, Dovidio, Nier, Banker, Ward, Houlette et al., 2000). Thus, progress might be made where doctors and patients are encouraged to see themselves as partners in a care team with a superordinate identity as well as a superordinate goal (Brewer, 2000). However, care must be taken to ensure that the categories do not actually reinforce each other such that conflict escalates (Brown & Turner, 1981). In other words, little might be gained if doctors self-define as expert team leaders, with the stereotypic female, ethnic minority, working-class patient as the team member!

6. Summary and Conclusions

Good communication is essential for effective healthcare because it is the means through which patients share their needs and concerns with doctors and doctors share expert help with their patients.

In the first section a common sense model of communication was suggested in which patients tell their doctors about symptom(s); doctors use the information to build a working model of the problem, on the basis of which they give relevant advice to the patient; and patients follow the advice.

In the second section, a corpus of empirical evidence and a case study challenged common sense, painting a rather bleak picture of the effectiveness of doctor–patient communication.

- Because of the professional status of doctors, the main responsibility accrues to them.

In the third section a working definition of communication as intentional sharing of meaning was developed.

- This usefully suggested that two sorts of miscommunication could occur, depending on whether information was unintentionally leaked or whether a different meaning to the one intended was understood.
- Subsequently, interactions were characterised as visible exchanges between people and relationships were characterised as mutual understandings between people, which take time to develop.

- Some doctor–patient interactions are embedded in relationships whereas others are not.
- The implication was that communication is likely to be easier, and less dependent on verbal language, in the context of relationships and that its effectiveness might be underestimated if based on observed elements. For example, a silence during which no action whatsoever occurs might score zero from the perspective of an outsider, but it might communicate megabytes to participants in a relationship.

In the fourth section social psychological influences were reviewed to help explain some of the ways in which the common sense model of doctor–patient communication fell short.

- Intrapersonal influences included lack of relevant background knowledge and opportunity to adjust communication channels on the part of the patient, together with schema-based heuristics and biases on both parts.
- Interpersonal influences were highlighted as the appropriate level of analysis for a discussion of communication. The thrust of the argument was that patients present symptoms as an on-line act, as opposed to passively reporting them. The dressing-up of symptom information to present important self-images and to negotiate status and affiliation vastly complicates communication and might account for many problems. One suspicion was that doctors' interruptions of patients might communicate status information, even though status differences between doctors and patients pre-exist.
- A group-level analysis suggested that a universal need for positive self-esteem might motivate doctors to interact with patients at an intergroup level, creating an inherent tension with a need for interpersonal relationships indicated by the demands of empathy and patient-centredness.
- A critical analysis suggested that doctors' communications might sometimes be to the advantage of the doctors, perhaps conveying normative messages over and above medical "facts".

In the fifth section, a social psychological model of doctor–patient communication was suggested.

- Its key feature was that the communicated schema of the patient's problem(s) belonged to interpersonal space, as opposed to the cognitive structures of either participant.
- The model incorporated not only social expectations, but also heuristics and biases arising from the personal worlds of both doctor and patient.
- Its outcome was the new illness schema taken away by the patient. This is more likely to match the shared schema constructed during the consultation, when the patient actively contributes. Such closeness, it was suggested might lead to better adherence.

- Although an important point was that communication could not be objectively measured, the model suggested seven visible communication skills likely to promote effective communication. The created match between doctor and patient, not the doctor's behaviour, underpinned them. These skills suggested ways in which doctors might gain insight into and improve their communications.

To acknowledge the dynamic complexity of communication is heartening. High numbers of miscommunications, interruptions, and bad manners can give the impression that communication is the exception rather than the rule. Perhaps it is, but this need not be catastrophic, because in the context of the multidimensional meanings and purposes that emerge from the interface between the personal worlds of doctor and patient, many other meanings might be shared and survive the ecological transition from the consultation. A social psychological model incorporating influences at all levels of analysis gives insights into the ways in which the process might be impeded and additionally suggests some likely strategies for improvement.

The ultimate point of improving doctor–patient communication is to help the patient through his or her illness so that s/he may more quickly become well and leave the patient role. The question arises therefore, just how does a person tell that s/he is well? Exactly this question is the topic of the next chapter.

6

"I'm Very Well Thank You". But How Do I Know I'm Well?

> I know when I'm healthy because I don't feel all drowsy and sleepy or sick and burpy
>
> *(Jack, aged 9)*

> . . . and I don't feel like I want to watch any more television like I do when I'm ill
>
> *(Harry, aged 5)*

This chapter begins a little after the last one ended. It begins when the individual is well again. More specifically, it considers the structures and processes that underpin this decision, or how people know they are well. Comparisons between lay judgements and professional approaches to measuring health feature throughout the chapter and this means that it especially emphasises the intergroup level of analysis.

In Section 1 the importance of evaluating positive health status is briefly discussed. Subsequently, not one but two common sense models of lay people's judgements of health status are suggested. Both assume that people evaluate themselves rationally with respect to their beliefs about health. However, the first model assumes that the underlying health schema is like the medical model and therefore conceptualises health as an absence of disease and symptoms, whereas the second assumes that the underlying health schema is more positive. The way these models seem to underpin professional measures of health status is also briefly considered.

In Section 2 both these common sense models are challenged by evidence that individuals with serious diseases often judge that they are well.

In the next two sections social psychological influences on wellness judgements are reviewed, in order to suggest some of the ways in which common sense models fall short. In Section 3, the focus is on the cognitive structures underpinning judgements. At the intrapersonal level of analysis, consideration of quality of life measures and subjective meanings of health suggests that individuals might base self-assessments on beliefs that are important in their personal worlds. At an intragroup level of analysis, meanings of health reflect normative functions expected of people and although individuals express these meanings, they "belong" to social groups or might be constructed during conversations and "belong", perhaps fleetingly, to a given social situation. These social psychological influences on health beliefs mean that subjective health status evaluations might be at odds with common sense ideas grounded in physical well-being.

In Section 4, the focus is on the cognitive process underpinning lay judgements of health status. At the intrapersonal level, denial and crisis theory suggest that individuals might not evaluate themselves in "rational" ways but in ways that inflate assessment. At an interpersonal level, social comparison theory suggests that self-evaluations of health status might be based on benchmarks drawn from other individuals and vary according to who is present, and since patients affiliate with each other, their self-assessments might be enhanced. At group levels, a social identity approach suggests a number of ways in which these ideas may be criticised and elaborated. In particular, judgements of subjective health status might be mediated by social creativity; a group-based strategy to preserve self-esteem.

In Section 5 a social psychological model of evaluating subjective health status is suggested in order to integrate the previous discussions and suggest some new possibilities for future research.

1. Introduction and Two Common Sense Models of Judging Positive Health Status

1.1 The importance of evaluating positive health

ACTIVITY 6.1 How are you?

Introspect upon the ways in which you made your judgement.
The likelihood is that you answered "Very well".
How did/would you distinguish between "Well" and "Very well"?
Compare your response to Activity 2.1.
Did you evaluate yourself as "well" here, even though you reported symptoms there? If so, how do you account for the mismatch?

Judgements of wellness are important. The individual needs to be able to judge that s/he is well in order to leave a patient role and resume normal duties. Judgements of wellness are also likely to underpin the decision to stop medication. They might also underpin many judgements that are not to do with leaving illness, such as persevering with a healthy regime or taking on a new challenge.

Health professionals also need to make decisions about health as opposed to illness. GPs might need to identify the end-point of treatment (Tapp & Warner, 1985). They might also need to evaluate the success of preventative programmes and prophylactic medication (R. Williams, 1983) and to know when to reassure anxious persons that they are well. Surgeons turn to positive health measures when there is no clinical basis to guide choices between treatments (Gilbar, 1991), and epidemiologists of lifestyle in well populations need to be able to distinguish degrees of health and well being (e.g., Blaxter, 1992; Fitzpatrick, 1993; Mercer, 1973; WHOQUAL, 1993).

More generally, increased prevalence of chronic as opposed to acute disease has created a need for positive measures of health. Because chronic disease might not have a definable onset, morbidity measures designed to count the sick are unreliable (Cartwright, 1983; Berkman & Breslow, 1983). Moreover, since chronic illness might last many years, mortality measures designed to count the dead also do not suffice. In other words, it is more important to add "life to years" than "years to life" (Bowling, 1997; Lalonde, 1974) and this means measures of positive "life" are needed as opposed to individual and group level measures of symptoms and signs.

1.2 Two common sense models of evaluating subjective health status

The judgement "I am very well" is taken as a convenient way of saying "I am healthy" (Murphy, 1996) and common sense simply assumes that individuals make this decision by evaluating themselves rationally with respect to a health schema or set of beliefs. However, given the importance of judgements about health, common sense is curiously elusive about the nature of the beliefs and the process. Two possibilities are suggested in the next subsections.

1.2.1 Evaluating health from a medical model perspective

Figure 6.1 shows a common sense model of the ways in which individuals decide they are well, which is underpinned by a biomedical perspective. Thus its cognitive structure is a default definition of health as an absence of disease, which is reflected in an absence of signs and therefore symptoms. Its cognitive process is a search for symptoms of disease. Thus the idea is that an individual who judges s/he is well has scanned for symptoms and found none. Strictly speaking, the model is categorical and perception of only one symptom means the criterion for health has not been satisfied.

Routine government health surveys typically focus on self-reported diseases and impairments and therefore assume a similar disease-based model of health (Bowling, 1997). However, these are not categorical, but ordinal in practice. They measure health in terms of something like "minus the number of symptoms", as opposed to an absence of symptoms. For example, the General Health Questionnaire, which is used in general household surveys in Britain, consists of checklists of symptoms and common conditions together with questions about service use (see Cartwright, 1983; Goldberg et al., 1984). Although a general question concerns

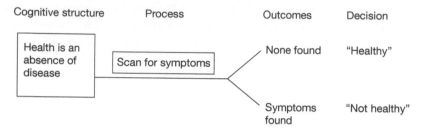

FIGURE 6.1 A common sense model of judging subjective health status (1).

respondents' perception of their health over the previous year, the emphasis is clearly on health problems, as opposed to positive health. Another example, the Cornell Medical Index is described by Bowling (1997) as consisting of 195 yes–no questions divided into 18 sections. A "yes" response indicates presence of a problem, and eight sections relate to physical systems, four to frequency of illness, and the remainder cover personal habits, moods, and feelings. Example questions are "Do you suffer badly from frequent severe headaches?", "Has a doctor ever said you have kidney or bladder disease?" Many other variations on this theme include the PILL (Pennebaker, 1982) and the McGill Pain Questionnaire (Melzack & Katz, 1992) which were both described in Chapter 3. Similarly, there are myriad indices relevant to individual diseases, such as the asthma symptom checklist (e.g., Hyland, 1990).

If the common sense model shown in Figure 6.1 is similarly "relaxed", the idea is that a lay man or woman who judges s/he is well has scanned for symptoms and found none, or just a few that are not too bad.

A serious problem inherent in judgements of wellness based on a medical perspective is that states such as "healthy" and "very healthy" cannot be distinguished because these, together with all positive states, score zero symptoms. In view of this and its negative emphasis, it is tempting to argue that the common sense model in Figure 6.1 is really about illness as opposed to health. Indeed, it is reasonable to speculate that it is underpinned by a high-level schema that incorporates everything an individual knows about the symptoms of disease and which has been assembled from his or her repertoire of illness schemata (see Chapters 3 and 4). The implication is that a more positive approach should be tried.

1.2.2 Evaluating health from a more positive perspective

The *Oxford English Dictionary* defines "well" as "in good health". The meaning of "health" derives from Old English and German forms of the word "whole". A positive definition of health that is closer to this meaning was famously suggested by the World Health Organisation in 1946: "a state of complete physical, mental and social well-being and not merely the absence of disease or infirmity" (WHO,

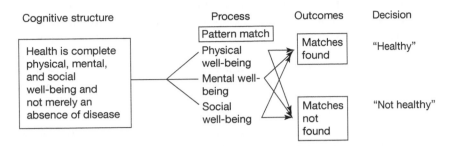

FIGURE 6.2   A common sense model of judging subjective health status (2).

1958). Figure 6.2 redraws the common sense model of subjective health status evaluations, replacing the medical model of health with the WHO's positive definition. This change implies that the process is now one of pattern matching. The individual who has judged him or herself well has compared physical, mental, and social states with stored ideals and established three "complete" matches. Intuitively, it seems even more difficult to pass the criteria needed to judge oneself "healthy" in this version of the common sense model, since to achieve perfect well-being in three spheres of life is rather a tall order. In addition, just what constitutes complete well-being is unspecified and poses great difficulty (Stacey, 1977).

In practice, measures of health status, which are underpinned by more positive definitions, avoid this problem by operationalising positive well-being in terms of statistical norms. For example, signs of physical well-being are measured by objective quantifiable parameters such as blood pressure, birthweight, handgrip strength, or physical fitness (e.g., Council of Europe, 1983; Hopkins & Walker, 1988; Tapp & Warner, 1985).

Relative ease of access to subjects as opposed to medical records, clinicians, or testing equipment is probably behind the development of measures of physical well-being based on health practices (DHSS, 1976), health risk attitudes (e.g., O'Rourke, Smith, Nolte, 1984), and symptoms. For example, the Physical Health Measure of the Alameda County Study assessed symptoms of health in terms of five categories: energy level compared with peers; recurrent symptoms; chronic illnesses; physical and sensory impairments; and disabilities (Berkman & Breslow, 1983). As this example shows, however, such positively named measures often turn out to be negatively oriented and therefore indistinguishable from symptom checklists.

To turn to measures of mental well-being, Holmes and Rahe (1967) attempted to quantify its signs in terms of the total adjustment thought likely to be necessitated by life events encountered by individuals during a given period. It is well known that the attempt was profoundly handicapped by variation in the human response to situations that were objectively the same (e.g., Cassidy, 1999). Later solutions to this problem involved building in reactions to events, thereby combining signs and symptoms (e.g., Brantley, Waggoner, Joncs, & Rappaport, 1987). Again these scales seem to be negatively oriented. The person who encounters relatively few disrupting events or hassles and/or does not mind about them is the one who is mentally well. A similarly negative emphasis is repeated across many scales purporting to measure mental well-being, which actually assess self-derogation and psychological distress to name just two (Kaplan, Robbins, & Martin, 1983; Kaplan & Porkorny, 1969). More positively oriented measures of mental well-being do exist, however, and they include self-esteem (Coopersmith, 1967); happiness (Bradburn & Caplovitz, 1965); the Satisfaction with Life Scale (Diener, Emmons, Larson, & Griffin, 1985); and positive affect (Pennebaker, 1982).

Ware (1984) thinks that social well-being might be the most important aspect of health. He also notes that it is one of the most difficult to define and measure, particularly as it is likely to depend on factors external to the individual, such as who is available in their community (Bowling, 1997). One useful definition is: "the degree to which a person's basic social needs are gratified through interaction with others" (Thoits, 1982, p. 147). Basic social needs include affection, esteem, approval, belonging, identity, security, and giving as well as receiving support. Signs of social well-being include counts of an individual's social contacts, and measures based on this approach are reviewed by Singer and Lord (1984). However, analogous to the situation concerning life events, perceived quality as opposed to objective quantity of social support is more important (Bartlett, 1998). Hence, examples such as the Social Support Questionnaire (Sarason, Levine, Basham, & Sarason, 1983) require respondents to list up to nine people to whom they can turn across a range of scenarios, and then to rate the amount of support they would expect from each. In this way, subjective and objective aspects are combined.

If the common sense model shown in Figure 6.2 is "relaxed" like these professional measures, statistical averages as opposed to ideal states can form the basis for lay assessments. In this case, individuals who judge they are well have confirmed their normal status on three constellations of dimensions, which represent the three global dimensions, physical, mental, and social well-being. Subsequently, they have somehow combined the result.

2. Challenges to Common Sense Models of Health

2.1 Empirical studies

For once, common sense suggested relatively little about the structures and processes that underpin subjective judgements about health status. However, it does suggest that people will not judge themselves well if they perceive serious symptoms. This follows by definition from the perspective depicted in Figure 6.1 in which health is defined as an absence of symptoms. In the more positive perspective of Figure 6.2, high levels of physical complaints seem grounds enough to rule out complete well-being.

The work of van Dam and his associates challenges this view. van Dam, Linssen, Englesman, Van Benthem, and Hanewald (1980) compared three groups of breast cancer patients. The first had advanced disease and was being treated with drugs. The second was being treated with radiotherapy and drugs, and amputation and/or radiotherapy had cured the third. To the authors' surprise, participants reported a "not inconsiderable degree of well-being" in spite of daunting levels of physical problems. A review of the quality of life in cancer patients comes to the same conclusions (de Haes & van Knippenberg, 1985) and after 10 years of review and research, Breetvelt and van Dam (1991) confirm the pattern, not only in different groups of cancer patients, but also in physically handicapped people, blind people, and even paralysed victims of traffic accidents.

A closer reading of the studies reviewed by Breetvelt and van Dam (1991) highlights that high levels of well-being are reported on *psychological* dimensions, in spite of a distressing array of *physical* disabilities. The point is illustrated in three earlier studies, in which levels of satisfaction with life of non-normal and normal people were compared. In the first study 64 individuals with paralysis, 37 with a muscular difficulty, 16 with deformed limbs, 12 with missing limbs, 11 who were blind, and 4 who were hearing impaired were participants. In the second 46 individuals from schools or workshops for the blind participated, and in the third the sample was 40 children with learning difficulties. For each study, matched "normal" controls were also recruited. Levels of happiness did not differ between groups of physically handicapped, blind, and able-bodied respondents, even though disabled groups did report more difficulties with their lives in general (Cameron, Titus, Kostin, & Kostin, 1973). Breetvelt and van Dam (1991) call this pattern "under-reporting". Clearly, under-reporting challenges common sense, which expects such individuals to be frustrated and upset by their conditions (Cameron et al., 1973).

2.2 Case study

Case studies such as the one below also challenge common sense by illustrating vividly that lay people can and do say they are well in the presence of serious and long-term signs, symptoms, pain, and disability.

Q   *"How are you and uncle?"*
A   *"Oh, very well, thanks. Mind you, your uncle had terrible 'flu. It was our John's little girl gave it to him. He was terrible with it, all over Christmas. And his hernia's been playing him up . . . the garden's too much for him now. My arthritis has got bad; it's in my knees so I can't drive like I used to . . . But I had my check last week. The cancer trouble is all clear now, but we've got to keep an eye on it. We just don't go out this weather. We've got plenty of groceries in, and we just don't go out. But we can't complain. We're very well really."*

2.3 Conclusions

A feature of the biomedical approach is that lay beliefs are often inaccurate. Thus, the possibility that lay people after all rationally use the common sense model depicted in Figure 6.1 cannot be ruled out, since inadequate knowledge might mislead them into scanning for the wrong symptoms! This was exactly the concern of Tissue (1972) who noted that elderly people's self-reported health frequently differed from their medical records. He concluded that clinical opinions should preferred, because lay people misjudged their own health. Not only might their beliefs be inaccurate, but also the ways in which they judge themselves might be irrational and haphazard.

Taken together, research and case studies challenge the common sense assumption that people evaluate their health status rationally with respect to health beliefs that resemble either a medical model of health or a more positive definition of health as complete physical, mental, and social well-being. The challenge is not detailed enough to reveal whether it is the underlying cognitive structure or the evaluative process that most flies in the face of common sense. Over the next two sections, social psychological influences on health beliefs and health evaluations will be reviewed in order to suggest some answers.

3. Social Psychological Influences on Structures Underpinning Judgements of Health Status

The purpose of this section is to consider the nature of the cognitive structures that might underpin lay judgements of health. These offer rival explanations to the common sense idea that they are based on structures that resemble a medical model of health as an absence of signs and symptoms, or a more positive model of health as physical, mental, and social well-being. To help in this attempt, professional measures of health status will be pirated as well as more social psychological approaches.

3.1 Intrapersonal influences on the cognitive structures underpinning judgements of health status

3.1.1 Quality of life

Quality of life focuses on what matters to the individual in the context of his or her own life. It is conceptualised as those qualities that make life and survival valuable to him or her (Bowling, 1997). Quality of life might hold the key to understanding the cognitive structures underpinning lay judgements of health status. This is because under-reporting could result if judgements are made on personally relevant as opposed to common sense meanings of health.

3.1.1.1 Approaches based on disability, discomfort, and distress

Unfortunately, just what constitutes quality of life is a source of debate (e.g., Perry & Felce, 1995). One important problem is how to limit the scope of the concept, which after all could be as wide as life itself. Since quality of life scales are typically designed to aid the allocation of resources, or to help clinicians evaluate the benefit of treatment options (Hyland et al., 1991), one solution is to limit their components to those for which the health system can be held accountable (e.g., Ware, 1984). A definition that fits this approach is the functional effect of an illness and its consequent therapy upon a patient as perceived by the patient (Schipper, Clinch, & Powell, 1990). The Sickness Impact Profile, for example, was designed comprehensively to evaluate the outcomes of alternative healthcare services and illustrates this tradition well (e.g., Bergner et al., 1981). Once again, however, the approach seems to encourage a negative focus more suited to states of illness than health. For example, Sugarbaker, Barofsky, Rosenberg, and Gianola (1982) tested the impact of different types of surgery on 26 cancer patients. Although their objective was to assess treatment in terms of the overall benefit to patients, they actually focused on the limitation of the adverse consequences of medical procedures. Specifically, they expected that the negative impact of high-dose radiation would be better tolerated than that of amputation (but to their surprise, they did not find that this was so).

More generally, the Index of Health Related Quality of Life, which is based on Rosser's (1991) Index of Disability, Discomfort and Distress, illustrates this negative orientation. Each of these three dimensions is broken down into subscales, and then sub-subscales. For example, one subscale of disability is "self-care" which includes the sub-subscales washing, dressing, and feeding. Each is scored from 0 to 1. Zero is defined as "dead" and 1 is defined as "health" or "no impairment". Although negative values are available to correspond to states worse than death, there are no values above 1 to represent performances that are better than not impaired. Thus the measure focuses on negative issues.

Furthermore the focus on impairments and healthcare issues means that items tend to be chosen by professionals. The result is that items of importance to patients can be omitted and this challenges validity, since it undermines the emphasis on patient perceptions. However, even when patient groups are used to generate items, the negative focus encourages the development of measures covering aspects of life most often affected by impairment. Thus, measures commonly used to assess quality of life for people with learning difficulties assess the physical environment in residential homes, community integration, and the opportunity to make personal decisions (Perry & Felce, 1995). Measures for use with people with rheumatological disorders, on the other hand, focus on walking mobility, employment, and their disruption by pain (Fitzpatrick, 1993). The Living with Asthma Questionnaire excludes items not relevant to the disease, but includes examples such as avoiding smoky rooms (Hyland, 1990; Hyland et al., 1991).

These and similar quality of life instruments allow for evaluations to differ from those predicted on the basis of the common sense models depicted in Figures 6.1

and 6.2. This means that they potentially offer insight into the nature of the cognitive structures that might underpin lay judgements of wellness and under-reporting. However, their negative focus means they are unlikely to be able to distinguish degrees of wellness. Moreover, they seem to encourage a focus on the needs of patient groups and are unlikely to be relevant to the well population. As such, they are unlikely to provide a truly successful rival to common sense.

3.1.1.2 A more positive approach

A more positive definition of quality of life is "an individual's perceptions of their position in life, in the context of the culture and value system in which they live and in relation to their goals, expectations, standards and concerns" (WHOQUAL Group, 1993). This is more promising because quality of life is no longer determined with reference to the healthcare system, but by interactions between the individual's "physical health, psychological state, level of independence, social relationships and their relationship to salient features of their environment" (WHOQUAL Group, 1993). From this perspective, a team of international researchers constructed 276 items to represent 29 facets collectively known as "quality of life". Items met rigorous psychometric criteria and there was worldwide agreement on their meaning and importance (WHOQUAL Group, 1995). Subsequent piloting allowed the facets to be assigned to one of six domains in order to construct a measure. These were physical, psychological, levels of independence, social relationships, environmental health, and spirituality. Two shortened versions of the measure were later developed. First, The WHOQOL-100 retained 24 facets, grouped into physical, psychological, social relationships, and environment domains, and supplemented with four questions about general life and health (WHOQUAL Group, 1995). Second, the further streamlined WHOQOL-BREF contains just 26 items, one for each of the 24 facets, supplemented with two general questions (WHOQUAL Group, 1998).

More important than these details for present purposes is the fact that focus groups of patients, professionals, *and well people* generated items for consideration. Hence, they were designed by the users, for the users (Skevington, 1998) and positive feelings, freedom, safety, and security feature in addition to negative feelings, pain, and discomfort.

If a schema resembling this version of quality of life underpins subjective health status, the lay individual who describes him or her self as well, self-assesses on a constellation of 24 facets and somehow combines the results. "Under-reporting" simply indicates that physical ailments play a relatively minor role in the whole. Indeed, pilot studies for the WHOQOL-BREF support this idea since the physical domain explained just under a third of the variance in quality of life (WHOQUAL Group, 1998). This version of quality of life therefore provides a useful candidate to rival the cognitive structure underpinning common sense models of how individuals judge "I'm well".

As an aside, an alternative possibility also deserves mention. In a representative sample of 252 ill people and 50 controls in Britain, Skevington (1998) investigated the relationship between pain and quality of life, using the full version of the WHOQUAL and other measures of pain. Although data showed that pain and discomfort were not synonymous with poor quality of life, they were significantly associated with all facets except three. For perceptions of the home environment and personal relationships correlations were significant, but weak. For spirituality, the correlation was insignificant. Further explorations suggested that it was the emotional dimensions of pain, as opposed to its somatic qualities, that most overshadowed quality of life. Thus, it is tempting to suggest that under-reporting will only occur in individuals with physical difficulties if they are free from pain.

The WHOQUAL was designed to have many uses. One is to assist clinicians in evaluating areas in which patients are most affected by disease, hopefully leading to improvements in doctor–patient communication as the doctor better understands the patient's needs and the patient finds healthcare more meaningful. Another is to assist treatment decisions and facilitate the identification of treatments appropriate in developing countries (WHOQUAL Group, 1993). Unfortunately, it was not designed to aid my speculations on the cognitive structures underpinning lay evaluations of subjective health status! Notwithstanding, patients are likely to be the beneficiaries rather than the users of the measure. The real users are more likely to be those involved in medical and political decisions. Furthermore, the international relevance of the approach suggests that it might be pitched at too general a level to allow insight into mundane idiosyncrasies used by individuals in everyday life.

Such idiosyncratic meanings are more likely to be revealed in studies that emphasise what individuals think or say. These form the topic of the next section.

3.1.2 Subjective approaches

3.1.2.1 Global measures

Researchers can avoid struggling to define and operationalise "health" and "quality of life" by leaving the defining to the subjects of their research. An added bonus is that this automatically allows for idiosyncratic responses. For example, Garrity's Health Ladder (Garrity, Somes, & Marx, 1980) simply depicts a ladder with its nine rungs labelled from "worst health" to "best health" and respondents indicate their status by choosing a rung. Such global measures are more successful than severity of disease in predicting outcomes such as service utilisation, relevant health practices, recovery from illness episodes, and even mortality (e.g. Bowling, 1997; Martini, Allan, Davison, & Backett, 1979; Segovia et al., 1989). However, because they mask an infinity of reasons for individual differences, they are unlikely to put forward a successful rival candidate to common sense for the cognitive structure underpinning lay judgements of health status because they offer no detailed clues to help solve the puzzle of under-reporting.

ACTIVITY 6.2 What does health mean to you?

Give six short definitions or descriptions.

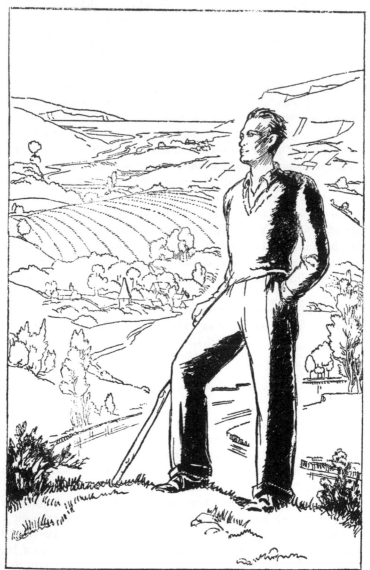

TOWARDS A HEALTHY AND CONTENTED LIFE

Compare and contrast your definitions with those you perceive to be objectified in the picture.

What have you learned about the meaning of health?

3.1.2.2 The Nottingham Health Profile

A more informative and better known subjective health measure is the Nottingham Health Profile (e.g., Hunt & McEwen, 1980). Its development was motivated by an acknowledgement of differences between lay and professional concepts of health, together with the realisation that the former might provide more useful guidelines in understanding human experience and demands on services. The original pool of 2200 items was collected during 1975, from interviews with 768 patients who were suffering from various acute and chronic ailments. Following inductive analysis, this was reduced to 82 items, covering 12 domains. Next, the instrument was shortened and items were simplified, which in practice meant focusing on unambiguous and frequently more serious complaints. Finally, six subscales remained to represent the constituents of subjective health. These were: physical mobility; pain; sleep; emotional reactions; social relationships; and energy levels. Each subscale is assessed by means of yes/no responses to simple statements such as "I have pain at night", affirmative responses being weighted to give a possible maximum score of 100 (McKenna, Hunt, & McEwen, 1981). Finally, and as a result of later research, seven statements relating to paid employment, jobs around the house, social life, personal relationships, sex life, hobbies, and holidays were added to complete the Profile (Hunt & McEwen, 1980). This was not always helpful because the questions were irrelevant to many groups of patients, and so they were subsequently removed (Bowling, 1997). Many studies demonstrate that it performs well. For example, it distinguishes between patients waiting in doctors' surgeries and controls (Hunt, McKenna, McEwen, Williams, & Papp, 1981). It is also sensitive to restrictions on daily life imposed by health problems (Hunt, McEwen, & McKenna, 1984).

Even from this brief description it is clear that, in spite of its name, the Nottingham Health Profile largely concerns self-assessment of morbidity and symptoms in populations of ill people. This means that it is unlikely to resemble the cognitive structures underpinning lay judgements of wellness.

3.1.2.3 More positively oriented approaches

In two more positively oriented though independent approaches to the measurement of subjective health status, brief interviews were carried out with many members of target populations in order to ascertain what "health" typically meant to them. The populations were well teenagers and adults, respectively (Norfolk, 1990; St. Claire, 1986b). A notable finding was that meanings relevant to the medical model accounted for only a small proportion of beliefs amongst teenagers (5–9%). Rather, positive and active meanings predominated. Two positive subjective health measures were constructed on the basis of item pools. The one designed for well adults has been published elsewhere (Norfolk, 1990). The second, for well teenagers, is illustrated in Table 6.1.

Behind this work, the motive was to construct a research measure analogous to the subjective model used by individuals who report they are well. Thus, to the

TABLE 6.1 *A subjective health status measure for UK teenagers*

Compared with an average teenager of my own age and sex:

1. I get the right amount of sleep　□........□........□........□........□........□........□

    　　much less　　　average　　much more

2. I get worried
    　　much less　　　average　　much more

3. I get worn out
    　　much less　　　average　　much more

4. I take care of myself
    　　much less　　　average　　much more

5. The physical condition of my body is ....
    　　much better　　average　　much worse

6. The amount of drugs I take is ....
    　　much less　　　average　　much more
    ("Drugs" can mean a lot of things. Use the meaning that's most important to you).

7. I look healthy
    　　much less　　　average　　much more

8. I am happy
    　　much less　　　average　　much more

9. The amount of alcohol I drink is
    　　much less　　　average　　much more

10. Physically I am able to do
    　　much less　　　average　　much more

11. I am fit
    　　much less　　　average　　much more

12. I am relaxed
    　　much less　　　average　　much more

13. I take exercise
    　　much less　　　average　　much more

14. The likelihood of my getting a job is
    　　much less　　　average　　much more

15. I get ill
    　　much less　　　average　　much more

16. I am alert
    　　much less　　　average　　much more

17. The number of good friends I have is ....
    　　much less　　　average　　much more

18. The amount of care I take over
    personal cleanliness is
    　　much less　　　average　　much more

19. The number of cigarettes I smoke is ....
    　　much less　　　average　　much more

20. I am happy with my sex life
    　　much less　　　average　　much more
    ("sex life" can mean a lot of things. Use the meaning that's most important to you).

21. I go out with friends
    　　ideal amount　　average　　much more or less

22. I am
    　　perfect shape　　average　　too fat or too thin

23. When exercising, I get out of breath ....
    　　much less　　　average　　much more

24. I am energetic (lively)	....		
	much less	average	much more
25. The amount of health foods in my diet is	....		
	much less	average	much more
26. I do sport	....		
	much less	average	much more
27. I feel well	....		
	much less	average	much more
28. I get fresh air and sun	....		
	much less	average	much more
29. My family life is stable	....		
	much less	average	much more

extent that pilot work successfully identified and represented relevant dimensions, the measures should characterise well the elements of the schema that underpin subjective judgements of health for the groups so far studied. In other words, a teenager who judges he or she is well has assembled self-assessments on a range of personally relevant continua similar to those in Table 6.1. As such these measures offer good rival candidates to the common sense idea that judgements are underpinned by something resembling a medical model of health, or a more positive model of health as complete physical mental and social well-being.

Clearly, many studies of health beliefs have been carried out for purposes other than to develop health status measures, and it is worth digressing briefly to consider some, for the insight they might offer into the beliefs underpinning health status judgements of other populations. Since these studies are typically pitched at interpersonal and group levels of analysis, they will form the topic of the next sub-sections.

3.2 Interpersonal-level influences on the cognitive structures underpinning judgements of health status

3.2.1 Discourse approaches

As discussed in Chapter 5 (Section 4.2) discourse approaches emphasise the functions language serves during interactions, and these can be entirely different from the meaning expressed in the words, as the goals of the speakers change. Discourse between two or more individuals offers a way of understanding interpersonal influences on the cognitive structures underpinning subjective judgements of health status. From this perspective, relevant models of health are not conceptualised as structures within individuals but as structures that emerge *between* them as a result of negotiation (see Potter & Wetherell, 1987).

Although it was carried out by a geographer, not a discourse psychologist, Cornwell's (1984) study of meanings relevant to health and illness expressed by people living in London's East End offers a good example (see also Chapter 5, Section 4.3.1). The study showed that meanings of health and illness were not abstract cognitions, but intimately entangled in everyday life. Two sorts of health beliefs labelled "public" and "private" accounts were discovered.

Public accounts entailed maintaining the appearance of an idealised family life and health status. Other features were respect for doctors and admiration of the puritan work ethic. Interestingly, a critical psychologist would notice that public accounts might not always be to the benefit of respondents, because one strongly held value, for example, was that individuals should accept social inequalities as "natural order" and should work hard and cheerfully to make the most of themselves. With effort, those who were intelligent might improve their lot (Cornwell, 1984). An individual judging his or her health with reference to a public account is likely to give judgements coloured by a veneer of stoicism and normality. This is likely to lead to under-reporting since s/he is likely to say s/he is well in spite of medical difficulties.

Private accounts, on the other hand, seemed more directly to reflect respondents' personal worlds, and the same individual judging his or her health with reference to a private account is likely to give idiosyncratic and perhaps contradictory judgements.

The important point for present purposes is that public accounts seemed to be triggered by respondents' need to put on a good face during interviews. In other words, they are constructed during the interaction between interviewer and interviewee. Moreover, since public accounts are most likely in research settings, a bias similar to under-reporting might arise because of demand characteristics in the research interview.

3.3 Group-level influences on the cognitive structures underpinning judgements of health status: A digression concerning health beliefs

There is an extensive literature on lay meanings of health and illness not only from psychological but also from anthropological and sociological traditions. It is far too wide to tackle here, but fortunately that Herculean labour has already been completed (Stainton Rogers, 1991), so only a few studies will be mentioned, which offer insights into the cognitive structures that might underpin lay judgements of positive health status.

3.3.1 Anthropological perspectives

According to Stainton Rogers (1991) contemporary medical anthropology stresses the rationality of health beliefs given the worldviews of the holders. For example, an early famous study of general practice patients found that most of respondents' beliefs about illnesses could be classified according to the way they made people feel and this informed beliefs about cause and treatment (Helman, 1978). For example, colds that made patients feel cold and shivery were thought to be caught as a result of sitting in draughts or going out into a cold damp place after a hot bath. Ways to avoid catching them included keeping one's feet dry or wearing a hat after a haircut. Treatments involved warming the body with hot drinks and so on.

From this perspective, an individual who judges he or she is well might base evaluations on a complex nexus of beliefs that are rational in the context of his or her social world, but which differ from the common sense beliefs that underpin Figures 6.1 and 6.2.

3.3.2 Sociological perspectives

Not surprisingly, sociologists gather lay beliefs about health and illness for different reasons from anthropologists. Frequently, the motive is to support one of two opposing themes. The first is the idea that social institutions evolve because they allow society to function smoothly. The second is the idea that they survive because they serve the interests and purposes of powerful others (Stainton Rogers, 1991).

3.3.2.1 Functional perspectives

From the first perspective, functional measures of health status concentrate on what people can do as opposed to what they are. To explain, society may be viewed as a network of interlocking social systems, each of which consists of social statuses, roles, and norms. Social statuses are positions that people occupy, either by virtue of behaviours (such as attending school; playing football) or personal characteristics (such as age) and many have titles by which the occupants are known, (such as "pupil"; "footballer"; or "Chelsea Pensioner"). A social role is the behaviours associated with a given social status, and the common expectations that constitute roles are known as social norms, which incidentally are typically pervaded by the cultural values of the most dominant political group (Mercer, 1973).

From this perspective, health is operationalised as the optimum capacity of an individual to perform the roles for which he or she has been socialised, and health status depends on the efficiency with which s/he performs them (Twaddle, 1974). In this way, functional measures side-step problems in defining states of health and identifying its constituent dimensions. However, identifying what roles people *should* perform presents a new set of difficulties. The most usual solution is to operationalise functions in terms of work or family roles (R. Williams, 1983), such as preparing meals; functioning sexually; caring for the self and others. Measures typically assess whether an individual can carry out these functions without help, with help, or not at all.

Important questions arise when roles are not adequately fulfilled because survival of any society depends on their continued performance. Techniques to contain deviance include punishment or ultimately exclusion from a society. Alternately, a devalued status might be created, to which the deviant individual may be assigned. The sick role (Parsons, 1951) is one such status, which "houses" individuals who cannot perform their roles because of ill health. Once an individual occupies it, his or her deviant behaviour is redefined as normal — normal for a sick person that is. Norms of the sick role include the temporary suspension of obligations to others and the right to be cared for. However, the sick person must co-operate with getting better; the problem must not be of his or her own making and it must be serious enough to merit help (Helman, 2000; Kleinmann, 1988). These obligations are epitomised in the "popular patient" who is cheerful, grateful, interesting to nurse, and has a physical diagnosis (Stockwell, 1972). On the other side of the coin, an alarming study discovered that doctors in several London hospital casualty departments punished individuals they thought were to blame for their own predicaments, who were not "really" unwell, or who otherwise violated norms of the sick role (Jeffery, 1984). A naughty, if understandable, example appeared in *New Woman*, in April 1998. A GP described working in a busy casualty department when she was a junior doctor. To deal with rude "obnoxious drunken City types", a competition evolved. The winner was the doctor who could cut up the most expensive suit during the night without the head nurse seeing.

A functional approach can lead to paradoxes, as for example when physical disabilities develop as a result of the efficient performance of work roles. However, the constellation of roles usually performed by an individual provides a promising candidate for the cognitive structures underpinning lay judgements of health status. From this perspective the individual who judges that he or she is well, simply ascertains that s/he is continuing to perform expected duties adequately. Since this might not reflect physical ailments, the perspective is well equipped to explain under-reporting and other divergences from common sense.

ACTIVITY 6.3 How do you expect to feel when you are "head over heels" in love? How do present-day expectations about this role differ from the "loveris maladye" of the late 14th century?

His slep, his mete, his drynke, is hym biraft,
That lene he wex and drye as is a shaft;
His eyen holwe, and grisly to biholde,
His hewe falow and pale as asshen colde,
And solitarie he was and evere allone,
And waillynge al the nyght, makynge his mone;
And if he herede song or instrument,
Thanne wolde he wepe, he myghte nat be stent.
So feble eek were his spiritz, and so lowe,
And chaunged so, that no man koude knowe
His speche nor his voys, though men it herde.

From Chaucer's *"Knight's Tale"*

3.3.2.2 Dominance perspectives

The second theme that motivates sociologists to collect health beliefs concerns dominance, and its perspective closely resembles that of critical social psychology which was described in Chapter 1 (Section 2.4). According to Stainton Rogers (1991) royal families, the church, politicians, and other powerful institutions have constructed and disseminated common sense beliefs about health in order to promote their own interests throughout history. Current examples might include the promotion of a view of the benefits of care in the community as opposed to care in National Health hospitals for those who cannot afford private healthcare. Alternatively, the rights of individuals to choose what they eat, and the consequences of such choices for chronic disease, might be emphasised rather than the need for health education or affordable and nutritious food. Although such emphases purport to be for the benefit of lay people, it can also be argued that the "real" beneficiaries are those who control and contribute most to government funds.

From this perspective, Pill and Stott carried out a famous series of studies of working-class women in Wales, collecting information about health beliefs, health knowledge, lifestyle, and variables such as Health Locus of Control. In one study (Pill & Stott, 1982) 41 mothers on a housing estate were asked what they thought were the main reasons for illness. The 73 responses were grouped into 10 categories, the most common being "germs, bugs, infection", "heredity and susceptibility", "being run down", "environmental factors", "self neglect", "stress and worry", "personality type", "diet", "hygiene", and "way of life" respectively. Most of these categories clearly exonerate the individual, in depicting causes of poor health that are beyond individual control. Even those that seem to be a matter of personal volition, on further probing transpired to depend on access to resources. For example, "being run down" was as a result of having to work extra shifts.

Another famous study of working-class mothers and grandmothers in Aberdeen supports this interpretation. Results showed that personal behaviours, such as a fondness for sugar, were seen as a cause of diabetes, but content analysis suggested little personal blame was involved, since respondents emphasised that such fondness was inevitable, given the circumstances (Blaxter & Patterson, 1982).

Dominance theorists emphasise that exoneration of the individual does not mean that those in poor health blame the state for their predicament (Townsend & Yeo, 1979). On the contrary, health beliefs expressed by underprivileged people are typically characterised by a stoical acceptance of poverty, which does not challenge unequal access to resources. Critical social psychologists would highlight exactly the same point and note that it was illustrated in the public accounts of health discovered by Cornwell (1984) and described above (Section 3.2.1).

The point emerges more vividly from intergroup contrasts. In one study, the meanings of health given by 30 working-class women emphasised "getting through the day" while those of 30 middle-class women placed emphasis on feeling fit and strong, active and energetic (Calnan, 1987). In fact, many studies report age, class, and gender differences in meanings of health, which can be interpreted in this way. A good example is a large-scale study of 15,000 people in two Western European populations which found two dimensions underpinned variation in meanings (d'Houtaud, Field, Tax, & Gueguen, 1990). The first dimension corresponded to social class. The most privileged individuals defined health in egocentric terms, such as "getting the most out of life" and self-actualisation; the middle classes defined it in terms of psychological well-being, hygiene, and importance, and manual workers defined it as an absence of disease, and in terms of functions needed to work. The second dimension concerned age. Younger respondents gave definitions that, like those of the higher social classes, concerned hedonic use of life, whereas elderly people gave meanings that paralleled those of manual workers. A final example is that British women construed vitality in terms of tackling jobs such as cleaning the oven (Blaxter, 1992).

Such data emphasise that meanings of health are not simply the results of individual cognitions. Rather they are also constructed by the social reality of hard lives (or easy ones). This provides a group-level rival to the common sense idea that judgements of health status are based on something like a medical model or a more positive view of health as physical, mental, and social well-being. This candidate is promising because an individual who judges that he or she is well might base judgements on beliefs that further the interests of powerful others and this can explain under-reporting. In fact, a further prediction is that under-reporting should more often occur in deprived people who should be more likely to soldier on cheerfully, in spite of physical ailments.

3.3.3 Psychological perspectives

To turn from anthropology and sociology, Stainton Rogers (1991) argues that the majority of psychological theorising on health beliefs is at an intrapersonal level of analysis, in which beliefs and explanations are constructed in the private inner world of the individual, and linked to other psychological variables and behaviour. The extent of the literature on social cognition models of health behaviour (see Chapter 4, Section 3.1) supports her view. Notwithstanding, Stainton Rogers (1991) continues that three approaches in social psychology *have* focused on beliefs that exist at social levels. These are social representations, everyday explanations, and discourse. Discourse approaches were briefly described earlier in Section 3.2. The next two subsections will discuss social representations and everyday explanations, respectively.

3.3.3.1 Social representations

In the theory of social representations, health beliefs belong to social groups collectively. Thus, although individuals might be studied, their individuality is not of significance. Rather their beliefs are pooled to build a shared belief or "social representation" that is current in their community. In 1981 Moscovici described social representations as:

a set of concepts, statements, explanations originating in daily life in the course of inter-individual communications. They are the equivalent, in our society, of the myths and belief systems in traditional societies. They might even be the contemporary version of common sense.

His idea is that social representations explain phenomena by anchoring them into a recognisable, existing ideology. This process gives social representations historical continuities, which lead to systematic differences between cultures. In addition, a second process called objectification expresses the idea that the anchoring of an abstract idea in a known image tends to lead to the image taking the place of the original idea (Augoustinos & Walker 1995; Farr and Moscovici, 1984).

The unexpected birth of a child with hydrocephalus provides an illustration. Some mediaeval European communities would have anchored their explanation in fairy lore, labelling the child "a changeling". The belief was then that the real baby had been stolen by fairies but would be returned some day, provided that the changeling was loved and nurtured. Other communities, however, anchored explanations in Christian dogma. The belief was then that the baby was an abomination sent by God as a punishment to the mother for her sexual excesses with the devil! In this case, the unfortunate family would most likely murder the infant before the church authorities arrived to burn the mother at the stake (Haffter, 1968).

A seminal study of health beliefs that was carried out from a social representation perspective is that of Hertzlich and Graham (1973) who conducted lengthy interviews with Parisians about health and illness. A number of health beliefs, which belonged to the sample as a whole, emerged. The first, "health in a vacuum", was analogous to the medical model since it conceptualised health as an absence of disease. In the second, "health as a reserve", health was construed like a bank account of physical robustness and resistance, which could be built up or expended through action. A third, "equilibrium", referred to health as a balance of physical, mental, and social well-being. Hertzlich and Graham (1973) concluded that Parisians' social representations of health and illness were not bipolar opposites but were better characterised as accounts, and during interviews they observed that participants drew on all of them.

The theory of social representations offers a way of understanding how members of a given community can come to share and use a common set of beliefs about health, which might have little to do with objective physical indicators and more to do with history and culture. An interesting example in the making, which has already been met in Chapter 1 (Section 1) and will be met again throughout Chapter 7, is the explanation of a liking for chocolate in women. This seems currently in the process of becoming anchored in existing views about premenstrual tension and women's behaviour, or more specifically in the view that "women's bodies send them mad" (Ussher, 1991). No one individual needs to have started the process. Rather, it might be imagined that it evolved from ideas about menstrual distress juxtaposed with ideas about chocolate as a comfort food. Alternatively, perhaps it evolved from ideas about premenstrual women losing control that merged with ideas about the needs of women to control urges to over-indulge in chocolate. Yet other possibilities are that bloating due to premenstrual fluid retention was misattributed to eating chocolate, or increased consumption of chocolate was misattributed to hormones. It might be speculated that many such juxtapositions and experiences are leading to a new social representation of premenstrual women who crave chocolate while out of control for a few days each month. However it began, the idea is gaining currency. For example, an increased need for potassium, triggered by hormonal changes, has been quoted as pseudo-scientific justification for it, even though there is no evidence that this is so (Jas, 1994).

A social representations perspective provides another group-level rival to the common sense idea that judgements of health status are based on something like a medical model or a more positive view of health as physical, mental, and social well-being. It predicts that individual group members will download the community's beliefs about health in order to judge their own wellness. Again, this is a fundamental departure from the common sense models depicted in Figures 6.1 and 6.2 because the relevant cognitive structures are not the results of individual cognitions and experience, but have evolved in the community.

The theory of social representations has been criticised for its vagueness, lack of testability, and circularity (Potter, 1996). To illustrate the problem of circularity, a group of Parisians might be targeted, and their beliefs about health examined in order to give a picture of their health social representations. However, it is assumed that the social representations derived both coincide with and define the boundary between Parisians and other groups. To answer this and other criticisms, Stainton Rogers (1991) suggested a different view of health beliefs based on the shared accounts used in everyday explanations.

3.3.3.2 Everyday explanations

Stainton Rogers (1991) used Q methodology in order to examine everyday explanations of health and illness. Q methodology is designed to enable individuals to express their own salient dimensions of meaning within a domain, or "Q-set", which is selected by the researcher in order to reflect the topic area of interest. Thus, Stainton Rogers (1991) gathered 327 beliefs about health and illness during formal interviews and informal conversations with an opportunity sample of 13 people over a period of 4 months. To these, she added a further 179 statements from an "immersion" in current media. By means of a series of pilot studies, these were reduced to a final set of 80 items, which represented the meanings of health and illness then current in British society. These 80 items constituted the Q-set.

A total of 70 men and women were asked to sort the Q-set into 11 categories. Category 1 was to contain items with which they agreed most strongly, and Category 11 the items with which they most disagreed. They were told how many items they were allowed to put into each category in order to produce a normal-shaped distribution of agreement, which allowed for statistical analysis. Subsequently, factor analysis revealed which items tended to group together and which participants especially agreed with each group. Stainton Rogers (1991) called these groups of items "accounts", and she devised a label for each and learned more about its meaning from scrutinising the items that contributed most strongly to it. Further information was gleaned from the comments and characteristics of people who most strongly agreed with it.

Seven accounts were identified. Stainton Rogers (1991) labelled the first "The cultural critique". This explained health in terms of status and wealth, which not only permits access to good nutrition, housing, and healthy habits but which also permits powerful people to construct and control the health of others. In contrast, the second account, "Willpower", located health within individuals. It explained it in terms of bodily resources that could be aided by willpower and positive thinking. Additional comments by individuals whose sorts showed they agreed strongly with this account, showed a further contrast with the first account, whose proponents tended to blame individuals for their ill health.

The third account, "Health promotion", emphasised the need for people to take on healthy lifestyles and not to rely on luck. It also stressed the benefits of health education and was critical of any reduction of medical resources in pursuit of monetarism. "The body as a machine" was the fourth account. Analogous to the biomedical model, this endorsed drug and surgical interventions as preferred therapies, although the importance of building constitution through good diet was also expressed. The fifth account, "Inequality of access", was similar to the first in stressing the injustices of health differences between rich and poor. However, it represented medicine as an effective, moral imperative in tackling disease, to which the poor have unequal access, whereas the first account had represented medicine as an instrument of power, often wielded to the disadvantage of the poor.

In the sixth account, "A body under siege", illness was explained in terms of viruses and other invaders including the upsetting actions of other people, the individual being construed as trying to cope in a hostile world. Finally, and as the name suggests, "Robust individualism" construed health in terms of individual freedom and responsibility, even if these entailed taking risks. It also represented health as an investment that could be saved, insured, or squandered.

An important finding was that individuals drew variously on accounts, using some and not others. This meant that data did not support the idea of group social representations of health that were shared by all group members. Rather, the accounts with which people agreed reflected their own social worlds. For example, a dietician was the only one who exemplified the fourth account and a teacher of health promotion was the only one who exemplified the third.

Stainton Rogers (1991) conceptualised accounts as dynamic structures that link items from an "encyclopaedia" of beliefs available in a community. The accounts that a particular individual draws on reflect his or her worldview on a topic. From this point of view the health beliefs an individual uses when assessing his or her subjective health status are a personal selection of patterns or accounts that are current in his or her community. This view provides yet another group-level rival to the common sense idea that judgements of health status are based on something like a medical model or a more positive view of health as physical, mental, and social well-being.

3.4 Summary and conclusions

This section discussed social psychological influences on the cognitive structures that might underpin lay judgements of wellness. Professional approaches to measuring health status together with anthropological and sociological studies were pirated in order to suggest rivals to the common sense view that they are based on something like a medical model or a more positive view of health as physical, mental, and social well-being.

At the intrapersonal level, the diversity of meanings and approaches to measuring health was immediately striking, although on closer examination many converged onto the medical model since they attempted to measure positive health in terms of an absence of morbidity, disability, distress, and discomfort! Such negative beliefs seemed to emulate rather than offer a rival to common sense. More positive approaches based on quality of life and subjective health measures suggested that health is better conceptualised as the opposite of illness, not of disease, because it is embedded in the individual's social world. This perspective suggested that individuals are likely to draw on a constellation of user-defined, personally relevant meanings when evaluating their health status. It explains under-reporting by acknowledging that the individual does not necessarily select the same evaluative dimensions as professionals. In this way it provides a rival explanation to common sense.

Interpersonal and group-level considerations moved away from the idea that individuals' health beliefs are intrapersonal structures. Meanings of health might be employed during conversations to achieve myriad goals. Alternatively, they might be constructed for individuals by wider institutions. Related self-evaluations might therefore reflect the interests of powerful others and under-reporting could well be to the advantage of those who pay for healthcare. Another idea was that people download social representations of health, and yet another was that they select and shape accounts that reflect their social worlds. Since relevant health beliefs do not necessarily focus on physical well-being but might have more to do with community history or impression management, these perspectives are also well equipped to explain under-reporting.

Such considerations portray the individual as active and greatly complicate the task of considering the meanings underpinning health status judgements, which are no longer right or wrong, but mercurial and purposive. They emphasise a need to understand how relevant beliefs are selected and why an individual might select beliefs that reflect one social world (such as dietician) but not another (such as British). In addition it is also necessary to understand how judgements are made on the basis of selected beliefs. Such evaluative processes are the topic of the next section.

4. Social Psychological Influences on the Processes Underpinning Judgements of Subjective Health Status

According to Skevington (1994), evaluative processes have attracted comparatively little attention in the health field. This position has changed with the publication of a substantial volume devoted to the subject (Buunk and Gibbons, 1997). Notwithstanding, a few predictions about the ways in which subjective health status is evaluated follow logically from assumptions about underlying cognitive structures. For example, where a medical model is the underlying structure (as depicted in the common sense model in Figure 6.1), the process is a search for symptoms. Identification of one terminates the search, but if none is found, then the categorical decision "healthy" is returned. Where a more positive approach to health as complete physical, mental, and social well-being is assumed (as depicted in the common sense model in Figure 6.2), the process is pattern matching against these three stored ideals. If successful, the decision "healthy" is returned.

The two common sense models were soundly challenged and in Section 3.1 the idea was developed that individuals use a constellation of personally relevant dimensions when evaluating subjective health status. If so, the process is a comparison between current state(s) and some benchmark on each relevant dimension. In fact, Sheridan and Radmacher (1992) propose a continuum with optimal wellness at one end, a neutral point in the middle, and premature death at the other end. This simple suggestion is powerfully useful because it allows for degrees of wellness or health as well as degrees of dysfunction. Since these are evaluated in relation to the neutral centre, further advantages are that the end states for dimensions do not need to be defined and the central benchmark can be a statistical norm or a personal average. In her epidemiological study of a representative sample of 9000 British people Blaxter (1992) adopted a similar approach. One of her aims was to evaluate the relative impact of living conditions and habits such as exercise and smoking on health status. Since most of the population was "well", she needed standardised health ratios as opposed to morbidity measures. Two of the four dimensions of health she developed were continua (unfitness vs fitness and psychosocial malaise vs well-being). Moreover, these could vary independently, so that an individual could be assessed as unfit yet psychosocially well.

From this perspective, an individual who judges that he or she is well has rationally evaluated his or her position on a range of continua and combined the results. "Under-reporting" can easily be explained by assuming physical dimensions play a small role in the constellation selected. Another possibility, however, is that the evaluative process is not rational. This idea is explored in the rest of Section 4.

4.1 Intrapersonal influences on the process of evaluating subjective health status

4.1.1 Denial

Breetvelt and van Dam (1991) suggest four explanations for under-reporting. The first is underpinned by the psychoanalytic theory, that faced with a threatening illness patients mobilise defence mechanisms, especially denial. The result is that symptoms, diagnosis, or consequences of a threatening experience, such as receiving the bad news that one has cancer, "hardly" become conscious.

From this point of view, under-reporting is explained because an individual who reports that he or she is well in the presence of physical disabilities has vanquished them from consciousness, so that they simply do not affect evaluations. In support of denial theory, Breetvelt and van Dam (1991) cite two studies of cancer patients which demonstrate (i) high levels of denial and repression of conflict and emotions compared with controls and (ii) a negative correlation between denial and anxiety and depression.

4.1.2 Crisis theory and coping

The second explanation suggested by Breetvelt and van Dam (1991) revolves around crisis theory and coping. The argument is that a crisis disturbs the balance between the perception of a problem and problem-solving ability. To reach a new balance, the patient mobilises extra problem-solving abilities. The effect of these is to reduce the perceived magnitude of the problem. Thus, under-reporting is explained because after a while the problem no longer appears so bad.

Crisis theory offers a better explanation than denial because it predicts an initial period of adjustment, (i.e., crisis) and therefore, unlike denial, it explains why under-reporting is not always found in acute or crisis situations during which victims of disasters might feel overwhelmed (see Wood et al., 1985). However, Breetvelt and van Dam (1991) criticise both explanations because they fail to explain why under-reporting is manifest selectively on psychological dimensions. Notwithstanding, crisis theory does seem to offer a convincing explanation of how levels of reported psychological *stress* might reduce after a period of emotion-focused coping.

4.1.3 Adaptation theory

Based on Helson's Adaptation Theory (1964), Breetvelt and van Dam (1991) offer a third explanation for under-reporting. The idea is that individuals store their experiences of health-related stimuli to make an internal rating scale. The adaptation level, against which they judge themselves, corresponds to its mid-point. Thus, the adaptation level of a person who has a run of negative experiences will shift in a negative direction. From this point of view, under-reporting in people such as cancer patients (who are assumed to have had many negative experiences) occurs because in comparison with their negatively recalibrated internal benchmark, the evaluation of any given state will be improved.

Although this theory is consistent with the idea that people make social comparisons with their own past states (Affleck & Tennen, 1991), it contradicts the usual finding that a deterioration results in negative evaluations, as the person perceives they are worse than before (Skevington, 1994). The theory also fails to explain why under-reporting is selectively manifest on psychological dimensions. If anything, it predicts that the daunting levels of physical problems described in cancer patients will lead to more under-reporting on these. Furthermore, it predicts that people who are extremely well would "over-report".

3.3.3 Conclusions

There are a number of weaknesses in the three intrapersonal influences outlined by Breetvelt and van Dam (1991), which makes them unconvincing rivals to the idea that evaluations are rational.

4.2 Interpersonal influences: Social comparisons and the recalibration of internal benchmarks

Based on Social Comparison Theory (Festinger, 1954), Breetvelt and van Dam (1991) suggest a fourth and final explanation for under-reporting. This time, the idea is that the individual's internal benchmark is recalibrated with respect to others. This proposal will be fleshed out and criticised in this sub-section, then modified and developed in the next.

In his seminal theory, Festinger (1954) argued that people have a drive to validate their opinions and abilities. The preferred method of evaluation is with respect to "physical reality" but if no objective means of validation is available, people turn to "social reality" and make social comparisons with others in order to evaluate themselves (Gruder, 1977; Kulik & Mahler, 1997). Later scholars added the functional explanation that the drive exists because accurate self-evaluations have survival value (Gruder, 1977; Suls, 1977). During the 1950s and 1960s researchers discovered that individuals also use social comparisons to assess internal states (Suls, 1977) and it is this that makes the theory relevant to symptom perceptions (see Chapter 3) and assessments of health status. This is well illustrated in a study of 418 patients who had received a diagnosis of cancer. The study showed that individuals wished to affiliate with other patients, in order to derive information from social comparisons, to the extent that information from experts (which represented something more "objective") was not available (Molleman, Pruyn, & van Knippenberg, 1986).

An important corollary of Festinger's theory was that the individual needs to make comparisons with relatively similar others in order for the information to be useful (Suls, 1977). Consistent with this idea, a range of studies have shown that self-evaluations are neither precise nor stable when individuals available for comparison purposes are widely diverse from the perceiver (see Gruder, 1977). More specifically, Molleman et al. (1986) also found that the value of information derived from comparisons with other cancer patients diminished as the similarity between the target and the evaluator grew less. The implication is that individuals will be motivated to affiliate with similar others, to the extent that they need to make social comparisons, and Turner (1991) has explained how this approach can form a general model of group formation and conformity. Supporting evidence is that blind people prefer to compare themselves with other blind people, as opposed to less similar others (Gruder, 1977).

The important implication for present purposes is that people who are ailing will affiliate with other sufferers and recalibrate their internal benchmark accordingly. Hence they are likely to judge themselves well in spite of the ailment. There are at least two difficulties with this argument. First, similar others might not be available, and Wood et al. (1985) hypothesise that individuals in this predicament might compare themselves with "supercopers" portrayed in the media, in comparison with whom they do badly. Second, the point is too general to explain why under-reporting is selectively manifest on psychological dimensions, or, strictly speaking, why it occurs at all. This is because an obvious point is that variation between the persons used for comparative purposes will affect the results of an individual's self-evaluations (Blalock, Devellis, & Devellis, 1989). Comparisons can be with people who are worse off. These are called "downwards comparisons", and they lead to relatively positive self-evaluations. Alternatively, comparisons can be with people who are better off. "Upwards comparisons" lead to relatively negative self-evaluations. On average, a patient who makes social comparisons with other patients might be expected to find some who are better and some who are worse off. Thus, a relatively narrow distribution of positive *and negative* self-evaluations reliably related to the patients available for comparative purposes would be expected. In other words, affiliation with other patients as opposed to well people might improve mean evaluations, but it does not explain under-reporting.

The missing notion is a "unidirectional drive upwards" (Festinger, 1954). Although its effects were not specified, and it was originally envisaged as characterising the evaluation of abilities, ego-enhancement has been accepted as a second general goal of social comparisons (Suls, 1977). In other words, in addition to a desire for accurate self-evaluation, the individual will desire "self-enhancement". S/he will want to possess the appropriate direction and degree of the attribute in question (Gruder, 1977).

The desire for self-enhancement predominates in situations of stress and those in which the individual's self-esteem is threatened (Gruder, 1977; Kulik & Mahler, 1997). Under such circumstances, s/he is not only willing to forego information in the interests of self-protection, but might also distort or construct it (Affleck & Tennen, 1991). Thus, a decrease in subjective well-being motivates a need to affiliate with fellow victims in order to make downwards comparisons. As a result, individuals can evaluate themselves more favourably, and restore subjective well-being (Wills, 1981). A number of early experimental studies in which participants were threatened by the prospect of receiving electric shocks supported this reasoning, since participants preferred to wait with others who were likely to suffer the same fate (see Kulik & Mahler, 1997, for a review).

Clearly, downwards comparisons have special relevance to individuals whose well-being is threatened by diagnosis of disease, and studies which show that patients usually prefer to make downwards comparisons support this general position. For example, women with lumpectomies compared themselves to women with mastectomies, and in another study of breast cancer patients there was an overwhelming preference for comparisons with other patients who were worse off in some respect (Taylor, 1983; Wood et al., 1985). Similarly, downwards comparisons far outweighed upwards ones in the unprompted descriptions of illness given by people suffering from arthritis (Affleck & Tennen, 1991). Further anecdotal support for the position was more recently found in focus groups of arthritis patients who compared themselves with the normal population and experienced envy and other negative emotions (Skevington, 1994). More recently, Wood and Vanderzee (1997) note a correlation between downwards comparisons and adjustment in cancer patients, which suggests that such comparisons are adaptive.

According to Breetvelt and van Dam (1991), introducing self-enhancement as well as self-evaluation as a motive for social comparisons completes the explanation for under-reporting and therefore offers a rival to the idea that evaluations are rational. While self-evaluation leads individuals to compare themselves with other patients, self-enhancement leads them to compare themselves with those who are worse off. As a result, they evaluate themselves as "well".

As it stands, the explanation is tantalisingly unsatisfactory. First, the nature of under-reporting has become unclear. Breetvelt and van Dam (1991) originally characterised it as the under-reporting of psychological stress. Metamorphosed, it now seems to represent psychological well-being which has been perked up as a result of downwards comparisons on another dimension(s), which has been recalibrated. Second, individuals should seek others who are similar on the attribute to be evaluated. This leads to a focus on diagnostic groups or victims of some common misfortune, which suggests that the evaluative dimensions that are recalibrated should be to do with diseases, physical impairments, or associated disabilities. However, the fact that under-reporting is manifest selectively on psychological dimensions (Breetvelt & van Dam, 1991), means that evidence of such recalibration has never been found. Indeed, one might ask why patients should affiliate with others with the same diagnosis as opposed to the same difficulties. Better still, why do patients not affiliate with depressed others with whom downwards comparisons would afford a direct opportunity to enhance psychological well-being? The focus on diagnostic groups not only reflects the direct power of the medical model, in the sense that services are organised on the basis of diagnostic labels that impose social grouping on patients, but it also reflects the stereotypic idea that those with the same label should have the same psychological experience and identity.

Another weakness is highlighted by Blalock et al. (1989) who point out that foregoing accurate self-assessments in the interests of protecting self-esteem might be dangerous and of questionable adaptive value. Their study of 75 women with rheumatoid arthritis allowed them to test whether downwards comparisons with other patients would lead to enhanced evaluation of ability and hence satisfaction and adjustment to illness, or whether just satisfaction and adjustment could be enhanced, leaving the evaluation of abilities *per se* unchanged.

The study is complex because it deals with two separate contexts, the establishment of desired performance standards and the experience of performance difficulties; and four classes of dependent variables: social comparison preferences; perceived ability; satisfaction with perceived ability; and psychological adjustment. Each class entailed various subscales and a range of scoring and treatment techniques, and was assessed across a range of relevant tasks.

Context had an important effect: when establishing standards for desired performance, comparisons with individuals not affected with arthritis predominated, but when experiencing performance difficulties, comparisons with other arthritis patients were preferred.

Overall, regression analyses showed that greater satisfaction with perceived ability was associated with better psychological adjustment. In turn, perceived ability was associated with greater satisfaction with perceived ability. However, no association between social comparison preferences and perceived ability or between social comparison preferences and psychological adjustment was found. Subsequently, hierarchical regression was carried out further to explore the importance of context in predicting satisfaction with perceived ability. In the context of performance difficulties, higher satisfaction was associated with social comparisons with other arthritis patients, even controlling for perceived ability. Consistent with this pattern of results, Affleck and Tennen (1991) found that arthritis patients who made positive social comparisons were better adjusted to their illness, irrespective of actual disease activity.

These results support the hypothesis that people use social comparisons adaptively to enhance psychological well-being, without "maladaptively" inflating perceptions of physical abilities. In other words, there is no evidence of a recalibrated internal benchmark leading to improved self-evaluations. In fact, the study moves away from the idea of internal benchmarks altogether, since the individual derives benchmarks from his or her social context, according to the task in hand. Thus, downwards comparisons might be the best choice when the task is self-enhancement, but for a task such as self-improvement, adaptation, or any circumstances that require cognitive clarity, upwards comparisons might be more useful. Empirical support for this position was found in a study of 73 patients awaiting coronary bypass surgery and 82 awaiting less threatening transurethral prostatectomy (see Kulik & Mahler, 1997). Under higher levels of threat, patients preferred room-mates who had already undergone surgery and could give them information about coping and what to expect, as opposed to individuals awaiting the same operation with whom emotions could be compared. More generally, the idea is supported by studies that show individuals might wish to evaluate themselves with respect to others who are worse off, although they prefer to avoid social contact with them (see Salovey et al., 1998, for a general discussion, and Tennen & Affleck, 1997, for a discussion in the context of chronic pain).

Another related challenge to the idea that self-enhancement motivates downwards comparisons among patients is that it can also motivate upwards comparisons (Skevington, 1994; Ybema & Buunk 1995). In this case, the need for self-enhancement in the first place, and interpretation of social comparisons to achieve it in the second, depend on perceived threat, current self-esteem, or a host of other factors (Gruder, 1977).

In a study of 112 people receiving disability payments in The Netherlands, Ybema and Buunk (1995) hypothesised that perceived control was the crucial variable that would determine the emotional impact of the direction of social comparisons. Participants heard about an interview with a (fictitious) disabled person, which contained either positive or negative information about the severity of their condition and the efficacy of their coping skills. Next, patients were given the opportunity to make social comparisons. Results showed that more positive emotions were experienced as a result of making upwards as opposed to downwards social comparisons, and confirmed that participants with high perceived control over their disease largely accounted for the relationship. The interpretation was that people with an internal locus saw the position of upwards targets as attainable and inspiring. Those with an external locus of control had been expected to experience negative emotions, perhaps seeing the predicament of a downwards target as their own future, but results only partly confirmed predictions for this group.

More recently Wood and Vanderzee (1997) have used a stress and appraisal approach to emphasise that individuals make both primary and secondary appraisals with relation to their own well-being and personal agendas, such that the choice of comparison and its result cannot be predicted from objective factors. They also observe that adjustment might not be a result of a comparison, since an individual who makes a downwards comparison and says s/he is better adjusted might simply be right on both counts! Notwithstanding, an interaction between intrapersonal factors and interpersonal social comparisons occurs. This again suggests that downwards social comparisons do not automatically occur to enhance self-esteem when available. This means they are not the complete explanation for under-reporting.

In summary, there are a number of weaknesses in the theory that (i) illness constitutes a threat and consequently (ii) triggers a self-enhancement motive that (iii) leads people with various ailments to compare themselves with others who are worse off, (iv) with the result that they evaluate themselves as well. The major weaknesses arise because there are individual differences in the experience of threat and the need for self-enhancement. Self-enhancement might lead to upwards as opposed to downwards comparisons, and in any case, patients might affiliate for other reasons. Furthermore, the presence of other patients does not necessarily mean individuals will affiliate, and perhaps the subjects of research do not necessarily adopt patient groupings "provided" by researchers. These weaknesses suggest that, although promising, the theory is not an entirely successful rival to the common sense idea that evaluations are rational.

A more social social psychological theory might better explain the link between illness, threat to self-esteem, and the ways in which social comparisons are strategically mobilised to deal with it. In the next section the level of analysis shifts to group levels, in search of such a theory.

4.3 Group-level influences on evaluating subjective health status

In the studies described in the previous section, a common assumption is that a social categorisation such as "cancer patients" or "asthmatics" is psychologically meaningful to participants. In this section a social social psychological model of evaluating subjective health status will developed, which considers what happens to an individual when he or she self-defines as a patient.

Plenty of research suggests that becoming an in-patient is a negative experience. For example, the individual is removed from friends and community at a time of personal crisis. Indeed, he or she is likely to experience such high levels of ambiguity, lack of comprehension, and uncertainty that it is difficult to disentangle emotions attributable to the symptoms from those attributable to the experience of going into hospital (Helman, 2000). In social psychological terms, hospitalisation is an example of ritual depersonalisation. The individual with his or her rich repertoire of social and personal identities completes the ecological transition to "patient" in a subordinate and dependent position, one among a ward of strangers, to whom s/he is assigned on the basis of age, organ, or illness (Helman, 2000).

A corpus of evidence assembled over almost half a century suggests that it is not merely the experience of becoming a patient that is negative. In addition, patient groups are negatively valued and sometimes stigmatised (e.g., Affleck & Tennen, 1991; Greenbaum & Wang, 1965). To extend this idea on the basis of self-categorisation theory (e.g., Turner, 1987), the suggestion is that the cognitive act of self-definition as a patient (or someone with an ailment), means joining a negatively valued social group and this constitutes a challenge to the individual's self-esteem. Anecdotal support for this idea is the use of words such as "humiliation", "defeat", and "shame" to describe the experience of illness (Baron, 1985).

Thus, in addition to threats and uncertainty associated with the illness itself, the individual who self-defines as a patient is likely to have a challenge to his or her self-esteem to overcome. The suggestion underlying the studies reviewed in the previous section was that a decrease in subjective well-being occasioned by the threat of a disease, leads to affiliation with fellow-sufferers (in order to afford an opportunity for downwards comparisons) and consequently, group formation. From the current perspective, things happen in a different order. It is the group formation, in the form of the psychological act of self-definition as a patient, that constitutes the blow to self-esteem.

Dependent on their beliefs about the nature of the intergroup relations, members of low-status groups may follow a number of strategies to protect self-esteem (e.g., Tajfel, 1978b; Turner & Brown, 1978). These strategies, it is suggested, offer an alternative explanation for under-reporting. The explanation also systematically incorporates the selection of evaluative dimensions. The first, common sense strategy is simply to leave, psychologically if not physically, the negatively valued group. "Individual mobility" can only occur if the individual perceives social boundaries as permeable. Individual mobility predicts that someone who has a disease or ailment will tend to avoid categorising him or herself in terms of it, but will use other well identities in order to protect self-esteem. Anecdotal evidence consistent with this is the frequently heard protest, "There is more to my identity than my illness". Similarly, categories such as "the elderly" might be handy for researchers but psychologically meaningless for the people to whom it is applied (R. Williams, 1983).

A study of 439 osteo-arthritis patients is intriguing from this view (Weinberger, Tierney, Booker, & Katz 1989, cited in Skevington, 1995). Participants were randomly assigned to three conditions. In one, extra information was given to them at outpatient clinics; in the second, participants were telephoned at home and given the information; and in the control condition no additional information was given. Results showed that the patients at home improved on physical health and pain measures, whereas those who had received information at the clinic actually showed poorer health status than controls. Although the study was not designed with these issues in mind, it is consistent with the possibility that attending outpatient clinic made salient an "osteo-arthritis patient" identity, conformity to which presented a challenge to well-being, which outweighed the benefits of extra information.

Under-reporting might represent the operation of individual mobility as the respondent self-assigns characteristics associated with a positively valued social identification as opposed to the low esteem and psychological distress associated with a disease label.

Where individual mobility is not possible, a series of group-oriented strategies are possible in order to preserve self-esteem. These come under the collective name of social creativity.

The first concerns the choice of reference group and predicts that individuals with a salient patient identity will compare themselves with groups who are worse off. For example, Skevington (1994) found that patients with rheumatoid arthritis made social comparisons with groups of patients with more serious diseases such as cancer. Second, individuals may also make intragroup comparisons and there is plenty of anecdotal evidence consistent with this strategy. Tissue (1972), for example, found self-rated health was more closely correlated to intragroup comparisons than to functional capacity or number of ailments. More recently, Skevington (1994) found that patients with rheumatoid arthritis made social comparisons with others with the same disease, but who were deteriorating more quickly, or who were younger yet more disabled, and so on, and Buunk, Gibbons, and Reis-bergan (1997) list nine more studies that show people generally prefer their group to include others with (more) serious problems. It is possible that an individual might use both the strategies at different times. For example, attitudes towards menopause become more positive with age, menopausal and postmeno- pausal women reporting positive characteristics such as increased confidence, calmness, freedom, and "feeling better" (Neugarten, Wood, Kraines, & Loomis, 1968; cited in Golub, 1992). This change might be underpinned by a change in identity: motivated by social competition, women who menstruate are likely to view menopausal women negatively, but once they enter menopause themselves, maintenance of self-esteem requires that the state is reinterpreted more positively. Finally, it is possible that both strategies may be used at the same time. For example, Affleck and Tennen (1991) found that arthritis patients categorised their own patient group into subgroups and then made downwards comparisons with their own stereotype of "the average person with rheumatic arthritis".

Both strategies are entirely consistent with Wills's point (1981) that downwards comparisons are relevant in negative situations that are "difficult to remedy through instrumental action". However, it is important to emphasise that in the current descriptions these are at inter- and intra-group levels as opposed to the interpersonal level (which seems to have been) assumed in previous studies.

A third strategy is to change the values of negative ingroup characteristics. This would entail valuing dimensions associated with the disease. Anecdotal support is provided by the personal narratives of breast cancer patients who construe their disease as an opportunity to take stock of their lives, and pursue "what really matters" or to find "peace and meaning" (Fallowfield, 1991; Wood et al., 1985). Similarly, Viner (1985, quoted in Murphy, 1996) describes how suffering a life- threatening illness, helplessly bedridden and hospitalised for 120 days, helped to make him a better doctor.

This strategy construes under-reporting in a similar way to crisis theory, but is better able to explain its selective nature, since it focuses on positive reinterpretation. This is most clearly illustrated in the example of a mother of a medically fragile baby, who reinterpreted her judgement that she was more upset than other mothers in terms of her superior understanding of the situation (Affleck & Tennen, 1991). Such emotion-focused coping strategies might be expected to bear fruit along psychological as opposed to physical dimensions, because these are likely to offer more opportunity for reinterpretation. This also accommodates the observation that people are more likely to report themselves as superior on dimensions that are vague (see Diener & Fujita, 1997, for a review).

In the fourth strategy, the idea is that the individual will "invest" in those evaluative dimensions along which he or she will do pretty well. This predicts that people will base their subjective health status on dimensions other than the signs and symptoms used by researchers. Consistent with the findings of Cornwell (1984) that were discussed in Section 3.2.1, the prediction is that meanings of health will be selected to represent "a best face" as opposed to a "true" medical history. There is plenty of evidence consistent with this idea. In their study of mothers of medically fragile infants, Affleck and Tennen (1991) noted that women made comparisons on dimensions selected to make their babies' condition less serious. For example, those whose babies were small made social comparisons with babies who were dependent on technological interventions such as ventilators, and mothers whose babies were larger, but otherwise seriously ill, made comparisons along dimensions of size. In another study, even women who were dying from breast cancer described ways in which they were better off than others, for example in being surrounded by loved ones (Wood et al., 1985). In other words, this strategy explains why the constellation of health beliefs selected to underpin judgements is likely to lead to under-reporting.

Preliminary evidence for this idea was found in a study of 48 patients with asthma, 48 matched well patients, and 34 general practitioners, each of whom gave up to six definitions of "health" (St. Claire, Watkins, & Billinghurst, 1996). The relevant hypothesis was that asthmatic patients would construe health in a manner biased to preserve their self-esteem. Compared with GPs, they were expected to define health more frequently in terms of abilities and actions and less frequently as an absence of disease (the medical model). The rationale was that they would choose dimensions of health along which they performed well, as opposed to freedom from signs and symptoms in terms of which they would be passive losers when evaluating their health. A subsidiary hypothesis was that well lay people would express meanings that fell between those of GPs and people with asthma.

Definitions were classified into nine categories of meaning, and in descending order of salience the meanings for general practitioners were "The Biomedical Model"; "mental well-being"; "general well-being", and "The World Health Organisation definition of health". The most important meanings for asthmatic patients were "being able"; "taking action"; "physical well-being", and "value of health", and for well patients, "taking action", "being able", "physical well-being", and "general well-being" (chi-squared between GPs and asthmatics was 98, $d.f. = 7, p < .0001$; chi-squared between GPs and well patients was 85, $d.f. = 7, p < .0001$). Results supported hypotheses, and it is also worth noting an interesting feature that the most salient dimensions to asthmatics were not ones that might be said to be vague, such as mental well-being for example. On the contrary, they included specific concrete actions.

Although the idea that people with asthma tend to define health in a way that protects their self-esteem was supported, the study suffers from a number of weaknesses. In particular, it was hoped that psychological salience of an "asthmatic patient" identity would be achieved by emphasising that the respondent had been recruited through their general practice because of their asthma. However, no manipulation check was carried out and it is possible that respondents had distanced themselves psychologically from this group. This reasoning might explain the lack of convincing support for the subsidiary hypothesis and the unexpected closeness of beliefs generated by the two lay groups. These shortcomings should be addressed in further research. However, the important point for present purposes is that individuals are selecting target dimensions as opposed to target people for comparative purposes, and therefore the emphasis on other individuals and "social" comparisons *per se* in the literature might be misplaced (Wood et al., 1985).

If generalisable, the implication is that people asked to evaluate their subjective health status will construct an underlying model of health on the basis of which to carry out the task, and the constellation of dimensions that constitutes the model will be selected in order that s/he does well. For people whose membership of patient groups is salient, this is likely to involve the selection of mental, social dimensions or dimensions other than those affected by their problems, leading to under-reporting.

An advantage of this explanation is that it can offer a more strategic understanding of which dimensions are likely to be conspicuously absent for a given patient group and why they might reappear for people with the same diagnosis but a different salient identification. A further advantage is that the explanation is also relevant to the "well" population, members of which might use medical, WHO, functional, and other models as needed, in order to put on a good face. Construction of health in terms of the vitality needed to clean an oven (see Blaxter, 1992) might not reflect the reality of working lives *per se*. Rather, the choice reflects a dimension on which a job has been well done.

Clearly more research is needed, but group-level social psychological influences on the ways in which people judge that they are well emphasise the possibility that individuals choose to base their evaluations on social comparisons, where this allows them to come off well. However, they might also disassociate themselves from a patient group or might construct models of health in a way that protects their self-esteem. The choice of strategy depends on their perception of their place in their current social context.

5. Towards a Social Psychological Model of Evaluating Subjective Health Status

Figure 6.3 depicts some likely elements in a social psychological model of the ways in which people evaluate their subjective health status. "How are you?" is likely to trigger a series of questions about interests and purposes, perception of the social context, and the individual's place in it. Perhaps the first issue to be settled is the individual's goal in carrying out the evaluation. The discussions in Section 4 began with accurate self-evaluation but converged on the maintenance of self-esteem as the more likely goal, particularly if the person is asked by a professional interviewer and/or feels threatened. Myriad other goals are possible. A few include leaving or entering the sick role; winning a compensation claim or passing a fitness test; gaining sympathy from friends or peace from over-solicitous relatives, and so on. During an interaction, a number of goals might take turns to predominate.

The next questions are about the person's perceived identity and social context. Some social identifications encountered in Sections 3 and 4 include "housewife"; "mother"; "working class"; "elderly"; "accident victim"; "cancer patient", and so on. The individual might self-categorise in one of these or an infinity of others. He or she also assesses the extent to which social boundaries are permeable. By

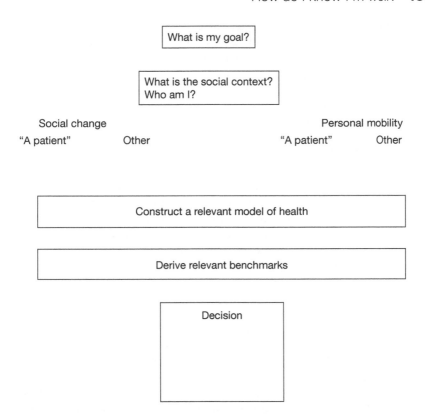

FIGURE 6.3 Towards a social psychological model of judging subjective health status: Some elements.

definition, a social identification should be salient when the perceived context is one of social change. Idiosyncratic personal identifications are also possible when it is not.

The person's goal is not only likely to determine answers to these questions, but is also likely to encourage active creation of an appropriate social context and choice of identity. For example, an individual who desperately wants to receive a "clean bill of health" so that an important match might be played, or longed-for world trip taken, is likely to self-define in anything other than "a patient" identification and to perceive the social context in a way that supports this goal. However, s/he is also likely to use discursive strategies to construct such an identification and context. In the reverse direction, the person's goals might be reordered so that the person invests in something that is perceived as within reach.

From the tapestry of health accounts and meanings to which the person has access, the next idea is that s/he selects those of relevance in order to construct a meaning of health upon which to make a self-evaluation. What is relevant is likely to shift and change as different goals or identities predominate. It is also likely to change if the perceived social context changes. Furthermore, others might actively shape it through their discourse strategies. However, meanings are likely to be structured into "accounts", and to include semantically related dimensions. Finally, the person derives appropriate benchmark(s) on the basis of intra- or inter-personal or group-level criteria before s/he makes a self-assessment and returns a decision that best promotes his or her interests and purposes at that moment.

Figure 6.4 attempts to sketch the model for an asthmatic schoolboy who is asked "How are you?" by a psychologist. It is hypothesised that this question will trigger maintenance of self-esteem as a major goal but this needs to be confirmed by future research. Such research could also attempt to manipulate goals by introducing incentives such as a prize for the most accurate assessment with respect to medical benchmarks. This is likely to release the respondent from the need to protect self-esteem from the damaging effects of reporting a low health status.

The next two issues are settled in interaction with each other. The boy should self-define as "an asthmatic" if he perceives a situation of social change in which his asthmatic identity is salient. Assuming that membership of any patient group is negative compared with being well, he should be motivated to self-define in terms of another identity if he perceives the context to be one of personal mobility. It might be that asthma is a part of his personal identity, but it might not. Again, role measures could be derived to research how different individuals self-categorise and many other interesting research possibilities arise. For example, "formal" decor in clinical settings or doctor-centred discourse might lead to a perceived context of social change, whereas use of the word "client" as opposed to "patient" might promote perceived personal mobility. There might also be interactions with disabilities. For example, an individual with a highly visible condition might be more likely to perceive a situation of social change than an individual with a disease like diabetes. However, since these make common sense from an outsider's perspective, they need sceptical research. Similarly, without measures of identity, the researcher who thinks s/he is studying a sample of asthmatics who, if plonked together, will affiliate, might be entirely misguided.

Next in the model, the boy goes on to construct and/or access a model of health. Many meanings are likely to be involved and consequently, the few examples depicted are oversimple. However, for a boy with a salient asthma identity a model of health might include meanings like the ones in box (1) in Figure 6.4. A medical professional interested in asthma is also likely to use such a model and in fact, items depicted include some that are included in health status measures designed for asthmatics. For the same boy with a school identity salient, the model might be more like the meanings in box (2). If his asthma is active, it might have fewer statements like the one suffixed (a) and more like the one suffixed (b). Again, to test this hypothesis is a challenge for researchers.

The last task is to derive benchmarks for evaluation. This is likely to be carried out in tandem with constructing a relevant model of health, so that constraints and losses on one can be recovered by adjusting the other. For example, if the boy is constrained to construe health in terms of box (1) he is likely to use benchmarks

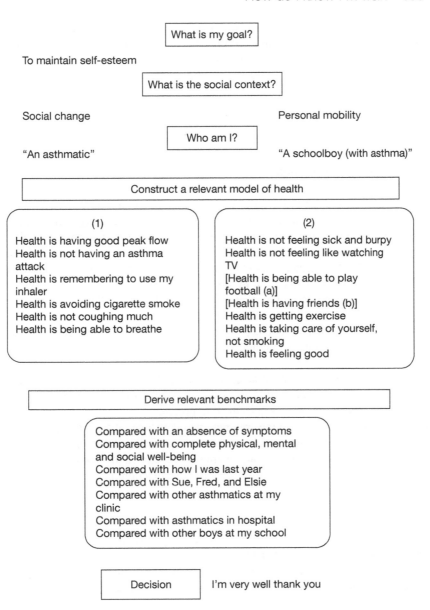

FIGURE 6.4 A social psychological model of judging subjective health status for a schoolboy with asthma, whose goal is to maintain self-esteem.

derived from social comparisons with other asthmatics or poorer personal states, leading to a high self-evaluation.

Under-reporting *per se* is likely to arise where he construes health in terms of meanings like the ones depicted in box (2), but with a preponderance of (b)-type statements, and makes comparisons with well people with whom he compares well. This is what is expected to happen if he is left to his own devices in a context of perceived social mobility. If directed to give self-evaluations based on (a)-type meanings however, under-reporting should not appear and the boy should report "expected" levels of disability.

Overall, the model offers a social psychological rival to the common sense models depicted in Figures 6.1 and 6.2.

6. Summary and Conclusions

This chapter was about the ways in which people judge that they are well. In the first section two common sense models of the way in which people make health status judgements were suggested. The models assumed that people evaluate themselves rationally with respect to their beliefs about health and that their beliefs might resemble the medical model of health or the World Health Organisation's more positive conceptualisation. In the second section evidence that individuals with serious diseases often judge that they are well challenged these common sense models.

In the third section many social psychological influences suggested rival models for the cognitive structures that underpin judgements of wellness.

- At the intrapersonal level of analysis, a discussion of quality of life measures and subjective meanings of health suggested that individuals might base self-assessments on beliefs of self-defined importance.
- At the interpersonal level the argument was developed that meanings of health expressed by individuals might emerge during discourse with interviewers.
- At the interpersonal level the argument was developed that meanings of health might belong to social groups, reflect normative functions or even be constructed by powerful others.

These social psychological influences offered rival explanations to the common sense idea that subjective health status evaluations are grounded in beliefs that reflect a medical model or a WHO model of health.

In the fourth section social psychological influences on the cognitive process underpinning lay judgements of health status were also found.

- At the intrapersonal level of analysis processes of denial and coping may lead to irrational evaluations.
- At the interpersonal level of analysis internal benchmarks against which judgements are made might be recalibrated and consequently, vary according to who is present. This led to the idea that patients affiliate with each other, in order to evaluate themselves more positively and protect self-esteem. Although this helped explain why evaluations might be positive in spite of serious signs

and symptoms, it was unsatisfactory because inflated self-evaluations might be maladaptive and there was no guarantee that a perceiver mingling with other patients will be better off than they.

● At group levels of analysis, a social identity approach offered a more systematic explanation based on social creativity. This suggested that strategic choices are made of both the meanings of health and the benchmarks used in self-evaluations. Moreover, these are likely to interact dynamically with the person's goals, perceived identity, and social context.

In the fifth section, a preliminary social psychological model of evaluating subjective health status suggested how some of these factors might operate for a hypothetical schoolboy with asthma. Possibilities worthy of future research were also suggested.

Overall, the simple question "How do I know I'm well?" turned out to have a complex, multifaceted answer, dependent on who wants to know and why as well as on the person's goals, identity, and the meanings of health that are employed.

A final point is that under-reporting indicates the medicalisation of the underlying model of health, because it takes for granted the common sense idea that physical complaints *should* cause low self-evaluations on mental dimensions. Indeed, the assumption is so strong that Breetvelt and van Dam (1991) suspect that patients fail to report the negative feelings "they are actually experiencing". Thus, there is a tension between what patients say and feel and what they are expected to say and feel.

The next chapter takes a more critical look at the ways in which menstruation is expected to cause many deficits in what menstruating women perceive, say, and do. More generally, it challenges the common sense idea that physical complaints cause deficits on mental dimensions and other problems.

7

Resisting Common Sense: Menstruation and its Consequences on Women's Health, Behaviour and Social Standing

> Because of her sex, woman is subject to certain nervous ailments to a greater extent than man. The chief reason for this lies in the fact that the transition periods in a woman's life are much more profound and much more sudden than the corresponding changes in the case of a man. At the age of eleven to fifteen, there is the onset of menstruation . . .
>
> *Somerville MD, DPM Medical Superintendent of the*
> *West Ham Mental Hospital (undated)*

> *Her:* I feel like I'm doing everything—the cooking, driving, childcare—plus of course, my own work. I think you should help more.
> *Him:* Is your period due?
>
> *After a cartoon cited in Golub (1992, p. 248)*

This chapter extends the emphasis on social context that was developed in the previous chapter. It also continues the emphasis on tension between what common sense expects of an individual with a health problem and the individual's own experience, particularly his or her capacity to resist. However, unlike the previous chapter, which focused on the ways in which the individual actively construes his or her social context, it focuses on the ways in which the social context shapes the behavioural and social consequences of the individual's health problems. Further than this, it also suggests that the social context can sometimes construct the health problems.

Because of its emphasis on social context, the chapter is pitched predominantly at group levels of analysis, with more emphasis on critical analysis and somewhat less on empirical studies than previous ones. Also unlike previous chapters, it focuses on a single example, namely women's menstruation. This example is ideally suited to a more critical analysis, which questions the common sense assumption that health problems associated with women's periods cause difficulties in many behavioural and social spheres. It is also chosen because of its conspicuous absence from most health and social psychology texts. Finally, this chapter seeks to revisit and integrate some of the themes that have appeared earlier.

In Section 1 a common sense model is suggested, in which menstrual pathology or dysfunction causes behavioural deficits, which in turn limit or interfere with the performance of roles and result in social disadvantages for women.

In Section 2 the common sense model is challenged. In Section 2.1 a logical challenge is described that is sufficient to disprove it. In Section 2.2 the stages of the common sense model and its underlying assumptions are challenged in greater detail.

In Section 3 social psychological influences on menstrual consequences in behavioural and social planes are briefly suggested. Sections 3.1 to 3.4 sketch influences at the four levels of analysis and Section 3.5 attempts a critical analysis in order to explain why beliefs about menstruation, and hence their impact, are medicalised and predominantly negative. These social psychological influences offer "top-down" sources of menstrual consequences on women's behaviour and social standing to rival the common sense idea that these consequences are caused by menstrual problems.

In Section 4, a social psychological model of the relationship between menstrual dysfunction and menstrual consequences on behavioural and social planes is suggested. Importantly, it shows how social influences can cascade between and integrate levels of analysis, so that cultural givens are reconstructed and reconfirmed.

In Section 5, it is emphasised that it could be otherwise.

1. Introduction and a Common Sense Model of Menstrual Pathology and its Consequences on Women's Behaviour and Social Standing

The previous chapter focused on the importance of the patient's perspective and social worlds in evaluating health status. Wood and Badley (1980) also emphasised the importance of the patients' world. However, their interest was in understanding how a given medical problem could have different impacts in different social ecologies. Their purpose was to use this understanding to develop new loci for interventions. Their idea was that medical interventions "miss the point" when patients experience most difficulty on behavioural and social planes, and that interventions designed to limit the impact of problems at these levels in an individual's world might be more beneficial.

To give a (stereotypic) example, a teenaged boy might suffer a serious long-term leg injury that causes difficulties on a range of complex behaviours including walking and running. These difficulties might cause him to be unable to perform the "footballer" role, which is normal for boys of his age in UK society today. Compared with boys who can, this would be a direct disadvantage, since he would miss the fun, exercise, and other benefits. Being teased or called names are further indirect disadvantages for him.

A major strength of the approach is that it accommodates the idea that a medical intervention, perhaps in the form of a ground-breaking operation, might be of interest and benefit to the boy's care team, but might miss the point as far as he is concerned. Hi-tech boots to compensate for difficulties with running, or extra coaching in order that the relevant football skills are after all acquired, might be of more value to him. A second strength is that the approach acknowledges that roles are defined by cultural norms. This means that other interventions of benefit to the boy might be to modify his social context by dealing with name-calling bullies. Alternatively, supporting an ecological transition to an alternative context, in which difficulty with football skills is no disadvantage, might be tried. For example the boy could be trained in swimming and provided with membership to a swimming club.

Based on Wood and Badley (1980), a common sense model of the relationship between a menstrual problem and its consequences in a woman's social ecology is in depicted in Figure 7.1. Its first stage is an objective menstrual pathology within the woman. At the second stage are (negative) consequences of the pathology on physical, psychological, and/or social behaviours. At the third stage are social disadvantages, which result when the pathology or its behavioural consequences limit or prevent fulfilment of a role that is normal for that individual. There are two sorts of these social consequences: women who can not fulfil a role are directly disadvantaged when compared with those who can. In addition, they are indirectly disadvantaged, because they are likely to attract censure. (Wood & Badley, 1980, coined the terms "impairment", "disability", and "handicap" to define difficulties at physical, behavioural, and social levels, respectively. For simplicity, and to avoid

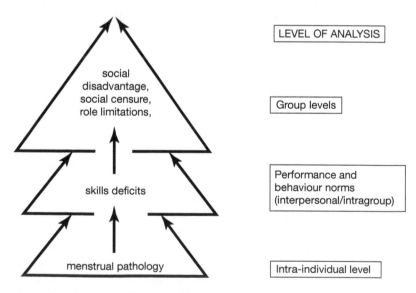

FIGURE 7.1 A common sense model of the relationship between menstrual pathology and related problems in a woman's life.

confusion with the terminology suggested in Section 4, these terms are not used in the common sense model.)

The common sense model is "bottom-up" in that the cause of difficulties is objective damage or dysfunction. Thus, whenever a health related consequence of menstruation is identified, it is assumed that a menstrual pathology or dysfunction has caused it. A second assumption is that a medical intervention to deal with the objective problem will "cure" these behavioural and social difficulties. However, where an intervention directed at the underlying problem is not possible or desirable, then other therapies might be devised to limit negative consequences of the pathology on physical, psychological and/or social behaviours. Likewise, therapies might be devised to enable women to fulfil normal roles or reduce censure if this is not possible. Such therapies are represented by the stepped edges of the levels in Figure 7.1, which although not drawn to any scale, are intended to convey the idea that behavioural and social consequences of menstrual pathology can be reduced or capped.

In the next section a general, logical challenge to the common sense model will be described, followed by more specific challenges to its stages and assumptions.

2. Challenges to the Common Sense Model of Menstrual Dysfunction and its Consequences on Women's Behaviour and Social Standing

2.1 A logical challenge

A logical argument is sufficient to challenge the common sense idea that social and behavioural consequences of menstrual dysfunction are necessarily caused by these health problems. Mercer (1973) pointed out that IQ tests and other evaluations of physical, psychological, and social behaviours are underpinned by statistical models of normality, which define subnormality in terms of sub-average performances on distributions of relevant characteristics. Yet common sense evaluations are medicalised to such an extent that statistical abnormality is frequently interpreted in terms of medical abnormality, although there is no logical connection between medical and statistical models of normality. Thus, a low IQ score is assumed to be caused by a pathology or dysfunction in the person.

Similarly, the evaluation of role performance is underpinned by sociological models of normality that define abnormality in terms of behaviour that deviates from role expectations (see Chapter 6, Section 3.3.2.1). Again, common sense evaluations are frequently medicalised so that difficulties in meeting role expectations are interpreted in terms of biological abnormality in the absence of any logical connection between medical and sociological models of normality. A striking illustration is "minimal brain dysfunction", a pathological condition often assumed to underpin children's failure to perform as pupils. Although there was no objective evidence for it and the problem frequently lay in teacher expectancies or political arrangements, it was confidently assumed that it would be confirmed when diagnostic procedures had progressed sufficiently.

Mercer's (1973) argument can be reformulated in terms of levels of analysis in social psychology. In essence, social disadvantage demands cultural or group levels of analysis, whereas pathology or dysfunction demands intrapersonal analyses. Depending on the performance norm in question, behavioural deficits can demand either, because as discussed in Chapter 6, the evaluative process, the selection of dimensions and benchmarks, and even the nature of the perceived social context are likely to vary according to who is doing the evaluating and why. In the common sense model, however, difficulties on behavioural and social planes are analysed in terms of intrapersonal dysfunction. This confounding of levels is a serious

ACTIVITY 7.1 Below is a page out of the health booklet that is given to new parents and in which their child's progress is recorded. Parents will remember the anxiety and/or pride about their baby's weight gains when first the midwife and then the health visitors made frequent visits, with scales. Give five reasons for a weight profile below that of the third centile. Are your reasons based on medical, statistical, or social expectations? What evaluation would you be likely to give, if you were that child's anxious parent?

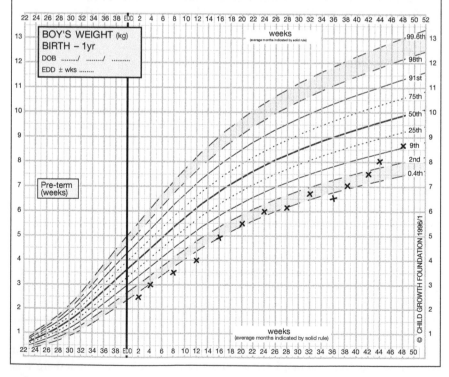

misunderstanding, which is characteristic of racism, sexism, ageism, and other biased modes of thinking (Jones, 1997).

To apply the argument to the example of menstrual periods, menstrual pathology or dysfunction cannot be the cause of a subnormal performance on a complex behaviour such as a performance on an IQ test or the amount of chocolate eaten because the definitions of normal IQ or chocolate consumption are independent of an individual woman's menstrual status. Rather, these depend on the performance of (selected populations of) other people. Furthermore, myriad variables such as motivation, availability of money, and access to chocolate supplies determine a woman's rank in such a behavioural distribution.

Likewise, a menstrual pathology or dysfunction cannot be the cause of failure to meet normal role expectations because medical and social models of normal are logically distinct. What roles are deemed normal for women and the behaviours that constitute role expectations are independent of an individual's menstrual status. They depend on "cultural givens", which might have been in place long before she was born. Furthermore, her performance of a selected role depends on myriad variables, including knowledge of appropriate norms and the opportunity to enact them.

In the next sections, this logical challenge will be elaborated more fully in the field of menstruation.

2.2 Challenging the identification of menstrual pathology and dysfunction

The first stage of the common sense model is a menstrual pathology or dysfunction. However, these are surprisingly difficult to identify with certainty. Around the middle of the last century, Crawford (undated) wrote:

> Women are particularly liable to neglect their health through lack of a clear understanding of what is normal and what is abnormal regarding their special functions. The female reproductive organs are liable to many disturbances of function and to various diseases, and this is not to be wondered at considering the changes and stresses which they normally undergo.

Contemporary writers complain that a clear understanding of menstrual pathologies and dysfunctions is still lacking, not only in lay women, but also in medical scientists (Walker, 1997). One reason for this is that the "normal" biology of the menstrual cycle is not well understood, since few have researched menstruation in healthy women (Golub, 1992; Scambler & Scambler, 1993).

The menstrual cycle is regulated by a complex hormonal feedback system. It is controlled by the hypothalamus, which stimulates the pituitary to produce two hormones that stimulate egg development and trigger ovulation. However, these processes result in the release of other hormones, which feedback to influence the action of the hypothalamus (see Golub, 1992; Scambler & Scambler, 1993). Day

1 is defined as the day menstruation begins. From then to day 14, an ovarian follicle ripens under the influence of follicle-stimulating hormone, which is released by the pituitary. The developing follicle secretes oestrogen, which stimulates the lining of the womb or endometrium to thicken. It also inhibits the release of follicle-stimulating hormone and influences the hypothalamus to stimulate the release of luteinising hormone, so that the oestrogen levels fall and luteinising hormone levels rise as the stage progresses.

Oestrus or ovulation is the end of this stage. It occurs when the pituitary gland produces a surge of luteinising hormone, which causes the ovarian follicle to rupture and release its egg. A peak in oestrogen production from the ripening follicle, followed by a steep decline as it exhausts its hormone-producing cells, triggers the surge itself. The egg is discharged into a fallopian tube. Subsequently, the empty follicle (corpus luteum) releases oestrogen and progesterone. The latter stimulates secretions that fill glands in the endometrium, in readiness for the fertilised egg to implant. If fertilisation occurs, ovulation is suppressed until after the pregnancy. If fertilisation does not occur, the corpus luteum regresses, oestrogen and progesterone levels fall, and the endometrium degenerates. The lowered levels of oestrogen and progesterone stimulate the pituitary to produce follicle-stimulating hormone and begin another cycle. Meanwhile, the egg remains in the womb for about 14 days, until it is lost with the endometrium during menstruation.

From this account four intrapersonal biological norm may be distinguished to provide benchmarks against which menstrual pathologies and dysfunction(s) can be identified. These are: an intact hypothalamic–pituitary axis; normal ovarian function; a functionally responsive uterus; and an intact outflow tract (Scambler & Scambler, 1993).

In practice, however, these are only investigated when a woman seeks help, but as discussed in Chapter 3, pathology and dysfunction are not reliably perceived as symptoms and there is a variable link between pain and pathology. These issues are particularly relevant here because the most common menstrual symptom for which women seek help is pain or dysmenorrhoea (Scambler & Scambler, 1993). Primary dysmenorrhoea is so frequent that it might almost be considered symptomatic of "normal" menstruation and about 50% of all women in the world are estimated to suffer from it at some time (Golub, 1992). For most women, dysmenorrhoea is unremarkable and does not have a significant impact on every day life (Walker, 1997). In severe cases, however, it is accompanied by vomiting, fainting, and headaches (Scambler & Scambler, 1993), but although these symptoms are serious they are not caused by pathology or dysfunction, because primary dysmenorrhoea is defined as painful periods in the absence of pathology or dysfunction. Thus, contrary to common sense, the most prevalent menstrual difficulty of all is not caused by an objective medical problem.

Secondary dysmenorrhoea is diagnosed when pelvic pathology leads to pain. One of its most common causes is endometriosis, which is estimated to affect 10–15% of premenopausal women (Golub, 1992). In this condition, fragments of the endometrium grow in other parts of the body, usually on organs in the pelvic cavity. The displaced patches continue to respond to the menstrual cycle and so bleed with the woman's menstruation. Since the blood cannot escape, it forms cysts and it is thought that these might be responsible for severe pain (Golub, 1992).

After pain, women most frequently seek help for amenorrhoea (absence of menstruation) and menorrhagia (excessive menstruation) (Scambler & Scambler, 1993). Of themselves, these symptoms are surprisingly difficult to verify. Moreover, like pain, their presence does not necessarily indicate pathology or dysfunction.

In the first instance, there are three types of amenorrhoea: apparent amenorrhoea, which occurs when menstrual blood fails to escape because of an obstruction; primary amenorrhoea, which occurs because menstrual periods have not started; and secondary amenorrhoea, which occurs when established menstrual periods stop (Scambler & Scambler, 1993). In many instances, the causes of primary and secondary amenorrhoea are the same, so there is doubt concerning the usefulness of the distinction (Scambler & Scambler, 1993). The age at which periods "normally" start provides a common sense, (albeit statistical) benchmark against which to identify primary amenorrhoea. On average, periods start at age 12 in the UK, but any time between 9 and 16 is "normal" (Golub, 1992). Exactly what triggers onset of periods is controversial, but skeletal and body growth, genetically programmed hormonal changes, nutrition, and lifestyle are all involved. For example, young women require 17% of their body weight to be fat in order to achieve menarche. Thus, it is normal for athletes to begin periods later than average or not to have them at all, probably because of a low fat:lean ratio or the effects of exercise-induced hormones. The "treatment" is simply to wait another year or two (Golub, 1992).

One reason secondary amenorrhoea is difficult to identify is that the idea that a 28-day cycle characterises "normal" is misleading. In fact, it characterises only 12% of cycles, and normal variations go from 15 to 52 days. Moreover, 16% of a sample of 465 women had such irregular periods that they could not predict when they were likely at all (Scambler & Scambler, 1993). This means that it is difficult to tell whether a period is absent or just late. Pregnancy is the most likely cause of secondary amenorrhoea and Helman (2000) provocatively points out that menstrual periods are currently more "normal" in Western industrialised countries than in the past because of social changes. For example, the average working-class woman in Britain in 1890 was either pregnant or nursing for a total of 15 years, compared with an average of 4 years today. Thus, the meaning and "diagnosis" of secondary amenorrhoea is also likely to vary according to secular change.

Overall, so many causes of secondary amenorrhoea lie in lifestyle choices or life events, including stress and poor nutrition, that it is difficult to decide whether it should be considered as dysfunctional, or as a functional response that protects the body from the work of pregnancy until more favourable conditions accrue.

To turn to menorrhagia, average blood loss is about 1 fl oz, or just over 30 millilitres, but again, there is great variation and one percent of normal women lose 200 ml or more (Scambler & Scambler, 1993). Surprisingly, objective assessment of blood loss is never carried out in clinical practice although it is known

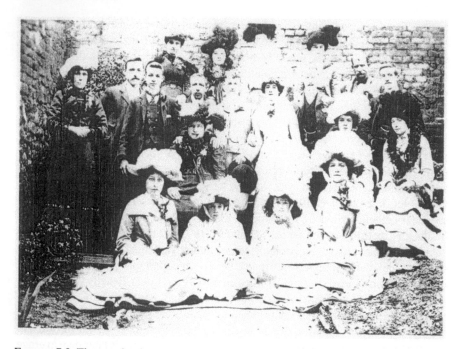

FIGURE 7.2 The matriarch seated is my great grandmother. She had 16 plus or minus 2 children who grew to adulthood. I can only identify one other person on the photograph. The woman in the back row on the left is her sister, who had 17 children, although only 5 survived. These women would have experienced far fewer menstrual periods than I, a woman with just two children. How do you suppose their attitudes to periods compared with those of women of today?

that women's assessments, the number of days of bleeding, or the number of sanitary towels or tampons used do not correlate with actual blood loss (Anderson & McPherson, 1983, cited in Scambler & Scambler, 1993). However, the extent of normal variation would in any case make it difficult to confirm the presence of an abnormally heavy flow. For these reasons, Scambler and Scambler (1993) question the rationality of the diagnosis of menorrhagia. Notwithstanding, causes cannot be found for up to 50% of cases, but the most common are uterine fibroids (benign growths); lesions of the cervix or ovary; abortion, ectopic pregnancy, intrauterine contraceptives, and other "foreign bodies"; blood disorders; thyroid disorders, and emotional shock (Scambler & Scambler, 1993).

To summarise in the words of Scambler and Scambler (1993), it is the foundation in medical science that gives authority to the concept of menstrual pathology and dysfunction, but in fact, the foundation is shaky. In fact, Laws (1990) reviewed modern gynaecology texts in order to build a picture of the medical view of menstruation. She was struck very strongly by the unscientific nature of the material in which circularity of logic was rife. Such arguments challenge the bedrock of the common sense model, namely menstrual pathology and dysfunction.

2.3 Challenging the identification of menstrual deficits

In the next stage of the common sense model, menstrual deficits are the expression of menstrual pathology or dysfunction in compound activities. They are characterised by deviations from performance norms in physical, psychological, or social behaviours, and they can be operationalised by objective measures or subjective reports. Many studies focus here and seek to characterise deficits associated with menstruation or other stages in the menstrual cycle in populations of women.

Whatever the choice of dimension and measurement strategy, there are a number of options for defining the norm against which deficits are to be distinguished. Some studies take premenarche as the norm and have demonstrated decreases in self-esteem and increases in depression following the onset of periods (Goleman, 1989, cited in Golub, 1992). These variables might be correlated with others in order to identify groups at special risk, such as girls who mature early (Petersen, 1983).

Other studies use benchmarks in, or averages across, the menstrual cycle as their norms. For example, Golub (1992) reviews studies that have found heightened visual and olfactory sensitivity around the time of ovulation. In addition, women eat more than normal for the 10 days after ovulation. Cravings are often experienced premenstrually and repeatedly focus on chocolate (Jas, 1994). In her review, Walker (1997) observes that the choice of benchmark in the menstrual cycle has an interesting history. Theorists from ancient times until the 19th century identified the activity of the womb at menstruation as the critical moment to search for madness or other deficits in women's behaviours. Following their discovery in the late 19h century, the ovaries were thought to control women's minds, but since ovulation was thought to occur during menstruation, menstruation remained the focus of research. The discovery of hormones, however, caused problems for researchers because it was no longer obvious which part of the cycle was the most dysfunctional and therefore the appropriate benchmark for research efforts. The concept of premenstrual tension provided a solution in the 1920s.

Myriad complex behaviours have been investigated. In particular, massive effort has been invested in seeking menstrual deficits in cognitive performance. Indeed, according to Golub (1992), the first study in this long tradition was carried out in 1877. The issue attracted urgent and sustained attention during the Second World War when (for example) the Allied Forces needed to know whether menstrual disabilities in code breakers would endanger their war effort. In a typical investigation, IQ scores and learning performance on solving equations of 96 unmarried college students were measured daily for a month in a so-called "learning study". Results showed no deficit in performance related to menstrual cycle (Lough, 1937, cited in Golub, 1992). In another series of studies, 29 women in an aircraft factory were observed assembling electrical equipment. A further 46 were observed making parachutes and 16 more were investigated in a garment factory. Their performance was analysed over a total of 3800 working days. No one phase of the menstrual cycle was associated with losses in speed or accuracy or with increased absence rates (Smith, 1950). Golub (1992) reviews many studies carried out over the following 40 years. These employed progressively more sophisticated methodology, larger samples (of up to 4000), and a plethora of cognitive variables including Raven's Progressive Matrices; mechanical comprehension; arithmetic; spatial skills; spelling; comprehension; assembly of models; verbal skills; and critical thinking. Other criteria such as honours degree results and medical school examination performances were also evaluated. While some individuals might suffer, Golub (1992) concludes that the notion that women are cognitively impaired during menstruation "just does not wash" and other reviewers such as Walker (1997) have come to the same conclusion.

In contrast, studies have found evidence of emotional deficits related to the menstrual cycle: anxiety, hostility, and depression increase premenstrually. Accidents, psychiatric hospital admissions, violent crimes, and suicide attempts are also more likely premenstrually and during menstruation (Golub, 1992). As many as 49% of women are distressed by irritability either before or during their periods (Scambler & Scambler, 1993). In one study, Golub (1976) gave a battery of tests to 50 women aged 30–45, which is the age at which such problems are most prevalent. Scores were broken down according to participants' stages in their menstrual cycles. The results are depicted in Table 7.1 and an important point is that although significant, the magnitude of deficits is small. In fact, they are comparable with mood changes associated with being in unfamiliar situations, and variation in mood associated with day of the week is much greater (Rossi & Rossi, 1977; Wilcoxon, Schrader, & Sherif, 1976; both cited in Golub, 1992).

This raises a general methodological question, namely how big and in what direction a deviation from a norm needs to be in order to qualify as a deficit. A practical solution is to use one standard deviation away from the population mean in the undesirable direction as cut-off point (see Haslum, St. Claire, & Morris, 1984). A frequent criticism, however, is that the statistical norm against which women are compared is derived from men and leads to inflated estimates of subnormality (Scambler & Scambler, 1993). Moreover, qualities that are desirable in men might be negatively evaluated in women (see Section 2.4 below for an example). Other problems with this line of research concern wide individual differences both between and within women, which means that averages over groups of women are likely to be misleading (Walker, 1997). Likewise, irregularity

TABLE 7.1 *Depression and anxiety scores in women (source: Golub, 1992)*

Group of women	Depression score	Anxiety score
Premenstrual	9.3	38.1
Mid cycle	6.8	33.6
Students	7.8	
Adults	7.8	
OAPs	6.2	
Depressed patients	16.0	54.4

is not taken into consideration, and feelings in the 5 days before a late period may well be coloured by the dread of an unwanted pregnancy rather than by hormones (Walker, 1997).

Golub (1992) also reviews a corpus of research that has investigated menstrual deficits in women's sexual behaviours. Overall, questionnaire studies seem to report pre- and post-menstrual peaks in desire and deficits around ovulation. Studies of sexual behaviour, on the other hand, indicate deficits in activity during menstruation, followed by an increase until around day 8, (about 6 days before presumed ovulation) and a subsequent decline until the next menstrual period. On top of this general pattern, some studies also show brief recoveries in activity just before menstruation and just after.

Such research is fraught with problems, not least because the critical variables are so difficult to operationalise. For example, female sexual desire has been measured by the content of dreams and fantasies; physiological arousal; uterine contractions; reported frequencies of masturbation or initiated sexual encounters; the speed with which orgasm is reached during intercourse by volunteers in laboratory settings; diary reports of sexual intercourse, and hosts of other variables. In addition, more fundamental conceptual problems arise, since it is frequently difficult to tell whether it is changes in the female's desire or the male's response that are being observed.

Another problem is that self-reports and behaviour measures of sexual desire and activity give different results. More generally, retrospective questionnaires frequently produce biased estimates of menstrual problems. In one study for example, women recorded their moods daily for 70 days. No changes related to menstrual cycle were found, but later, women *recalled* more unpleasant moods in premenstrual phases (McFarlane, Martin, & Williams, 1988). Similarly, women who complete symptom checklists throughout their menstrual cycles typically report similar symptoms to control groups of men, unless they are aware of the focus of data collection in which case they report more symptoms during menstrual periods and when they are expected (e.g., AuBuchon & Calhoun, 1985).

Perhaps the most difficult problem underpinning the search for menstrual deficits lies in the methods used to determine cycle phase, which are varied, expensive, and often invasive in a manner that reveals the focus of the study (Golub, 1992). Less invasive methods such as counting backwards from the first day of menstruation are simply unreliable (Jas, 1996; Walker, 1997).

Overall, the reliability of menstrual deficits can be challenged. Many seem to be entirely unfounded while others are of such small magnitude that the term does not seem justified. Moreover, the search for them is replete with methodological difficulties.

2.4 Challenging the identification of roles that women are normally expected to do, which are limited by menstruation

To identify menstrual consequences on women's role performances and social standing first entails identifying the roles that women are normally expected to do. This difficulty has been met before in Chapter 6 (Section 3.3.2.1) and its usual solution is to use work or family roles to define them (R. Williams, 1983). The next task is to distinguish those roles that are limited by menstruation. Beyond this is the intriguing difficulty of identifying just whose opinion matters as far as being regarded as unusual is concerned. Neither Wood and Badley (1980) nor common sense offer answers to these difficult questions.

One reason why answers are so hard to find is that they are embedded in cultural givens, which are embodied in the very fabric of any society, including its physical architecture, language, and discourse (Hardy, 1998; Wetherell, 1996b). Cultural givens are extremely difficult for members of a society to discover because they are taken for granted as an aspect of social reality. They are more likely to be discerned by outsiders who have different social expectations. This means that it is easier to identify roles that are limited by menstruation in other cultures and/or times. In fact, a vast anthropological literature has been devoted to this task (see Golub, 1992, and Scambler & Scambler, 1993, for reviews). Indeed, so many roles normally performed by women are limited by menstruation that a special status for menstruating women has been defined in many societies. Typically this devalued role entails separating menstruating women from the rest of the population, and in some areas such as Ethiopia the practice continues today (Scambler & Scambler, 1993). Menstrual prescriptions concerning clothing have also been common. For example, North American Indians living in the Hudson Bay Territory were required to wear long hoods that covered their heads and breasts. In addition, violation of menstrual roles could lead to punishment. For example, menstruating longer than the prescribed 4 days incurred 100 lashes and a second banishment to a menstrual hut in ancient Persia. A woman who menstruated for longer than this second period would receive a further 400 lashes (see Scambler & Scambler, 1993).

To contemporary Western eyes such cultural givens seem to belong to an unequal and superstitious world in which the roles that are limited by women's menstruation seem especially constructed for the purpose, so that they are an effect as opposed to a cause of social disadvantage. In other words, to wear certain clothing seems clearly to be a limit imposed by a social requirement, not by a menstrual problem. It is not necessary to be a critical social psychologist to question whether things need to be so. However, a critical approach does question whether similar cultural givens also exist in Western society. Early texts provide many interesting examples that suggest they did. One cultural given literally built into the fabric of Western society was embodied in women's lavatories (Crawford, undated):

> Frankly acknowledging that menstruation is an inconvenience and often a strain, we should endeavour to minimise the discomforts, and to smooth the difficulties, which

undoubtedly do exist. .... In all women's lavatories, receptacles should be provided for soiled sanitary towels. An excellent form is an enamelled box with a slot in the lid. .... It is an easy matter for a business woman to carry a fresh napkin with her, but without some means of disposing of the soiled one, a day from home may be one of inconvenience amounting to actual suffering.

This example shows that menstruation was likely to interfere with the role performance of travelling businesswomen and no doubt contributed to many social disadvantages. However, the problem lay in the facilities provided in public "conveniences" as opposed to women's menstrual pathologies. Not only did the design of women's lavatories reflect the cultural given that (menstruating) women did not travel from home, but it also discouraged deviation from this norm and hence helped maintain the status quo. It need not be so, and in the third millennium where disposal units may be taken as given in women's lavatories, this particular menstrual limitation no longer exists. However, contemporary critical psychologists might ask why menstrual facilities are provided in lavatories as opposed to more esteemed and less secret settings. They might also search for current examples of the ways in which women's roles are limited by their menstruation. Dalton (1983, p. 116) gives the following example:

> The lowering of mental ability during the paramenstruum accounts for unnecessary typing errors and more than one secretary has been referred for treatment when her boss could no longer put up with those few days in each month when letters had to be returned for retyping . . .

Dalton (1983) also notes that premenstrual irritability may show itself in bad-tempered service by shop workers, receptionists, and waitresses, and further remarks that an honest teacher described herself as simply not worth the salary her employers paid her on one or two days each month. In the absence of empirical evidence of relevant cognitive deficits, attention is drawn to the subordinate positions of the women described, and the possibility that these indicate social disadvantage, out of which bad-tempered service might arise.

The case of Jane Couch, the world champion boxer, provides an example covered in the media (e.g., *Guardian*, 1998, see later in Section 2.6). Her professional licence was withheld because of menstrual deficits, on the grounds that premenstrual hormones might make her unfairly aggressive, and her "female anatomy", especially her breasts, needed to be protected from damage inflicted by punches. This example is interesting because aggressiveness seems likely to be a desirable quality in a boxer. Thus it suggests menstrual deficits can be constructed as reasons to limit women's access to roles that they are *not* normally expected to do. In other words, to keep them in their place. Again, this seems to indicate that social disadvantages are often a cause rather than an effect of role limitations.

Overall, the identification of roles that women are normally expected to do, which are limited by menstruation, may be challenged. This is because women's roles are themselves a matter of social construction. Thus, special menstrual roles reflect social rather than objective prescriptions. Furthermore, rather than interfering with cultural givens, menstrual dysfunctions and deficits seem to function as illusory "facts" which justify and maintain them.

2.5 Challenging the causal link between menstrual pathology and menstrual deficits

In the common sense model of menstrual problems depicted in Figure 7.1, the assumption is that menstrual pathology or dysfunction causes menstrual deficits. This has already been logically disproved and the discussions in the previous section suggest that paradoxically, menstrual pathology seems more often to be a causal attribution for, rather than a demonstrated cause, of menstrual deficits. Thus, irrespective of whether they are verified, an implicit interpretation of menstrual deficits is that they indicate something dysfunctional about menstruation itself. By generalisation, deficits associated with other stages in the cycle can also be taken to indicate something pathological about the menstrual cycle or women's biology *per se*. Such an interpretation is supported by a focus on the rhythm of women's hormones (Walker, 1997).

Perhaps the best known and most controversial candidate for such a status is premenstrual syndrome (PMS). Indeed, Laws (1990) points out that an increase in public discussion about it stands in stark contrast to the silence that surrounds menstruation. PMS refers to physical, emotional, cognitive, and behavioural symptoms reported to occur in the week or so before menstruation, and which are relieved on its arrival (e.g., Dalton, 1983). According to the *Concise Oxford Dictionary*, a syndrome is "a group of concurrent symptoms of a disease". Since no relevant disease has yet been found, Golub (1992) reasons that PMS does not exist. Notwithstanding, many contested attempts have been made to ontologise it. A notable compromise was reached by including it in the appendix of DSM-III-R, the diagnostic manual of the American Psychiatric Association. In this way, "it" could be used as a basis for classifying and treating patients while further research evidence is gathered (Golub, 1992).

Between 2% and 5% of women are sufficiently distressed to diagnose themselves as suffering from PMS and seek help. Usually the most bothersome symptom is depression followed by lethargy, sleep disturbance, and craving for carbohydrate (Golub, 1992). However, many women report other symptoms and a bewildering array includes aches, pains, and cramps; bloating and weight gain; changes in energy levels; skin disorders; decreased co-ordination; tearfulness, anger, irritability, and mood swings; lowered performance; changes in routines, eating, or sexual behaviours, and many others. In fact, Dalton (1977) begins her book by listing asthma, herpes, tonsillitis, acne, baby battering, epilepsy, and alcoholic bouts. Walker (1997) reviews 65 measures, which between them cover 199 symptoms. With such variation, and in the absence of an agreed definition, it is not possible to present accurate morbidity figures and estimates of women suffering from PMS range from 20% to 95% (Scambler & Scambler, 1993). Furthermore, variables such as stress, depression, use of oral contraceptives, pregnancy, marriage, low self-esteem, anger, genetic factors, and age 34–44 have all been reliably associated with increased PMS symptom reporting (Golub, 1992).

Much research has attempted to establish the cause of PMS and Golub (1992) reviews the key theories. Based on studies that have found a tranquillising effect of progesterone and an excitatory effect of oestrogen, many researchers suspected an abnormal ratio between the ovarian hormones progesterone and estradiol was to blame. However, studies have failed reliably to support this hypothesis. Moreover, progestin therapy has had variable and disappointing results. For example about 60% of patients report improvements whether they receive progesterone or a placebo (Sampson, 1979). Other researchers investigated the relationship between hormones such as aldosterone and water and electrolyte balance. Again, reliable associations between these variables and PMS symptoms could not be established. Notwithstanding, diuretics and dietary changes designed to reduce fluid retention often feature in treatments designed to alleviate PMS.

Golub (1992) explains that another approach was based on observed overlaps in the functions of neurotransmitters such as serotonin and ovarian hormones. Since both are involved in the regulation of "biological clocks", some theorists postulated abnormalities in hypothalamus function as the cause of PMS. Again, attempts to gather empirical evidence for this view have been unsuccessful. Yet another research initiative investigated prostaglandins, which are synthesised by the body from fatty acids and which, amongst other functions, regulate smooth muscles, including those that are thought to cause dysmenorrhea by contracting too much. However, their role in PMS has not been clarified.

Next, Golub (1992) considers nutritional theories, which have identified vitamin and/or mineral deficiencies as the cause of PMS. Again, she concludes that many large-scale interventions have proven neither effective nor even convincing because the role of vitamins in hormone metabolism is so poorly understood. Finally, Golub (1992) reviews psychological studies, which have also failed to establish a reliable association, let alone a causal link, between variables such as early experiences with menstruation, anxiety, neuroses, and PMS symptoms.

In the absence of a known aetiology for PMS it is not surprising that there is no agreed treatment for it. Rather an individualised programme to relieve specific symptoms and stress together with lifestyle changes such as reducing caffeine, sugar, and sodium, and eating regular and frequent small meals is generally recommended.

Recently, Crossley (2000) expressed the critical argument that diagnostic classification systems do not simply name a pre-existing disorder as a starting point for theory and practice. Rather, the existence of the disorder is "partly a result of such practices". In other words conditions might be reified because naming a condition can create the illusion that it exists as part of objective reality, independent of its name. In the absence of an agreed definition, reliable symptom clusters, a known cause, and an effective treatment plan, PMS seems to fit this picture well.

More generally, even if links are established between the menstrual cycle and behavioural deficits, Golub (1992) points out that the direction of causality might be opposite to that assumed in the common sense model because stress-related hormone changes and even exposure to male scents can trigger ovulation (Golub, 1992). Similarly, low incidence of intercourse during menstruation and increases shortly before and after it are more easily explained by cultural taboos and attitudes, including a partners' squeamishness or "making up for lost time" than by dysfunctional stages in women's menstrual cycles.

Empirical data consistent with this position are to be found in a study of 52 women who were using the contraceptive pill. This minimised hormone fluctuation, but conveniently had inconsistent effects on the volume and duration of menstrual bleeding so that some women reported increased flow, some decreased, and some no change (Paige, 1973). The hypothesis was that menstrual deficits are linked to the volume of bleeding as opposed to hormonal fluctuations. Thus, it was predicted that women who reported their flow had reduced since using the pill should have fewer complaints than those who reported increases or no change. If hormone fluctuations are to blame, the null hypothesis was that no differences in complaints between these groups would be found. Dependent measures were levels of hostility and anxiety in premenstrual women, which were measured using an interview technique. Results supported the experimental hypothesis. The interpretation was that women who do not anticipate as much "mess, worry, and fuss" because of menstruation are less apprehensive about it. In the opposite direction to common sense, it was "fuss" or social disadvantage as opposed to "raging hormones" pathology or dysfunction that "caused" menstrual deficits in complex psychological behaviours such as anxiety and hostility.

Most often in everyday life it is a woman's husband who attributes changes in her behaviour to a menstrual impairment or dysfunction (Scambler & Scambler, 1993). Medicalised common sense discourse encourages a fundamental error in attributing deficits in women's behaviour to their menstrual cycles. Moreover, it is likely that pathological conditions will be reified in both everyday life and science.

Thus, the common sense idea that menstrual pathology causes menstrual deficits can be further challenged. It also seems fair to argue that, contrary to Wood and Badley's (1980) positive vision, there seems to be a conspicuous lack of efforts to develop interventions on behavioural levels to support supposed deficits. Rather, the emphasis seems to be on discovering whether women are fit to work or driven mad during their periods, and on treating reified underlying conditions.

2.6 Challenging the causal link between menstrual deficits and difficulties in meeting normal role expectations

An assumption of the common sense model of menstrual problems, illustrated in Figure 7.1, is that a woman is socially disadvantaged because of menstruation when a menstrual pathology (or the menstrual cycle *per se*) causes deficits that interfere

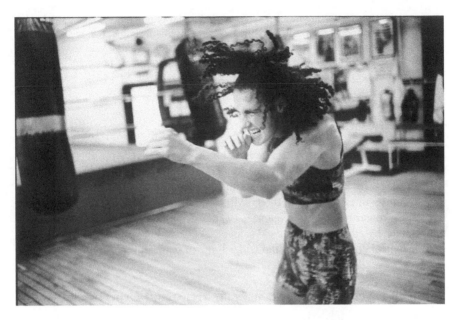

FIGURE 7.3 Jane Couch. Photograph by Antonio Olms. Copyright © Antonio Olms.

with the performance of a role she is normally expected to do. This has already been logically disproved and the discussions in the previous section suggest that menstrual deficits seem more often to be a causal attribution for, rather than a demonstrated cause of, social disadvantage, and serve to maintain the status quo.

Another reference to the case of the boxer, Jane Couch (Figure 7.3) makes the point vividly. It will be remembered that her licence was withheld because premenstrual hormones might make her too aggressive. However, this medicalised imperative was irrelevant, because as a trained athlete her muscle to fat ratio was high, so she had no menstrual cycles (personal communication from an Early Childhood Studies student, who prefers to remain anonymous). Another reason given was that her female anatomy, especially her breasts, needed to be protected. Rather than modifying the "no hitting below the belt" rule or suggesting she should wear protective underwear, the solution was simply that she had better not be allowed to box professionally, for her own good.

Again, it also seems fair to argue that, contrary to Wood and Badley's (1980) positive vision, there seems to be a conspicuous lack of efforts to develop interventions on social levels to support supposed limitations in women's performance of normal roles. Rather, the emphasis seems to be on commercial sanitary products to conceal menstruation and allow normal role performance, or on treating reified underlying conditions when normative expectations are violated. The latter is well illustrated in the following quotation (Dalton, 1969, p. 132):

Fortunately an increasing number of larger industrial organizations are supplying luxurious rest rooms for women. While these are highly desirable, one wishes that instead their industrial medical advisors would sift out those employees to whom a new lease of life could be given by the correct administration of hormone therapy and arrange for them to receive treatment.

2.7 Conclusion

Although some individuals suffer, neither logic nor evidence supports the common sense idea that social disadvantages associated with menstruation result when women have difficulty performing roles that they are usually expected to do because menstruation interferes with their skills and behaviour. Yet common sense frequently construes the consequences of menstruation as "women's problems", to be solved by advances in medical science. As Crossley (2000) argues critically, such technical emphasis leaves the wider issue of its moral worth unquestioned.

3. Social Psychological Influences on Menstrual Experiences

In this section, social psychological influences offer rivals to the common sense idea that the limiting effects of menstruation on women's emotions, skills, and behaviours, and their performance of roles are a direct consequence of menstrual pathology.

3.1 Intrapersonal influences on menstrual experiences

Accuracy of lay beliefs has been a recurring theme in previous chapters, and although they perceive themselves as knowledgeable, many women and girls have sketchy understandings about menstruation, which are not only inaccurate but also negative (Whisnant & Zegans, 1975, cited in Golub, 1992).

In one study, about half of a sample of 9 to 12-year-old girls thought women should not swim when menstruating and 27% believed menstruation to be disgusting (L. R. Williams, 1983). In addition 85% and 40% felt they should not talk about menstruation with boys or their own fathers, respectively. In 1998 *Company* magazine asked readers if they would tell their fathers when their periods "got them down". Half of the respondents replied "no way", 14% adding that they would be teased. Just under two-thirds of respondents in Scotland and the south of England and 95% in the midlands, said they could not even tell their fathers about their periods. This is a recent example of a menstrual "etiquette". Laws (1985) describes etiquette as rules of behaviour that govern relationships between people of unequal status. Her research revealed a menstrual etiquette that women should keep their menstruation hidden from all men except their heterosexual partners, even though men would frequently attribute women's behaviour to menstruation.

Such etiquette can contribute to a stigmatising attitude that there is something to be ashamed of and concealed, and it helps to create an atmosphere in which fear, shame, and negative misconceptions can thrive. Laws (1985) further remarks that it helps reconstruct an image of women's lives as circumscribed by men.

Surprisingly, such studies indicate little change in beliefs from those of a famous earlier study in which a representative sample of 1000 American men and women aged 14–65 were interviewed by phone (Tampax Report, 1981, cited in Golub, 1992). One third of women thought they should conceal the fact that they are menstruating, even when in their own homes. Nearly two-thirds thought it unacceptable to talk openly about their periods and 30% thought women cannot think or function normally when they have a period. A similar number thought physical activities should be restricted.

Although menstruation is neither rare nor unusual, it is private and hidden in our culture. Walker (1997) notes that references to it are seldom made in our literature and even women's diaries either do not mention it, or have had the references edited out. As a result, very little is known about women's experiences of menstruation, and following her review Walker concludes that women have very little to say about their experiences of menstruation apart from medicalised views of its pain, distress, or mess. For example, high percentages of adult women remember experiencing negative emotions at menarche. In one study, 74% remembered fear and 82% remembered embarrassment (Woods, Kramer Dery, & Most, 1982). Disappointment and misunderstandings are also common. For example, one young woman thought her first period was the only one she would have and was shocked to learn they would recur monthly, and another woman had eaten a caramel the night before her first period, and thought it had "come out of the wrong opening" (Weideger, 1975). In a more recent study of attitudes, only 25% of a community sample of 79 women regarded their periods positively, giving responses such as, "It's a normal, healthy thing; everybody has one"; 27% were characterised as "Fatalists" giving comments such as "I'm indifferent: I know I've got to have them so I put with them". However, at 48% the highest proportion showed antipathy: "I don't like them. I'd rather not have them. It's messy and I don't like mess. It's not a thing I enjoy talking about" (Scambler & Scambler, 1993).

The negative views depicted in these studies are likely to represent a negative intrapersonal-level influence on the behaviour and experiences of menstruating women. This is because (as discussed in Chapters 2 and 3) schema-based processing is likely to fulfil expectations, creating negative symptoms. That this can happen was demonstrated in an early study in which women were told that they were in premenstrual or intermenstrual phases, although in fact they were randomly allocated to these conditions (Ruble, 1977). Next women completed menstrual distress questionnaires and results showed that beliefs about menstrual phases, rather than the phases themselves, accounted for the amount of distress reported. Many later studies have also concluded that cognitive expectations as opposed to biological status affect the experience of menstrual symptoms (e.g., Olasov & Jackson, 1987; Scambler & Scambler, 1985; see Jas, 1996, for a review).

Such processes are social psychological rivals to common sense, although paradoxically they are likely to fulfil its predictions.

3.2 Interpersonal influences on menstrual experiences

Adolescent girls usually learn about periods from their mothers (Scambler & Scambler, 1993). Hence, it might be hypothesised that negative expectations and misconceptions are passed interpersonally from mother to daughter. In support of this idea, Whitehead, Busch, Heller, and Costa (1986) found that students whose mothers had provided models of menstrual distress reported significantly more menstrual symptoms.

On the basis of discussions in Chapters 4 and 5, further hypothetical examples within heterosexual couples, friends, and doctor–patient relationships may be readily imagined. For example, an oversolicitous spouse might exacerbate the experience of menstrual pain. Alternatively, medical problems might go untreated if overshadowed by a misdiagnosis of primary dysmenorrhoea. More likely, however, relationship problems might be reified into PMS and treated with progesterone, without considering why a woman is upset with her partner. These possibilities would be interpersonal rivals to common sense, which again would tend to confirm it. However, much of the literature dealing with meanings of menstruation emerging in relationships seems to focus on power and gender differences and is therefore characterised by social influence and intergroup relations. These are discussed in the next two subsections.

3.3 Intragroup-level influences on menstrual experiences

Intragroup-level influences that are likely to contribute to limited role performance and other difficulties arise when women conform to disadvantageous norms once they begin menstruating. More generally, Golub (1992) argues that women learn a range of terms for periods, around the time of menarche. They typically know more terms than men and often use obscure ones in order to maintain a "secret language". In societies where marriage bargains are important, enforced obedience to new rules designed to guard chastity might also occur, and an interesting feature is that these arrangements are often organised and maintained by women themselves. (Golub, 1992). Perhaps more relevant in the West today, Golub (1992) reviews a number of studies which suggest that families treat their daughters differently to their age peers once they start menstruating.

In Chapters 3, 4, and 5 a recurring theme was that salience of a social identification leads to the enhanced perception of associated symptoms, even controlling for impairments. By extrapolation, it can be hypothesised that menstrual symptoms are more likely to be perceived when a relevant "female" role is salient. Impressive, if anecdotal, evidence for this hypothesis is to be found in a study of

87 girls aged 14 who were asked to draw female figures on two occasions, 6 months apart (Koff, 1983). The two drawings of 34 girls who had not yet started their periods were compared with the two drawings of 23 who had. Striking differences were apparent. Compared with those who had not started, post-menarchial girls drew curvaceous figures wearing make-up and high-heeled shoes. Especially interesting, however, were the drawings of the 30 girls who began their periods between testing sessions. Their drawings were transformed between the two occasions, suggesting changes in self-image that were far more rapid than any physical changes. The speculation is that menarche is the moment when a new "woman" social identity becomes operational in a girl's repertoire of identities, ready to mediate symptom perceptions and other relevant experiences when salient. To the extent that the evaluative direction of these perceptions and experiences is negative, they construct menstrual limitations.

3.4 Intergroup-level influences on menstrual experiences

Scambler and Scambler (1985) argue that women acquire attitudes and beliefs about menstruation at an early age and that the beliefs generally reflect the prevailing cultural stereotype. Intergroup-level limitations arise when women are stereotyped by others and assigned negative characteristics associated with menstruation, irrespective of their individual status and skills. In Chapter 5 (Section 4.3) it was argued that a need for positive self-esteem might motivate doctors to self-categorise as medics in order to establish a positive differential in favour of themselves compared with their patients. This applied especially to women patients. By generalisation, many types of self-categorisations might create menstrual limitations and social disadvantages. For example, individuals who categorise themselves as employers might be more likely to attribute a woman's typing errors to her menstrual status than to her poor working conditions. In such a way, employers could benefit both by keeping women workers' pay low and by maintaining their own self-esteem through justifying this state of affairs with reference to employees' natural unreliability.

3.5 Cultural "givens" about menstruation. A critical analysis

Cultural givens about menstruation include expectations that menstrual pathology, or simply women's hormones, cause deficits in women's emotions, behaviours, and skills that go on to interfere with their performance of roles. They are important not only because they describe the social reality of disadvantages for (menstruating) women but also because they are a "bank account" of knowledge that is likely to shape discourse and information processing about women. Anecdotal evidence for this idea is a study in which 75 men and 197 women used bipolar attitudes to profile the typical man, woman, themselves, and the typical premenstrual woman.

The two important points for present purposes were that the typical premenstrual woman was given more extreme and negative ratings especially on items relating to irritability, tenseness, and being under the weather. Secondly, her profile was thought to resemble representations of premenstrual women portrayed in the media (Hill, McKinlay, & Walker, 1994, cited in Walker, 1997).

In addition, women are likely to use and conform to cultural givens themselves. From this point of view, words about menstruation are of interest because these influence the process of representation, by predisposing users towards certain types of observation, choices, and interpretations (Montgomery, 1986). In addition, language plays a crucial role in constructing the "order of meaning" because it is through language that people render their experiences meaningful and so construct themselves and each other, and indeed, reconstruct cultural givens (Crossley, 2000). In the folklore archives at an American university, Golub (1992) was surprised to find as many as 128 terms for this one biological event. The most common of these are given in Table 7.2, which suggests that Western language about menstruation employs many euphemisms. It focuses on cyclicity, sexual unavailability, discomfort, and inconvenience.

Few studies have concerned men's talk about menstruation (Scambler & Scambler, 1993). However, Laws (1985) interviewed British men and found their talk typically entailed jokes about sanitary towels which, interestingly, they reported using in order to "get at girls" during school years, before they knew what the terms meant. Menstruation simply did not exist as a theme in men's fantasies about women, but another common theme was sexual unavailability. The latter discourse defines women as existing for men's sexual convenience, since it presents time and effort spent "chatting up the wrong one" as wasted.

Similarly, medical discourse about menstruation is coloured by the idea that the female reproductive system exists purely to nurture embryos (Martin, 1989; Walker, 1997). From this functional perspective, menstruation indicates failure of

TABLE 7.2 *Common words for menstrual periods in American Folk Speech (source: Golub, 1992)*

Cyclicity	*Positive terms (mostly relief at not being pregnant)*
Monthlies	Safe again
Time of the month	I've got my flowers
Old faithful	Women's friend
Visitor	*Reference to sanitary wear*
My friend	Riding a white horse
Tante Anna (German)	Jam rag
	Cotton bicycle
Negative terms	
The curse	*Sexual unavailability*
Weeping womb	Tide's in
Indisposed	Tide's out
	The red flag is up

conception or pregnancy. For example, Dalton (1969) writes: "the endometrial lining which, being no longer required, disintegrates and flows out . . . Thus menstruation represents a failed pregnancy, and may be seen as a monthly spring-clean in preparations for the next potential pregnancy." In this discourse, it is described in negative terms such as "loss". In lay language, this discourse is reflected in phrases such as "weeping womb".

The question still arises as to why cultural givens about menstruation are predominantly negative in our culture and therefore likely to be a source of disadvantage when it need not be so. Discourse surrounding menstruation could revolve round renewal, closeness to nature's rhythms, female fertility, and a host of positive ideas, and in some cultures it does (Walker, 1997). According to Golub (1992), one important reason is the Christian myth that periods were "the curse" inflicted on Eve as punishment for tasting forbidden fruit from the tree of knowledge. Over two millennia, Golub continues, Christian philosophers have tried to decide whether menstruation is unclean and sinful or just unclean. For example, as late as the 1960s, men studying to become priests were advised that women who were having periods were unclean but not so unclean that Holy Communion should not be given.

Negative beliefs about menstruation also have historical roots in medical science, although these are of surprisingly short duration, reflecting the critical point that alternatives are possible. During medieval times for example, medical men believed menstrual blood was beneficial because it washed away spoiled and toxic substances that accumulated in women's bodies because of their sedentary lives (men were not believed to have such impairments because they took more exercise) (Fidell, 1980). It was during the 19th and early 20th centuries that menstruation was reconstructed as pathological processes. Rewritten medical texts included lurid descriptions of menstrual losses, and marvelled that such extreme events could heal without surgical intervention (Scambler & Scambler, 1993). Again, common sense might argue that this is not surprising, because blood loss is always potentially dangerous and therefore frightening. However, during those times bleeding was widely accepted as a general therapy and routinely carried out.

It was in the 19th century that many physicians became concerned about the vulnerability of women. This was when the question of female education became an issue (Walker, 1997). Mental effort, especially during menstruation, was feared to damage reproductive capacity and to produce a range of problems including: an "unfeminine" frame of mind (Fidell, 1980); stunted growth, nervousness, childbirth problems, and insanity (Scambler & Scambler, 1993); or even "repulsive and useless hybrids" (Moebius, undated, cited in Ehrenreich & English, 1978, p. 131). In the context of such frailty, it was common sense that education in general and medical education in particular should be withheld from women.

Golub (1992) points out that physicians' talk about women's frailties grew in spite of the ready availability of evidence to the contrary. The critical evaluation is that medical opinion about periods changes in a manner that has less to do with science and more to do with social history, from which "truth", duly influenced by power relations, emerges. Thus, the discourse that (upper-class) women needed to be protected against education for their own good grew with the rise of female emancipation and in effect justified traditional feminine roles and the status quo. When educated women were needed for economic reasons or war efforts, the discourse disappeared (Bullough & Voght, 1973; Golub, 1992; Scambler & Scambler, 1993).

A perceptive evaluation is that "women's roles" typically entail deskilled or routine labour, and that contrary to the predictions of frailty, women frequently worked long hours in dangerous and debilitating conditions (Martin, 1989; Walker, 1997). Fidell (1980) observes that the view of women's frailties depended on their social class. Since it was mental as opposed to physical work that was felt to be damaging, lower-class women were perceived as robust and well suited to punishing labour. Yet at the same time middle-class women could be perceived as needing to be protected from the dangers of education (Scambler & Scambler, 1993).

In addition to justifying and maintaining traditional roles, critical writers have argued that medicalised reification of menstrual deficits also provides an intrapersonal level explanation for the violation of feminine role expectations (Scambler & Scambler, 1993). Thus, aberrations in a woman's behaviour become a treatable, personal problem and causes in other locations, including cultural givens, need not be addressed. Moreover, after "treatment" normative behaviours may be restored, and cultural givens, preserved. The cases of Phyllis and an anonymous wife seem to illustrate this well (Dalton, 1983, p. 89):

> Phyllis, 17 years old, had been captain of her form at 12 years and her work was the envy of others. But she gradually went downhill in work and behaviour. She became slovenly, rude and bored with everything, gave up any attempt at O levels and left school at the first opportunity. She first worked in a hairdresser's shop . . . her next job was a filing clerk, where her work was not appreciated . . . the mother noted the correlation of awkwardness and menstruation and asked for medical help. With treatment her daughter brightened up again, restarted her social life which had been absent for five years and later returned to evening classes, obtaining higher qualifications in shorthand and typing.

> Last Saturday, I deliberately smashed all the dishes after clearing the table. I started menstruating in the evening. My general practitioner puts it down to my Irish temper. I get so depressed, hateful, horrid, tired, I stay in bed, shout and I could go on and on like this. It is my husband who asked me to write for help.

The "naughtiness" of Phyllis and others like her is cured by progesterone treatment after which she becomes "a normal, well-behaved woman" (despite the anonymous wife's GP's racist as opposed to sexist attributions).

Overall, a critical analysis concludes that the negative content of menstrual beliefs serves the interests and purposes of powerful others in society. These include drug companies who sell remedies for menstrual dysfunctions and manufacturers who sell feminine hygiene products to maintain menstrual etiquette, together with anyone who dismisses a woman's anger and pain as due to her hormones as opposed to the realities of her social world (Walker, 1997). Further than this, Laws (1985) sees men not as puppets of an abstract "society" but as individuals who benefit personally and specifically from their unequal relationships with women. Thus, if women did not menstruate, it seems likely that behavioural deficits and limitations would still be sought out and attributed to some other unchangeable female characteristic.

Steinem (1978) hilariously pursued this line of thought, considering what would happen if men, as opposed to women, menstruated. One hypothesis was that women would be disbarred from any sphere in which an understanding of space, time, or measurement was required, because without the biological gift for measuring cycles of the moon, they would be deemed incapable of mastering them. Their disconnection from the rhythm of the universe would also render women naturally unsuited to philosophy and religion.

A final example illustrates the point from a different perspective: testosterone levels are higher during the morning, but no researchers have sought male deficits in men's physical, psychological, and social skills and behaviours caused by lower testosterone levels later in the day (Golub, 1992). It is tempting to speculate further that such a daily pattern in women would provide scientific justification for their natural suitability for early morning cleaning jobs.

To borrow Steinem's (1978) words, the logic of the common sense model is "in the eye of the logician".

3.6 Conclusion

Social psychological influences cascade top-down to construct and exacerbate menstrual problems on behavioural and social planes and even reify menstrual dysfunctions. They offer rival explanations to the common sense model.

Of course, my intention is not to imply that all menstrual problems are "in the mind" or even in social relationships. It is women who have painful messy periods who are likely to develop negative attitudes to menstruation, just as surely as the other way round. The term "handicap" captures the spirit of my intention. A point that bears repeating is that the *Oxford English Dictionary* describes "handicap" as a word of obscure origin, thought to have its roots in "hand in the cap", a 17th-century game in which competitors put stake money into a cap and then made chance draws for it. Later, the term was used in horse racing, when "a handicapper" would assign extra weights to horses by chance, to make things more exciting. Still later, the meaning of the term changed again, when extra weights for the best horses to carry were calculated in order to even the odds at races. In general, the term simply means to place someone (or something) at a disadvantage (see St. Claire, 1989, 1993). Its spirit is characterised by (bad) luck, human agency, and (un)fairness, as opposed to an inevitable effect of "objective reality".

In keeping with this spirit, the term "menstrual handicap" usefully refers to socially constructed disadvantages for menstruating women or more generally, social disadvantages constructed for women in the name of their menstrual cycles. These can exacerbate or create role limitations, deficits, and dysfunctions over and above the objective levels of these problems. Although the relative contributions of social and physical influences could never in practice be distinguished, the logic is clear. The former need not be so.

4. Towards a Social Psychological Model of Menstrual Pathology and Menstrual Consequences on Complex Behaviours and Role Performances

Figure 7.4 depicts the foundation for a social psychological model of menstrual problems. Three conceptually distinct spheres represent menstrual pathology or dysfunction; menstrual deficits on physical, psychological, and social skills and behaviours; and role performances that are limited by menstruation. Based on the discussion in the previous section and earlier work in the field of "mental retardation" (St. Claire, 1986a, 1989, 1993), there is no bottom-up causal imperative. Rather the three spheres can overlap in any permutation.

Area 1 refers to menstrual pathology or dysfunction *per se*. Examples include women with pre-clinical cancers; mild cases of endometriosis that involve no discomfort or "fuss"; or girls with Turner's syndrome (who have no ovaries) who are treated with hormones so they look, develop, and perform as normal.

Area 2 refers to menstrual deficits *per se*. Examples include menstrual pain, but no pathology or dysfunction and no interference with role expectations. As discussed earlier, this probably characterises almost half the women in the world at some time or other.

Area 3 refers to interference with the performance of a role *per se*. An example would be a woman with superior sales skills whose performance as "travelling

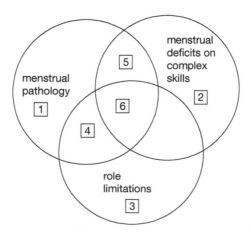

FIGURE 7.4 Towards a social psychological model of menstrual problems.

salesperson of the month" is limited because a lack of sanitary disposal units away from home. This might mean she does not pursue her career while menstruating, and therefore has difficulties meeting her sales targets. Golub (1992) describes another relevant example: as recently as 1982, menstruating women workers in south Portugal were excluded from preparing pork sausages, because it was thought that they turn meat sour simply by looking at it.

Area 4 refers to menstrual consequences, which interfere with meeting role expectations, accompanied by menstrual pathology or dysfunction but no performance deficits. The case of Jane Couch described earlier provides a good example. Because she was denied her licence upon menstrual grounds, her menstrual cycle interfered with her becoming a professional boxer. Ironically, her dysfunction was amenorrhoea (absent periods) and far from evincing relevant performance deficits, she possessed world-class boxing skills.

Area 5 refers to menstrual pathology or dysfunction accompanied by behavioural deficits but no interference or limitations in role performance. An example would be a woman who has endometriosis and experiences pain, difficulties with walking, depression, irritability, and other performance deficits, but who nevertheless continues to fulfil the roles normally expected of her. Although menstruation *per se* was not discussed, this pattern is typical of women in Cornwell's (1984) study (see Chapter 6, Section 3.2.1). Some of these women had serious medical conditions and many difficulties on behavioural planes, yet "could not" be ill because their families depended upon them meeting their duties as wives and mothers.

Finally, area 6 refers to presence of all three types of problem.

In the social psychological model, overlaps of menstrual dysfunction, behavioural deficits, and difficulty in meeting role expectations do not occur because all are caused by the same underlying pathology. Rather, they reflect a synchronicity between levels of analysis, which is supported by cultural givens and other social psychological factors. For example, even severe menstrual pathology in a woman need not be associated with behavioural deficits because she could be compared with similar others and perform as average. Alternatively, her deficits would not be an issue if dimensions on which she does comparatively well were evaluated. Likewise, there would be no role limitations if the roles she is normally expected to perform were chosen or designed to be precisely those with which her pathology does not interfere. However, such a social ecology would be unrecognisable. Rather than focusing on what is logically possible, the purpose is to focus critically on contemporary cultural givens. The question is how and why these support an illusion that biological aspects of menstruation cause so many menstrual deficits and limit role performances of (menstruating) women when this need not be so. One answer lies in the medicalisation of common sense in which women tend to be construed as passive victims of health problems. Another lies in the politics of power.

5. Summary and Conclusions

Unlike medical pathology, social psychological influences *can* permeate between levels of analysis. Crossley (2000) notes that multiple levels of analysis are often acknowledged but not integrated. A social identity approach provides a way to understand how a cascade of cultural givens can become self-fulfilling.

The point of the social psychological model of menstrual distress is to challenge the common sense idea that menstrual social disadvantages for women are caused by menstrual deficits in complex physical, psychological, and social behaviours, which in turn are ultimately caused by menstrual dysfunction. Without such a causal imperative, social psychological ways can be identified, not just to alleviate menstrual deficits and disadvantages but also sometimes to eliminate them. Such benefits can occur irrespective of medical interventions. Individual women might attempt to resist negative beliefs, stigma, and secrecy about menstruation. Other women might continue to resist social pressure to conform to disadvantageous social norms or not to enter other ones. Perhaps a change in self-definition from "feminine" to "female" might relieve many menstrual symptoms. A provocative point in this respect is that improvements in attitudes towards menstruation on menarche are taken to mean that young women discover the reality is not as bad as they had anticipated. However, the improvement could reflect the strategies of social creativity as discussed in the previous chapter as opposed to a reflection of "the truth". Thus, an intriguing question is why "menstrual under-reporting" is not an issue. At more social social levels, employers, doctors, and politicians (for example) might resist stereotyping. However, Crossley (2000) argues that the major function of a critical analysis is not to give definitive answers, but to ask questions that challenge the status quo. Perhaps, therefore, the best way to alleviate menstrual deficits in complex physical, psychological, and social behaviours and to alleviate negative effects on women's performances and social standing is to question why it has to be so.

In the first section of this chapter a common sense model of menstrual problems was suggested in which menstrual pathology directly causes related menstrual deficits in behavioural, psychological, and social spheres, which in turn limit or interfere with the performance of related roles and thereby result in social disadvantages. An assumption of this model is that the presence of a behavioural or social consequence is underpinned by a relevant pathology.

In the second section the common sense model was challenged.

- Mercer's (1973) argument showed that it was logically flawed because evaluations of complex skills depend on statistical norms and evaluations of role performances depend on social norms, and there is no logical connection between medical, statistical, and sociological models of normal.
- The identification of menstrual pathology and dysfunction is frequently unscientific and unreliable.
- The identification of menstrual deficits in complex behaviours is also fraught

with difficulty. Much research effort has been invested in establishing menstrual deficits in cognitive behaviour, with little or no success. Deficits on emotional variables are of small magnitude. Methods to determine cycle phase are either unreliable or expensive and invasive. Correlations between menstrual deficits and cycle phase do not establish the direction of causality. Underlying causes for deficits, such as premenstrual syndrome are likely to be reified.

- Anthropological studies describe many women's roles that are limited by menstruation, but these seem to be a result of social disadvantage rather than a cause of it. A critical analysis identifies similar influences in contemporary Western society but, embedded in cultural givens, these are difficult to discern. Surprisingly, menstrual pathology is frequently a causal attribution for consequences rather than a demonstrated cause of them.

In the third section social psychological influences on menstrual consequences on behavioural and social planes were suggested as rivals to the common sense idea that they are caused by menstrual pathology.

- A critical analysis attempted to explain why beliefs about menstruation, and hence their impact on women's behaviours and social standing are predominantly negative.

In the fourth section a social psychological model of menstrual dysfunction and menstrual consequences on behavioural and social planes was suggested.

- Different combinations of problems at different levels of analysis provide a rival to a common sense causal chain with objective pathology as its source.
- A reconceptualisation of "handicap" represents social psychological influences as a "top down" source of menstrual consequences on women's behaviour and social standing. This provides an alternative to assuming that menstrual consequences coincide on different levels because they are caused by a single underlying pathology.

It was concluded that handicap is self-fulfilling when women conform to handicapping beliefs about menstruation. A critical stance emphasises that it could be otherwise.

More generally, to argue that illness may be alleviated and health promoted irrespective of common sense biological facts was the main purpose of all the preceding chapters. This will be briefly reviewed and future directions suggested in the concluding chapter.

8

Deconstructing Common Sense: Review and Future Directions

Common sense is commonly nonsense

(Old saying)

In Chapter 1, four main purposes of this book, embodied in four aspects of common sense views of health and illness, were outlined. The purposes overlapped and are best understood as facets of a single challenge to those common sense views, which I argued emulate a scientific, medicalised style. The aims of this final chapter are briefly to review the four purposes, to highlight some of the ways in which they were (I hope) successfully addressed, and to suggest some directions to pursue them in the future.

1. "The Facts Are the Facts"

The phrase, "the facts are the facts" was intended to represent the idea that objective, publicly verifiable biological facts are what matters in health and illness. The common sense models that featured in Chapters 2 to 7 embodied this view. They were challenged by empirical and case studies. Subsequently, social psychological analyses suggested the rival truths that social cognitions as opposed to facts frequently determine health status and behaviours.

Without denying the importance of biological facts, one purpose of this book was to challenge their primacy further by tracing the permeability of human biology to social psychological meanings and influences. Perhaps Chapters 2 and 3, which were about the private world of symptom perceptions and appraisals, were most relevant to fulfilling this purpose. The common sense position was that symptoms are a reasonably accurate reflection of bodily signs and form the building blocks of rational symptom appraisals, but case studies and empirical data showed that people are generally inaccurate in perceiving what goes on inside their bodies. Social psychological analyses revealed the rival truth that symptom perceptions can reflect external stimuli as well as, and sometimes instead of, internal signs. Thus, humans are likely to perceive their hearts leaping with joy or pounding with fear, but they are unlikely to perceive it beating similarly fast as a result of pedalling on an exercise bicycle before they carried out a distractor task. This is because the former two represent significant experiences that emerge in interaction with social contexts, whereas the latter is simply a fact.

Contrary to common sense therefore, symptoms might sometimes be a reasonably accurate reflection of an individual's social ecology, but not of the relevant biological facts. This picture was further complicated by the finding that symptom appraisals and perceptions could vary in response to group-level influences and changes in the perceived social context, which trigger changes in the perceiver's salient self-image. Thus, rather than objective signs forming the building blocks of symptom perceptions and appraisals, influence also flows top-down.

To turn to the permeability between the individual's physical boundaries and the social world in a more literal sense, Chapter 4 considered the ways in which people respond to symptoms in the context of their social worlds. In this case, the common sense position was that people would seek professional medical advice if they appraised a symptom as serious or bothersome. This was challenged by studies that showed how irrational delays characterise the progression to help. Subsequently, social psychological analyses revealed the rival truth that responses to symptoms reflect attempts to manage the threat to well-being, as well as or instead of biological dangers. Moreover, a stress response to a symptom experienced in the absence of any underlying signs can effect physical changes, including inhibition of the immune system. This meant that the individual might fall prey to opportune infection and therefore develop signs. Furthermore, maladaptive coping behaviours might exacerbate or create signs. Such influences cross and re-cross the boundaries between psychological and physical worlds and, contrary to common sense, they demonstrate that signs can be an effect rather than the cause of illness.

In summary, the rival truth to emerge from social psychological analyses was that meanings rather than facts are what matter in health and illness. From this perspective, a focus on the accuracy of symptom perceptions, the precision of appraisals, or the timeliness of the decision to seek help miss the point. This is because human perceptions and actions depend on social cognitions, and therefore to strip symptoms and responses from meanings and the social ecology is to attempt the impossible.

Future directions for research might acknowledge that medicalised ways of thinking, which lead to seeking an internal cause for symptoms, are themselves socially constructed, and might aim to understand their role in patients' lives, and the ways in which they are supported by the social environment. New therapies to reduce symptoms might involve helping patients to develop self-images in which symptoms are aschematic, perhaps targeting a range of images in order to maintain improvements across different social settings. Other therapies might target not the patient, but significant others in his or her life, who might inadvertently have been encouraging symptom perceptions. Yet other therapies might seek to develop designs of hospital environments that distract from symptom perceptions.

However, such externally oriented strategies might rekindle old tensions, as illustrated by two examples. In the first, Dalton (1969) describes receiving letters from men who were literally nauseated by the experience of seeing sanitary products in women's bathrooms. At the beginning of the third millennium, the more acceptable cure is for such men to take an antiemetic or to change their attitude, than for women to conceal the fact that they menstruate. In the second example, Shakespeare depicted the cause of Hamlet's symptoms as the political and moral corruption of his uncle, the King of Denmark, who had usurped the throne by murdering Hamlet's father. The cure was for Hamlet to avenge his father by killing his uncle—but clearly an antidepressant or a passive coping strategy is likely to be the more acceptable cure today! Of course, tensions between social and personal causes and therapies for symptoms are likely to arise. Other tensions are likely to concern the extent to which it is safe or justifiable to distract individuals from perceiving their symptoms; how to develop public awareness of symptoms for signs currently considered to be potentially dangerous; and who chooses which signs fall into which category.

2. "Given Time and Resources, Science Will Accumulate a Full Understanding of the Facts About Disease"

The phrase "given time and resources, science will accumulate a full understanding of the facts about disease" was intended to express the common sense idea that medical advances are built on a smooth and progressive growth of scientific truth. This was challenged in Chapter 7, which showed that medical advances could sometimes reflect social arrangements as opposed to scientific discoveries.

Without denying the reality and importance of medical advances, a second purpose of this book was to argue that the beliefs and practices of medical practitioners are not always based on them, but often reflect social constructions. Chapter 5, which focused on doctor–patient communication and considered doctors' practices, was perhaps most relevant to fulfilling this purpose. Four common sense assumptions about communication were that patients tell their doctors about symptom(s); that doctors use the information and their scientific expertise in order to build a working model of the underlying problem; that doctors give relevant advice to patients; and that patients follow the advice. Each of these assumptions was challenged by empirical and case studies.

Social psychological analyses offered rival truths to common sense. One paradoxical truth was that the common sense model of communication was grounded at an intrapersonal level because it conceptualised doctor and patient as creating, sending, and decoding meanings in turn. From this perspective, the work of communication is carried out in each person's cognitive structures and messages are sent fully formed. This means that objective features such as the words that are spoken should map onto intentions and understandings. On the contrary, an interpersonal-level analysis revealed that patients do not passively report symptoms, but actively present them, together with many other meanings that are interwoven with their views of what is decent, meaningful, or important. This means that what they say might be inconsistent with the symptoms they had intended to mention, but is not necessarily an irrational failure to say what is wrong. Rather, it might reflect the need to put on a best face, which emerged unexpectedly during an encounter. Likewise, what matters in relationships and what is communicated cannot be observed, but is shared between individuals in context. This means that violations of common sense expectations need not indicate a failure of doctors to listen properly or to tell their patients the truth. Rather, effective communication might have occurred through a mutually understood reference to a past incident, but might not have been shared by an outside researcher.

One direction for future research is to seek to identify the nexus of patients' meanings and purposes that emerges during doctor–patient communication, rather than the clinical facts that were exchanged. Another is to focus on the created match between doctor and patient, as opposed to the doctor's static abilities. As well as providing welcome relief from the dogma that doctors "should be better trained", this should lead to better tailoring of consultations to patients' needs, and hence more effective communication.

Since the communicated schema of the patient's problem "belongs" to shared interpersonal space, as opposed to the cognitive structures of participants, interpersonal analyses also suggested that failure of the patient to follow the doctor's advice need not be a function of patient forgetfulness or dissatisfaction, nor of the doctor's bad manners. Rather, it might be a function of the ecological transition from the surgery and a patient identification to a different social context and self-category. Thus, future researchers might find that efforts spent on comparing social contexts and supporting ecological transition between them might be more fruitful than trying to improve patients' and doctors' capacities and skills.

A group-level analysis suggested that well-criticised characteristics of doctors' communications, such as their frequent interruptions of patients, reconstructed the history of intergroup relationships between doctors and patients; surgeons and apothecaries; men and women; and other relevant social categories. The idea was that doctors gained positive self-esteem when interactions with patients were conducted at an intergroup level because of a positive status differential in their favour. It follows that a direction for future research is to develop strategies that reduce the salience of doctors' clinical social identifications. Unfortunately, however, there are at least two ways in which this suggestion might be overly naïve. First, doctors' need for positive self-esteem is likely to trigger (not to be triggered by) intergroup relations and therefore is likely to sabotage attempts to personalise relationships between doctors and patients. Second, professional expertise is the *sine qua non* of the doctor–patient relationship, and therefore to attempt to deprofessionalise it is likely to have other, unwanted effects.

In fact, this second point indicates a more general tension inherent in doctor–patient communication. In order to fulfil clinical and relational functions, the doctor is simultaneously expected to interact at intergroup *and* interpersonal loci, which is not possible in terms of Tajfel's (1978a) interpersonal–intergroup continuum. One direction that future theorists might therefore pursue is to develop other conceptualisations. For example, several identity concerns might act simultaneously (Worchel et al., 2000), multiple continua might exist within a consultation, rapid switches between relevant identities might be possible, or perhaps doctor and patient can recategorise into a superordinate group such as a care team.

More critical reflection on Chapter 5 suggests that doctor–patient communication is assumed to be about "real" diseases that it is the doctor's job to identify in spite of the vagueness of the patient's symptoms and communications. This picture fits closely the medical model of acute disease. From this perspective, what the patient says *per se* is relatively unimportant compared with the clear and quick exchange of the facts necessary for accurate diagnosis. In some ways, this should come as no surprise, because a focus on acute disease was one reason why doctors stopped listening so much to patients' talk and started using stethoscopes and other instruments to listen directly to their organs (Hardy, 1998).

This conceptualisation of communication is less relevant in the context of chronic disease, in which the technical armoury of what the doctor can do might be relatively restricted, and what the patient says, relatively more important. For example, clues to diagnosis and management might lie in descriptions of past lifestyles, family history, or other events buried deep in patients' narratives.

Future directions for research might focus especially on communication in the context of chronic disease and seek to understand whether hallmarks of effective communication include "unfathomable and embarrassing" (Crossley, 2000) dimensions relevant to healing and spirituality. If so, it follows that investment in counselling and communication skills might facilitate changes in doctors' behaviours that offer quick, effective, and cheap ways to enhance patient health status that need not wait for medical breakthroughs.

3. "Medical Advances Offer the Most Effective Way to Combat Disease"

The phrase "medical advances offer the most effective way to combat disease" is perhaps the common sense assumption about health and illness that is most often taken for granted. Without denying their effectiveness, a third purpose of this book was to challenge the idea that they are always so. Chapter 4 was most relevant to fulfilling this purpose. The common sense idea that people make rational use of available medical care was challenged with case studies and research, which showed that people typically delay seeking help. This was sufficient to show that developing a full understanding of a given disease, together with an advanced medical therapy to cure (or prevent) it, will be ineffective if people do not take advantage of these advances. Social psychological analyses suggested that rival ways of combating disease might be based on understanding such decisions.

In Chapter 4 a range of social cognition models was reviewed in order to consider what progress has been made in predicting health behaviours. The scientific effectiveness of medical advances played no role in these models. Their appraised effectiveness, like symptom appraisals, failed to predict medical help seeking but was one of a relatively small number of core variables that in combination predicted up to 60% of variance in relevant behaviour. A moment spent considering the epistemology of social cognition models, however, suggests that they are underpinned by scientific determinism, which means they have little place for human reflexiveness or creative free choice. It follows that one direction for future research is to move away from refining models of the variables thought to cause health behaviours and towards more hermeneutic studies of individuals' interpretations, experiences, emotions, and reasons for health-related actions. These might provide new ways to combat disease, because even if use of medical advances can be predicted, their use might not be understood (Banister et al., 1994; Sutton, 1998). Based on understanding, techniques such as negotiation might be developed in order to help health professionals and lay people to agree on situations where risk of disease is acceptably low and those in which the decision will be to embrace medical advances.

In spite of their name, however, social cognition models are paradoxically asocial, in the sense that they are grounded at the intrapersonal level. Thus, an individual's subjective norm about combating a given disease could include beliefs about significant others' approval, and his or her attitude could accommodate relevant meanings, which emerged in the context of a relationship. However, this is unsatisfactory because interpersonal meanings, by definition, emerge between people and might not pertain to individuals. Likewise, group-level factors also influence the individual's intention via his or her subjective norm, but this does not capture examples when the group's intention is different from his or her own. Similarly, a health-relevant self-identity might become an aspect of perceived behavioural control if the individual's knowledge of repeated behaviours is internalised (Sparks Guthrie, 1998) but this conceptualisation fails to allow for rapid changes in identity, as a result of changes in salient reference groups and social context.

In summary, the notion of collective behaviour is missing from social cognition models. It follows that another direction for future research is to discover whether the relationships between intra-individual cognitions and health behaviours are recalibrated by changes in salient self-categorisations. If they are, it might be possible to construct optimum social contexts for the performance of behaviours to combat disease.

Crossley (2000) points out another way in which the social context is missing from social cognition models. She argues that risky behaviours, such as over-indulgence in food, alcohol, or drugs, which are carried out instead of embracing medical advances to combat disease cannot be analysed in terms of individuals because they are related to social forces in complex ways. Under the influence of consumerism, for example, individuals are constantly tempted to be impulsive and self-indulgent. Under the influence of the work ethic, on the other hand, they are required to aspire to self-control, denial, and respectability. Crossley makes the interesting point that fattening foods, such as chocolate, are represented as especially dangerous and frightening to women, who might gorge themselves if they "lose control". Thus, it is no coincidence that the research reviewed in Chapter 7 found that women frequently crave chocolate at times during their menstrual cycles, when putative raging hormones provide a reason for aberrant behaviour. Similarly, the values implicit in defining what constitutes a medical advance or the health it is designed to achieve are also entangled with middle-class cultural givens about morality, responsibility, and self-denial. Crossley (2000) observes that social groups that attract the attention of health psychologists because of their risky behaviours are frequently minority groups whose members hold different values, in relation to which the risky behaviours make more sense. For example, smoking might be an adaptive behaviour. For a lonely unemployed person it might afford a means to establish social support and friendships which are of far more value than a medical advance that allows him or her to build a disease-free body that will compare well on the beaches of St. Tropez. Smoking might also represent values such as personal power, rebellion, freedom, and resistance to mainstream culture. To seek to promote an acceptance of medical advances in such individuals might undermine important values upon which their lives are built and deny them crucial survival strategies. However a real tension arises, since not to promote such advances encourages health inequalities.

Finally, Crossley (2000) poses the critical question as to whether a healthy, long-lived population, in whom medical advances have banished disease, would be denied the experiences of pain and pleasure that define them as human. Reflection suggests that people want health and longevity as well as, not instead of, rich, varied, happy, and meaningful lives. In other words, the ultimate goal against which medical advances are defined is physical survival, which omits much of what it means to be a person, for whom quality of life might be more important than quantity. At the time of writing, a sad case in the media is that of conjoined twins "Mary" and "Jody". Their parents believed that they should be left to live and die together. Their doctors believed the stronger twin, Jody, should be given the chance of life, and they went on to win a court appeal for permission surgically to "remove" Mary. Whether this appears as a ghoulish experiment condemning Jody to a life of painful treatments, difficult relationships, and agonising reflections on her sister, or whether this appears as a joyous, technical triumph that has rescued a spark of life from religious bigotry depends on the perceived value of prolonging life in comparison with other human values.

Clearly, a direction future research might take is to adopt a more critical social psychological approach and try to identify the ways in which social forces have constructed the meanings and values underpinning not only medical advances but also risky substances and behaviours. This might enable a fuller understanding of human behaviour than that which is based on their scientific nature, chemical compositions, or rationality. This understanding might be used to empower individuals to make more informed choices between risky and safe behaviours. It might even contribute to a new common sense in which goals of treatment include health, well-being, and joy.

4. "Medical Treatment Is the Best Remedy for Ill People"

It was the fourth purpose of this book to attempt some critical analyses by challenging the idea that medical treatment is the best remedy for ill people. Without accusing medical professionals of deliberate attempts to impose their explanations upon the public in order to advance themselves, the aim was to raise awareness that the root of health problems might sometimes lie outside patients' biology and inside social arrangements. A related aim was to point out that lay people often adopt medicalised common sense ideas about health, which are to their *own* disadvantage. Under such circumstances, the best remedy is not medical treatment of individuals but a social intervention. This could range from large-scale political change to small-scale changes in personal beliefs or self-concepts that empower individuals to resist common sense.

Most relevant to this purpose, Chapter 7 focused on the ways in which medical views on menstruation have been shaped by cultural givens, as well as or as opposed to science, in a manner that served to justify and maintain the social disadvantage of women. This meant that menstrual impairments often turned out to be a causal attribution for out-of-role behaviour and not a biological dysfunction. It followed that efforts medically to treat menstrual problems were often to the advantage of doctors and men rather than the patients, since in localising the problems in women's biology, as opposed to social arrangements, they helped maintain the high status of doctors and the oppression of women (Crossley, 2000).

Chapter 6 was about the ways in which people judge that they are well and it is also relevant to the present discussion. The common sense position was that people evaluate themselves rationally with respect to beliefs about health and that these beliefs resembled a medical model of health or a more positive model of health as mental, physical, and social well-being. Evidence that individuals with serious diseases often judge that they are well challenged common sense. While an intrapersonal-level analysis suggested that individuals might base self-assessments on beliefs of self-defined importance, a more critical social psychological analysis suggested that meanings of health expressed by individuals might "belong" to social groups. These might have been constructed by powerful others and be disadvantageous to group members who hold them. For example, deprived individuals might believe themselves healthy as long as they can work cheerfully on, in spite of medical problems. They might not link their health problems that do arise with punishing and debilitating work, poor housing, and impoverished opportunity in life. It follows that medical treatment of such oppressed individuals is likely to maintain the status quo and be of more advantage to their oppressors.

Because cultural givens are taken for granted, they are extremely difficult to discover and so a challenging avenue for future research will be to discover the ways in which common sense assumptions about health and disease are socially constructed. This might enable the development of relevant social therapies to deconstruct common sense.

Chapter 6 is also relevant to the present discussion in a more positive way. Striking case studies and research showed that patients' self-evaluations are often positive in spite of serious signs and symptoms. Social psychological analyses showed that patients could resist negative self-evaluations of health status even in a context of daunting medical evidence to the contrary. At group levels of analysis, a social identity approach suggested that strategic choices are made both of the meanings of health and of the benchmarks used in self-evaluations in order to maintain positive self-esteem. This analysis offers many future directions for research, which might develop pathways to alleviate debilitating or demoralising self-appraisals by affording individuals the opportunity to make intragroup social comparisons, for example by facilitating support groups. However, such approaches will need careful handling, since some individuals might prefer to protect self-esteem through personal mobility and might have no desire for contact with similar others.

Other practical applications could include the development of "home services" (Relton, 2000) in which the individual is treated in his or her own home, or even in a public place, enabling him or her to circumvent the challenges to self-esteem caused by entering a more conventional patient role. Guidelines for hospital design or the organisation of patients might also be developed by helping to identify the circumstances in which single or shared accommodation is more beneficial, or those in which a recovering companion as opposed to one awaiting the same procedure has the more positive effect. Clearly, however, a critical eye will need to ensure that multiple occupation of hospital rooms or care in the community is not imposed as a cost-saving substitute for medical treatment.

5. Conclusion

Overall, each chapter of this book confirmed the importance of biological facts but challenged the common sense idea that they are all that really matters in health and illness, because health and illness turned out only to make sense in the context of human experience, and human biology could be permeated by social psychological meanings and influences. Indeed, the ability to "distort" (sic: Taylor & Brown, 1988) facts by denying a life-threatening disease might be beneficial because it can help preserve self-esteem, promote happiness, and allow the individual to continue a productive and satisfying life even at the cost of shortening it. The reality and importance of medical advances were also acknowledged, but the common sense assumption that the beliefs and practices of medical practitioners are always predicated upon them was challenged because these often turned out to reflect social constructions and the status quo instead. Likewise, the common sense ideas that medical advances are the most effective way to combat disease and the best remedy for ill people were challenged. In the first case this was because people do not make rational use of available care, and in the second it was because the sources of "medical" problems often lie in social arrangements, not biology. This meant that understanding human health behaviours and the social construction of medical problems might lead to more effective and equitable treatments.

My purpose was to challenge the primacy of biological facts, not to assert that social psychological meanings are prime instead. Another example taken from the magical world of Harry Potter (e.g., Rowling, 1997) provides an illustration of what might happen if meanings as opposed to biological facts were to be accorded this primary status. It also provides an amusing and thought-provoking note on which to end. The example is about the only ghost to teach at Hogwarts School. Professor Binns, who gave the most boring lessons, had fallen asleep in front of the staff-room fire one night. He got up to teach the following morning, having died without noticing, and simply left his body behind! No matter how boring and devoid of meaning, it is inconceivable that a biological death could have so little impact on an individual in this world. Thus, although we have seen that common sense medicalised views of health and illness were commonly nonsense, the real challenge to future researchers will be to understand the interplay between social psychological meanings and biological facts.

References

Aarrts, H., Verplanken, B., & van Knippenberg, A. (1998). Predicting behaviour from actions in the past: repeated decision making or a matter of habit? *Journal of Applied Social Psychology, 28*, 1355–1374.

Affleck, G., & Tennen, H. (1991). Social comparisons and coping with major medical problems. In J. Suls & T. A. Wills (Eds.), *Social comparison: Contemporary theory and research*. Hillsdale, NJ: Lawrence Erlbaum Associates Inc.

Ajzen, I. (1985). From intentions to actions: A theory of planned behavior. In J. Kulh & J. Beckmann (Eds.), *Action-control: From cognition to behaviour* (pp. 11–39). Heidelberg: Springer.

Ajzen, I. (1988). *Attitudes, personality and behaviour*. Milton Keynes, UK: Open University Press.

Ajzen, I., & Fishbein, M. (1977). Attitude–behaviour relations: A theoretical analysis and review of empirical research. *Psychological Bulletin, 84*, 888–918.

Ajzen, I., & Timko, C. (1986). Correspondence between health attitudes and behaviour. *Journal of Basic and Applied Psychology, 42*, 426–435.

Andersen, B. L., Cacioppo, J. T., & Roberts, D. (1995). Delay in seeking a cancer diagnosis: Delay stages and psychophysiological comparison processes. *British Journal of Social Psychology, 34*, 33–52.

Anderson, A., & McPherson, A. (1983). Menstrual problems. In A. Anderson & A. McPherson (Eds.), *Women's problems in general practice*. Oxford: Oxford University Press. [Cited in Scambler, A., & Scambler, G. (1993). *Menstrual disorders*. London & New York: Tavistock/Routledge.]

Anderson, D. B., & Pennebaker, J. W. (1980). Pain and pleasure: Alternative interpretations for identical stimulation. *European Journal of Social Psychology, 10*(2), 207–212.

Appleton, P. L., & Pharoah, P. O. D. (1998). Partner smoking behaviour change is associated with women's smoking reduction and cessation during pregnancy. *British Journal of Health Psychology, 3*(4), 361–374.

Archer, J. (2001). Evolutionary social psychology. In M. Hewstone & W. Stroebe (Eds.), *Introduction to social psychology* (3rd ed, pp. 23–46). Oxford: Blackwell.

Argyle, M., & Dean, J. (1965). Eye-contact, distance and affiliation. *Sociometry*, *28*, 289–304.

Armstrong, D. (1983). *Political anatomy of the body*. Cambridge: Cambridge University Press. [Cited in Beattie, A. (1992). *Health as a contested topic*. *Workbook 1; K258. Health and wellbeing, a second level course*. Milton Keynes, UK: Open University Press.]

AuBuchon, P., & Calhoun, K. (1985). Menstrual cycle symptomatology: The role of social expectancy and experimental demand characteristics. *Psychosomatic Medicine 47*, 35–45.

Augoustinos, M., & Walker, I. (1995). *Social cognition*. London: Sage.

Banister, P., Burman, E., Parker, I, Taylor, M., & Tindall, C. (1994). *Qualitative methods in psychology: A research guide*. Buckingham, UK: Open University Press.

Baron, R. J. (1985). An introduction to medical phenomenology: "I can't hear you while I'm listening". *Annals of Internal Medicine*, *103*, 606–611.

Bartlett, D. (1998). *Stress: Perspectives and processes*. Buckingham, UK: Open University Press.

Baum, A. (1990). Stress, intrusive imagery and chronic distress. *Health Psychology*, *9*, 653–675.

Beattie, A., & Jones, L. (1992). *Prologue to health and well-being course. A course at second level*. Milton Keynes, UK: Open University Press.

Becker, G. S. (1976). *The economic approach to human behaviour*. Chicago, IL: University of Chicago Press. [Cited in Stroebe, W., & Stroebe, M. (1995). *Social psychology and health*. Buckingham, UK: Open University Press.]

Beckman, H. B., & Frankel, R. M. (1984). The effect of physician behaviour on the collection of data. *Annals of Internal Medicine*, *101*, 692–696.

Beecher, H. K. (1959). *Measurement of subjective responses*. New York: Oxford University Press. [Cited in Taylor, S. E. (1995). *Health psychology* (3rd ed). New York: McGraw Hill.]

Bergner, M., Bobbitt, R. A., Carter, W. B., & Gilson, B. S. (1981) The Sickness Impact Profile: Development and final revision of a health status measure. *Medical Care*, *19*(8), 787–805.

Berkman L. F., & Breslow, L. (1983). *Health and ways of living: The Alameda County Study*. New York & Oxford: Oxford University Press.

Bierhoff, H. W. (2001). Prosocial behaviour. In M. Hewstone & W. Stroebe (Eds.), *Introduction to Social Psychology* (3rd ed, pp. 285–311). Oxford: Blackwell.

Bishop, G. D., & Converse, S. A. (1986). Illness representations: A prototype approach. *Health Psychology*, *5*(2), 95–114.

Blalock, S. J., Devellis, B. McG., & Devellis, R. F. (1989). Social comparisons among individuals with rheumatoid arthritis. *Journal of Applied Social Psychology*, *19*(8), 665–680.

Blaxter, M. (1992). *Health and lifestyles*. London: Routledge.

Blaxter, M., & Patterson, L. (1982). *Mothers and daughters*. London: Heinemann Educational Books.

Boer, H., & Seydel, E. R. (1996). Protection motivation theory. In M. Conner & P. Norman (Eds.), *Predicting health behaviour* pp. 95–121. Buckingham, UK: Open University Press.

Bogdan, R., & Taylor, S. (1976). The judged, not the judges. Outsiders' view of mental retardation. *American Psychologist, 31*(1), 47–52.

Bohner, G. (2001). Attitudes. In M. Hewstone & W. Stroebe (Eds.), *Introduction to social psychology* (pp. 239–284). Oxford: Blackwell.

Booth, T. A. (1978). From normal baby to handicapped child. *Sociology, 12*, 203–221.

Bowling, A. (1997). *Measuring health: A review of quality of life measurement scales* (2nd ed). Buckingham, UK: Open University Press.

Bradburn, N. M., & Caplovitz, D. (1965). *Reports on happiness: A pilot study of behaviour related to mental health*. Chicago: Aldine Publishing.

Brantley, P. J., Waggoner, C. D., Jones, G. N., & Rappaport, N. B. (1987). A daily stress inventory: Development, reliability and validity. *Journal of Behavioural Medicine, 10*, 61–74.

Breetvelt, I. S., & van Dam, F. S. A. M. (1991). Under reporting by cancer patients. *Social Science and Medicine, 32*(9), 981–987.

Brewer, M. (2000). Superordinate goals versus superordinate identity as bases of intergroup cooperation. In D. Capozza & R. Brown (Eds.) *Social identity processes* (pp. 117–132). London: Sage.

Brewer, W. F., & Treyens, J. C. (1981). Role of schemata in memory for places. *Cognitive Psychology, 13*, 207–230.

Brickman, P., Rabinowitz, V. C., Karuza, J., Coates, D., Cohn, E., & Kidder, L. (1982). Models of helping and coping. *American Psychologist, 37*, 368–384.

Brierley, L., & Reid, H. (2000). *Go home and do the washing! Three centuries of pioneering Bristol women*. Bristol, UK: Broadcast Books.

Broadstock, M., & Borland, R. (1998). Using information for emotion-focused coping: Cancer patients' use of a cancer helpline. *British Journal of Health Psychology, 3*(4), 319–332.

Bronfenbrenner, U. (1979). *The ecology of human development*. Cambridge, MA: Harvard University Press.

Brown, H. (1996). Themes in experimental research on groups from the 1930s to the 1990s. In M. Wetherell (Ed.), *Identities, groups and social issues* (pp. 11–59). London: Sage, in association with the Open University.

Brown, R. (1996). Intergroup relations. In M. Hewstone, W. Stroebe, & G. M. Stephenson (Eds.), *Introduction to social psychology* (pp. 530–562). Oxford: Blackwell.

Brown, R. J., & Turner, J. C. (1981). Interpersonal and intergroup behaviour. In J. C. Turner & H. Giles (Eds.), *Intergroup Behaviour*. Oxford: Blackwell.

Buckman, R. (1993). Communication in palliative care: A practical guide. In D. Doyle, G. Hanks, & N. MacDonald (Eds.), *Oxford textbook of palliative medicine*. Oxford: Oxford University Press.

Bullough, V., & Voght, M. (1973). Women, menstruation and nineteenth century medicine. *Bulletin of the History of Medicine*, *47*, 66–82

Buunk, B. P. & Gibbons, F. X. (1997). (Eds.). *Health, coping and wellbeing*. Mahwah, NJ: Lawrence Erlbaum Associates Inc.

Burnett, A. C. & Thompson, D. G. (1986). Aiding the development of communication skills in medical students. *Medical Education*, *20*, 424–431.

Bush, J. P. (1987). Pain in children: A review of the literature from a developmental perspective. *Psychology and Health*, *1*(3), 215–236.

Buss, A. H., & Portnoy, N. W. (1967). Pain tolerance and group identification. *Journal of Personality and Social Psychology*, *6*, 106–108.

Butt, D. S., & Signori, E. I. (1976). Social images of disadvantaged groups. *Social Behaviour and Personality*, *4*(2), 145–151.

Buunk, B. P., Gibbons, F. X., & Reis-bergan, M. (1997). Social comparison in health and illness: A historical overview. In B. P. Buunk & F. X. Gibbons (Eds.), *Health, coping and wellbeing* (pp. 1–24). Mahwah, NJ: Lawrence Erlbaum Associates Inc.

Byrne, P. S., & Long, B. E. L. (1976). *Doctors talking to patients*. London: HMSO.

Cacioppo, J. T., Andersen, B. L., Turnquist, D. C., & Petty, R. E. (1986). Psychophysiological comparison processes: Interpreting cancer symptoms. In B. L. Andersen (Ed.), *Women with cancer* (pp. 142–171). New York: Springer-Verlag.

Calnan, M. (1984). The health belief model and participation in programmes for the early detection of breast cancer: A comparative analysis. *Social Science and Medicine*, *19*, 823–830.

Calnan, M. (1987). *Health and Illness: The lay perspective*. London: Tavistock.

Cameron, D., McAlinden, F., & O'Leary, K. (1988). Lakoff in context: The social and linguistic functions of tag questions. In J. Coates & D. Cameron (Eds.), *Women in their speech communities: New perspectives on language and sex*. London: Longman.

Cameron, P., Titus, D. G., Kostin, J., & Kostin, M. (1973). The life satisfaction of non-normal persons. *Journal of Consulting and Clinical Psychology*, *41*, 207–214.

Cannon, W. B. (1942). Voodoo death American. *Anthropologist*, *44*, 169–181.

Cartwright, A. (1983) *Health surveys in practice and in potential: A critical review of their scope and methods*. London: King's Fund Publishing Office.

Carver, C. S., DeGregorio, E., & Gillis, R. (1981). Challenge and Type A behaviour among intercollegiate football players. *Journal of Sport Psychology*, *3*, 140–148.

Cassidy, T. (1999). *Stress, cognition and health*. London: Routledge.

Centeno-Cortes, C., & Nunez-Olarte, J. M. (1994). Questioning diagnosis disclosure in terminal cancer patients: A prospective study evaluating patients' responses. *Palliative Medicine*, *8*, 39–44.

Clark, A. (1991). What is breast cancer and how is it treated? A surgeon's experience of breast cancer. In L. Fallowfield & A. Clark (Eds.), *Breast cancer*. London: Tavistock/Routledge.

Clark, D. M. (1986). A cognitive approach to panic. *Behaviour Research and Therapy, 24*, 461–470.

Clark, H. H., & Murphy, G. L. (1982). Audience design in meaning and reference. In J. F. Leny & W. Kintsch (Eds.), *Language and Comprehensions*. London: North Holland.

Cochrane, A. L. (1971). *Effectiveness and efficiency: Random reflections on health services*. London: Nuffield Provincial Hospitals Trust [1972].

Cohen, S., & Herbert, T. B. (1996). Health psychology: Psychological factors and physical disease from the perspective of human psychoneuroimmunology. *Annual Reveiw of Psychology, 47*, 113–142.

Cohen, S., Tyrrell, D. A. J., & Smith, A. P. (1991). Psychological stress and susceptibility to the common cold. *New England Journal of Medicine, 325*, 606–612.

Cohen, S. Tyrrell, D. A. J., & Smith, A. P. (1993). Negative life events, perceived stress, negative affect and susceptibility to the common cold. *Journal of Personality and Social Psychology, 64*, 131–140.

Conner, M., & Armitage, C. J. (1998). Extending the theory of planned behaviour: A review and avenues for further research. *Journal of Applied Social Psychology, 28*, 1429–1464.

Conner, M., & Norman, P. (Eds.) (1996). *Predicting health behaviour*. Buckingham, UK: Open University Press.

Conner, M., & Sparks, P. (1996). The theory of planned behaviour and health behaviours. In M. Conner & P. Norman (Eds.), *Predicting health behaviour* (pp. 123–162). Buckingham, UK: Open University Press.

Cooper, C. L., Cooper, R. D., & Eaker, L. H. (1988). *Living with stress*. London: Penguin.

Coopersmith, S. (1967). *Antecedents of self-esteem*. San Francisco, CA: W. H. Freeman.

Cornwell, J. (1984). *Hard earned lives*. London: Tavistock.

Council of Europe (1983). *Testing physical fitness: Eurofit Experimental Battery*. Strasbourg: Council of Europe.

Crawford, B. (undated) Women's special problems. In Sir W. Arbuthnot Lane (Ed.), *The Modern Woman's Home Doctor* (pp. 15–29). London: Odhams Press Ltd.

Crossley, M. L. (2000). *Rethinking health psychology*. Buckingham, UK: Open University Press.

Croyle, R. T., & Jemmott, J. B. (1991). Psychological reactions to risk factor testing. In J. A. Skelton & R. T. Croyle (Eds.), *Mental representations of health and illness* (pp. 85–107). New York: Springer-Verlag.

Dalton, K. (1969). *The menstrual cycle*. Harmondsworth, UK: Penguin.

Dalton, K. (1977). *The premenstrual syndrome and progesterone therapy*. London: Heinemann Medical Books.

Dalton, K. (1983). *Once a month* (2nd Ed). Glasgow: Fontana.

Deary, I. J., Clyde, Z., & Frier, B. M. (1997). Constructs and models in health psychology: The case of personality and illness reporting in diabetes mellitus. *British Journal of Health Psychology, 2*(1) 35–54.

de Haes J. C. J. M., & van Knippenberg, F. C. E. (1985). The quality of life of cancer patients: A review of the literature. *Social Science and Medicine, 20,* 809–817.

De Monchy, C. (1992). Professional attitudes of doctors and medical teaching. *Medical Teacher, 14*(4), 327–331.

Department of Health and Social Security (1976). *Prevention and health: Everybody's business.* London: HMSO.

Devalle, D. (1996). Science and social psychology. In R. Sapsford (Ed.), *Issues for social psychology* (pp. 117–142). Buckingham, UK: Sage, in association with the Open University.

d'Houtaud, A., Field, M. G., Tax, B., & Gueguen, R. (1990). Representations of health in 2 Western European populations. *International Journal of Health Sciences, 1*(4), 243–255.

Diener, E., Emmons, R. A., Larson, R. J., & Griffin, S. (1985). The satisfaction with life scale. *Journal of Personality Assessment, 49,* 71–75.

Diener, E., & Fujita, F. (1997). Social comparisons and subjective well-being. In B. P. Buunk & F. X. Gibbons (Eds.), *Health, coping and wellbeing* (pp. 329–358). Mahwah, NJ: Lawrence Erlbaum Associates Inc.

DiMatteo, M. R., & Friedman, H. S. (1982). Health care as an inter-personal process. *Journal of Social Issues, 35*(1), 1–11.

Doise, W. (1978). *Groups and individuals: Explanations in social psychology.* Cambridge: Cambridge University Press.

Durkin, K. (1996). *Developmental social psychology: From infancy to old age.* Oxford: Blackwell.

Eagly, A. H., & Chaiken, S. (1993). *The psychology of attitudes.* San Diego, CA & Fort Worth, TX: Harcourt Brace Jovanovich.

Ehrenreich, B., & English, D. (1978). The "sick" women of the upper classes. In J. Ehrenreich (Ed.), *The cultural crisis of modern medicine* (p. 131). New York: Monthly Review Press.

Elliot-Binns, C. P. (1973). *An analysis of lay medicine.* [Cited in Helman, C. G. (1994). *Culture, Health and Illness* (3rd ed). London: Wright.]

Engel, G. L. (1977). The need for a new medical model: A challenge for biomedicine. *Science,* 1977, 129–136.

Engel, G. L. (1980). The clinical application of the biopsychosocial model. *American Journal of Psychiatry, 137*(5), May.

Epstein R. M., Campbell, T. L., Cohen-Cole, S. A., McWhinney, I. R., & Smilkstein, G. (1993). Perspectives on patient–doctor communication. *Journal of Family Practice, 37*(4), 377–388.

Essau, C. A., & Jamieson, J. L. (1987). Heart rate perception in the Type A personality. *Health Psychology, 6,* 43–54.

Evans, P., Clow, A., & Hucklebridge, F. (1997). Stress and the immune system. *The Psychologist, 10*(7), 303–307.

Ewan, C. E. (1987). Attitudes to social issues in medicine: A comparison of 1st year medical students with first year students in non–medical faculties. *Medical Education, 21,* 25–31.

Fallowfield L. J. (1988). Counselling for patients with cancer. *British Medical Journal, 297,* 727–728.

Fallowfield, L. J. (1991). *Breast cancer.* London: Tavistock/Routledge.

Farr, R., & Moscovici, S. (1984). *Social representations.* Cambridge: Cambridge University Press.

Fernandez, E., & Turk, D. C. (1989). The utility of cognitive coping strategies for altering pain perception: A meta-analysis. *Pain, 38*(2), 123–136.

Festinger, L. (1954). A theory of social comparison processes. *Human Relations, 7,* 117–140.

Festinger, L., & Carlsmith, J. M. (1959). Cognitive consequences of forced compliance. *Journal of Abnormal and Social Psychology, 58,* 203–210.

Fidell, L. S. (1980). Sex role stereotypes and the American physician. *Psychology of Women Quarterly, 4*(3), Spring.

Fields, H. L., & Levine, J. D. (1981). Biology of placebo analgesia. *American Journal of Medicine, 70*(4), 745–746.

Fillingim R. B., & Fine, M. A. (1986). The effects of internal versus external information processing on symptom perception in an exercise setting. *Health Psychology, 5*(2), 115–123.

Fillingim, R. B., Roth, D. L., & Haley, W. E. (1988). The effects of distraction on the perception of exercised-induced symptoms. *Journal of Psychosomatic Research, 33*(2), 241–248.

Fishbein, M., & Ajzen, I. (1975). *Belief, attitude, intention and behaviour: An introduction to theory and research.* Reading, MA: Addison-Wesley.

Fiske, S. T., & Taylor, S. E. (1984). *Social cognition.* New York: McGraw Hill.

Fitzpatrick, R. (1993). The measurement of health status and quality of life in rheumatological disorders. *Ballière's Clinical Rheumatology, 7*(2), 297–306.

Flowers, P., Smith, J. A., Sheeran, P., & Beail, N. (1997). Health and romance: Understanding unprotected sex in relationships between gay men. *British Journal of Health Psychology, 2,* 73–86.

Floyd, D. L., Prentice-Dunn, S., & Rogers, R. W. A. (2000). Meta-analysis of research on protection motivation theory. *Journal of Applied Social Psychology, 30*(2) 407–429.

Fortune, D. G., Richards, H. L., Main, C. J., & Griffiths, C. E. M. (2000). Pathological worrying, illness perceptions and disease severity in patients with psoriasis. *British Journal of Health Psychology, 5*(1), 71–82.

Friedman, M., & Rosenman, R. H. (1974). *Type A behaviour and your heart.* New York: Knopf.

Friedson, E. (1986). *Professional powers: A study of the institutionalization of formal knowledge.* Chicagago: University of Chicagago Press. [Cited in Stainton Rogers, W. (1991). *Explaining health and illness.* Hemel Hempstead, UK: Harvester Wheatsheaf.]

Frijda, N. H., Kuipers, P., & ter Schure, E. (1989). Relations among emotion, appraisal and emotional action readiness. *Journal of Personality and Social Psychology, 57*(2), 212–228.

Gaertner, S., Dovidio, J. F., Anastasio, P. A., Bachevan, B. A., & Rust, M. C. (1993). The common ingroup identity model: Recategorization and the reduction of intergroup bias. In W. Stroebe & M. Hewstone (Eds.), *European review of social psychology* (pp. 1–26). Chichester, UK: Wiley.

Gaertner, S. L., Dovidio, J. F., Nier, J. A., Banker, B. S., Ward, C. M., Houlette, M., et al. (2000). The common ingroup identity model for reducing intergroup bias: Progress and challenges. In D. Capozza & R. Brown (Eds.) *Social identity processes* (pp. 133–148). London: Sage.

Garrity, T. F., Somes, G. W., & Marx, M. B. (1980). Factors influencing self-assessment of health. *Social Science and Medicine, 12,* 77–81.

Gergen, K. J. (1985). The social constructionist movement in modern psychology. *American Psychologist, 40,* 266–75.

Gilbar, A. (1991). The quality of life of cancer patients who refuse chemotherapy. *Social Science and Medicine, 22*(12), 1337–1340.

Gill, L. J., Shand, P. A. X., Fuggle, P., Dugan, B., & Davies, S. C. (1997). Pain assessment for children with sickle cell disease: Improved validity of diary keeping versus interview ratings. *British Journal of Health Psychology, 2*(2), 131–140.

Girdano D. A., & Everly, G. S. Jr. (1986). *Controlling stress and tension: A holistic approach.* Englewood Cliffs, NJ: Prentice Hall.

Goldberg, D. P., Hobson, R. F., Maguire, G. P., Margison, F. R., O'Dowd, T., Osborn, M. M. et al. (1984). The clarification and assessment of a method of psychotherapy. *British Journal of Psychiatry, 144,* 567–580.

Goldsen, R. K., Gerhard, P. R., & Handy, V. (1957). Some factors related to patient delay in seeking diagnosis for cancer symptoms. *Cancer, 10,* 1–7.

Goleman, D. (1989, January 10th) Pioneering studies find surprising high rate of mental ills in young. *The New York Times,* C1. [Cited in Golub, S. (1992). *Periods: From menarche to menopause.* New York: Sage International Edition.]

Golub, S. (1976). The magnitude of premenstrual anxiety and depression. *Psychosomatic Medicine, 38,* 4–14.

Golub, S. (1992). *Periods: from menarche to menopause.* New York: Sage International Edition.

Gottlieb, J., & Gottlieb, B. W. (1977). Stereotypic attitudes and behavioural intentions towards handicapped children. *American Journal on Mental Deficiency, 80,* 376–381.

Graumann, C. F. (2001). Introduction to a history of social psychology. In M. Hewstone & W. Stroebe (Eds.), *Introduction to social psychology* (3rd ed, pp. 3–23). Oxford: Blackwell.

Greenbaum, J. J., & Wang, O. D. (1965). A semantic differential study of the concepts of mental retardation. *Journal of General Psychology, 73,* 257–272.

Greene, J., & Coulson, M. (1995). *Language understanding: Current issues* (2nd ed). Buckingham, UK: Open University Press.

Greenfield, S., Kaplan, S. H., & Ware, J. E. (1988). Patients' participation in medical care: Effects on blood sugar control and quality of life in diabetes. *Journal of General Internal Medicine, 3*, 448–457.

Greenwald, H. P., & Nevitt, M. C. (1982). Physician attitudes toward communication with cancer patients. *Social Science and Medicine, 16*, 591–594.

Gruder, C. L. (1977). Choice of comparison persons in evaluating oneself. In J. M. Suls & R. L. Miller (Eds.), *Social comparison processes* (pp. 21–41). Washington: Hemisphere.

Hackett, T. P., Gassem, N. H., & Raker, J. W. (1973). Patient delay in cancer. *New England Journal of Medicine, 289*, 14–20. [Cited in Helman, C. G. (1994). *Culture, health and illness* (3rd ed). London: Wright.]

Haffter, C. (1968). The changeling. *Journal of the History of Behavioural Sciences, 2*(1), 55–61.

Hampson, S. E., Glasgow, R. E., & Strycker, L. A. (2000). Beliefs versus feelings: A comparison of personal models and depression for predicting multiple outcomes in diabetes. *British Journal of Health Psychology, 5*(1), 27–40.

Hannay, D. R. (1979). *The symptom iceberg: A study of community health.* London: Routledge & Kegan Paul.

Hardy, M. (1998). *The social context of health.* Buckingham, UK: Open University Press.

Harris P., & Middleton W. (1994). The illusion of control and optimism about health: on being less at risk but no more in control than others. *British Journal of Social Psychology, 33*, 369–386.

Harrison, J. A., Mullen, P. D., & Green, L. W. (1992). A meta-analysis of studies of the Health Belief Model with adults. *Health Education Research, 7*, 107–116.

Hart, K. E. (1983). Physical symptom reporting and health perception among Type A and B college males. *Journal of Human Stress, 9*, 17–22.

Haslum, M., St. Claire, L., & Morris, A. (1984). *A profile analysis of the abilities of children with impairments.* Report to DHSS Department of Child Health, London.

Helman, C. G. (1978). Feed a cold, starve a fever—folk models of infection in an English suburban community, and their relation to medical treatment. *Culture, Medicine and Psychiatry, 2*, 107–137.

Helman, C. G. (1994). *Culture, health and illness* (3rd ed). London: Wright.

Helman, C. G. (2000). *Culture, health and illness* (4th ed). London: Wright.

Helson H. (1964). *Adaptation level theory.* New York: Harper & Row. [Cited in Breetvelt, I. S. & Van Dam, F. S. A. M. (1991). Under reporting by cancer patients. *Social Science and Medicine, 32*(9), 981–987.]

Hertzlich, C., & Graham, D. (1973). *Health and illness.* London: Academic Press.

Herz, M. J., Kahan, E., Zaleveski, S., Aframian, R., Kuznitz, D., & Reichman, S.

(1996). Constipation: A different entity for patients and doctors. *Family Practice*, *13*(2), 156–159.

Hewstone, M., & Fincham, F. (1996). Attribution theory and research: Basic issues and applications. In M. Hewstone, W. Stroebe, & G. M. Stephenson (Eds), *Introduction to social psychology* (2nd ed, pp. 167–204). Oxford: Blackwell.

Hewstone, M., Manstead, A. S. R., & Stroebe, W. (Eds.) (1997). *The Blackwell reader in social psychology*. Oxford: Blackwell.

Hill, Y., McKinlay, A., & Walker, A. (1994). *Man, woman and premenstrual woman: Stereotypes of British students*. Paper presented at the British Psychological Society, Social Psychology Section, Conference, Oxford, September. [Cited in Walker, A. E. (1997). *The menstrual cycle*. London: Routledge.]

Hindmarch, I. (1981). Too many pills in the cupboard. *New Society*, *55*, 142–143. [Cited in Helman, C. G. (1994). *Culture, health and illness* (3rd ed). London: Wright.

Hochbaum, G. M. (1958). *Public participation in medical screening programs: A socio-psychological study. Public Health Service Publication No. 572*. Washington, DC: United States Government Printing Office.

Holmes, T. H., & Rahe, R. H. (1967). The social readjustment rating scale. *Journal of Psychosomatic Research*, *11*, 213–218.

Hopkins, W. G., & Walker, N. P. (1988). The meaning of "physical fitness". *Preventive Medicine*, *17*, 764–773.

Horn, S., & Munafo, M. (1997). *Pain: Theory, research and intervention*. Buckingham, UK: Open University Press.

Hunt, S., McEwen, J., & McKenna, S. P. (1984). Perceived health: Age and sex comparisons in a community. *Journal of Epidemiology and Community Health*, *38*(2), 156–160.

Hunt, S., McKenna, S. P., McEwen, J., Williams, F., & Papp, M. (1981). The Nottingham Health Profile: Subjective health status and medical consultation. *Social Science and Medicine*, *15*A, 221–229.

Hunt, S. M., & McEwen, J. (1980). The development of a subjective health indicator. *Sociology of Health and Illness*, *2*(3), 231–245.

Hyland, M. E. (1990). The Living with Asthma Questionnaire. *Respiratory Medicine*, *85*, Supplement B, 13–16.

Hyland, M. E., Finnios, S., & Irvine, S. H. (1991). A scale for assessing quality of life in adult asthma sufferers. *Journal of Psychomatic Research*, *35*(1), 99–110.

Ingham, J. G., & Miller, P. M. (1986). Self-referral to primary care: Symptoms and social factors. *Journal of Psychosomatic Research*, *30*(1), 49–56.

Jarvinen K. A. J. (1955). Can ward rounds be a danger to patients with myocardial infarction? *British Medical Journal*, *1*, 318–320.

Jas, P. (1994). The menstrual cycle, mood and appetite. *Nutrition and Food Science*, *2*, 23–25.

Jas, P. (1996). *Changes in food intake and mood across the menstrual cycle*. PhD

Thesis submitted to the Department of Psychology, University of Reading, UK.

Jeffery, R. (1984). Normal rubbish: Deviant patients in casualty departments. In N. Black, N. Boswell, A. Gray, S. Murphy, & J. Popay (Eds.), *Health and disease: A reader* (pp. 249–254). Milton Keynes, UK: Open University Press.

Jewson, N. (1976). The disappearance of the sick-man from medical cosmology, 1770–1870. *Sociology, 10,* 224–244. [Cited in Beattie A. (1992). *Health as a contested topic. Workbook 1; K258. Health and wellbeing, a second-level course.* Milton Keynes, UK: Open University Press.]

Jones, J. M. (1997). *Prejudice and racism.* New York: McGraw-Hill.

Kahney, H. (1993). *Problem solving: Current issues. Open guides to psychology.* Milton Keynes, UK: Open University Press.

Kalat, J. W. (2001). *Biological psychology* (7th ed). Belmont: Wadsworth.

Kaplan, H. B., Robbins, C., & Martin, S. S. (1983). Antecedents of psychological distress in young adults. *Journal of Health and Social Behaviour, 24,* 230–244.

Kaplan, R. M., & Porkorny, A. D. (1969). Self-derogation and psychosocial adjustment. *Journal of Nervous and Mental Disease, 149,* 421–434.

Kaplan, S. H., Greenfield, S., & Ware, J. E. (1989). The impact of the doctor–patient relationship on the outcomes of chronic disease. In M. Stewart and D. Roter (Eds.), *Communicating with medical patients* (pp. 228–245). Newbury Park, CA: Sage.

Kaye, K. (1984). *The mental and social life of babies.* London: Methuen.

Kendrick, A. H., Higgs, C. M. B., Whitfield, M. J., & Laszlo, G. (1993). Accuracy of perception of severity of asthma: Patients treated in general practice. *British Medical Journal, 307,* 422–424.

Kerns, R. D., Turk, D. C., & Rudy, T. E. (1985). The West Haven–Yale Multidimensional Pain Inventory (WHYMPI). *Pain, 23,* 345–356.

Key, S. (2001). Fighting the fear that feeds a killer. *Bristol Evening Post,* 4th December, pp. 8–9.

Kleinmann, A. R. (1988). *The illness narratives: Suffering, healing and the human condition.* New York: Basic Books.

Knapp, M. L., & Hall, J. A. (1992). *Nonverbal communication in human interaction* (3rd ed). Fort Worth: Harcourt Brace Jovanovich.

Koff, E. (1983). Through the looking glass of menarche. What the adolescent girl sees. In S. Golub (Ed.), *Menarche* (pp. 77–86). Lexington, MA: Lexington Books.

Korsch, B. M., & Negrete, V. F. (1972). Doctor–patient communication. *Scientific American, August,* 66–74.

Kuhn, M. H., & McPartland, T. S. (1954). An empirical investigation of self-attitudes. *American Sociological Review, 19,* 68–76.

Kulik, J. A., & Mahler, H. I. M. (1997). Social comparison, affiliation and coping with acute medical threats. In B. P. Buunk & F. X. Gibbons (Eds.), *Health, coping and wellbeing* (pp. 227–263). Mahwah, NJ: Lawrence Erlbaum Associates Inc.

Lakoff, R. (1975). *Language and woman's place*. New York: Harper & Row.

Lalljee, M. (1996). The interpreting self: An experimentalist perspective. In J. R. Stevens (Ed.), *Understanding the self* (pp. 89–146). London: Sage, in association with the Open University.

Lalljee, M., Lamb, R., & Carnibella, G. (1993). Lay prototypes of illness: Their content and use. *Psychology and Health*, *8*, 33–49.

Lalonde, M. (1974). *A new perspective on the health of Canadians*. Ontario: Government of Canada.

LaPierre, R. (1934). Attitudes versus actions. *Social Forces*, *13*, 230–237.

Lau, R. R., Bernard, T. M., & Hartman, K. A. (1989). Further explorations of common-sense representations of illness. *Health Psychology*, *8*, 195–219.

Lau, R. R. & Hartman, K. A. (1983). Common sense representations of common illnesses. *Health Psychology*, *2*, 167–185.

Lau, R. R., Hartmann, K. A., & Ware, J. E. (1986). Health as a value: Methodological and theoretical considerations. *Health Psychology*, *5*, 25–43.

Laws, S. (1985). Male power and menstrual etiquette. In H. Thomas (Ed.), *The sexual politics of reproduction*. London: Gower.

Laws, S. (1990). *Issues of blood: The politics of menstruation*. Basingstoke, UK: Macmillan Press.

Lazare, A., Eisenthal, S., Frank, A., & Stoeckle, J. D. (1978). Studies on a negotiated approach to patienthood. In J. D. Stoeckle (Ed.), *Encounters between patients and doctors* (pp.?????). Cambridge, MA: MIT Press. [Cited in Murphy, J. (1996). *Trigger Unit for social psychology: Personal lives, social worlds. A third level social sciences course*. Milton Keynes, UK: Open University Press.

Lazarus, R. S. (1966) *Psychological stress and the coping process*. New York: McGraw Hill.

Lazarus, R. S. (1999). *Stress and emotion: A new synthesis*. London: Free Association Books.

Lazarus, R. S., & Folkman S. (1984). *Stress, appraisal and coping*. New York: Springer.

Levenson, H. (1981). Differentiating among internality, powerful others and chance. In *Research with the locus of control construct Vol. 1: Assessment methods*. New York: Academic Press. [Cited in Stainton Rogers, W. (1991). *Explaining health and illness*. Hemel Hempstead, UK: Harvester Wheatsheaf.]

Leventhal, H., Nerenz, D. R., & Steele, D. J. (1984). Illness representations and coping with health threats. In A. Baum, S. E. Taylor, & J. E. Singer (Eds.), *Handbook of psychology and health IV* (pp. 219–249). London: Lawrence Erlbaum Associates Ltd.

Leventhal, H., Shacham, S., & Easterling, D. V. (1989). Active coping reduces reports of pain from childbirth. *Journal of Consulting and Clinical Psychology*, *57*, 365–371.

Levine, F. M., & De Simone, L. L. (1991). The effects of experimenter gender on pain report. *Pain, 44,* 69–72.

Levine, F. M., Krass, S. M., & Padawer, W. J. (1993). Failure hurts: The effects of stress due to difficult tasks and failure feedback on pain report. *Pain, 54,* 335–340.

Levine, R. M. (1999). Identity and illness: The effects of identity salience and frame of reference on evaluation of illness and injury. *British Journal of Health Psychology, 4*(1), 63–80.

Levine, R. M., & Reicher, S. D. (1996). Making sense of symptoms: Self-categorisation and the meaning of illness and injury. *British Journal of Social Psychology, 35,* 245–256.

Levy, S. M. (1986). Behaviour as a biological response modifier: Psychological variables and cancer prognosis. In B. L. Andersen (Ed.), *Women with cancer.* New York: Springer-Verlag.

Levy, S. M., Herberman, R. B., Whiteside, T., Sanzo, K., Lee, J., & Kirkwood, J. (1990). Perceived social support and tumor estrogen/progesterone receptor status as predictors of natural killer cell activity in breast cancer patients. *Psychosomatic Medicine, 52,* 73–85.

Ley, P. (1990). *Communicating with patients.* London: Chapman & Hall.

Lough, O. M. (1937). A psychological study of functional periodicity. *Journal of Comparative Psychology, 24,* 359–368. [Cited in Golub, S. (1992). *Periods: From menarche to menopause.* New York: Sage International Edition.]

Lowery, B. J., Jacobsen, B. S., & Murphy, B. B. (1983). An exploratory investigation of causal thinking of arthritics. *Nursing Research, 32*(3), 157–162.

Lupton, D. (1994). *Medicine as culture: Illness, disease and the body in Western societies.* London: Sage.

Lyus, J. (1999). *Menstrual distress, femininity and identity salience: The effects of female identitiy salience on menstrual distress.* Third year research project, Department of Experimental Psychology, University of Bristol, UK.

Maguire P., Fairbairn S., & Fletcher, C. (1986). Consultation skills of young doctors. I: Benefits of feedback training persist. *British Medical Journal, 292,* 1573–1576.

Maguire P., & Faulkner A. (1988). How to do it: Communicate with cancer patients: 1 Handling bad news and difficult questions. *British Medical Journal, 297,* 907–909.

Maguire P., Roe P., & Goldberg D. (1978). The value of teaching interviewing skills to medical students. *Psychological Medicine, 8,* 695–704.

Malone, A. B. (1996). The effects of live music on distress of pediatric patients receiving intravenous starts, venipunctures, injections and heel sticks. *Journal of Music Therapy, 33,* 19–33.

Markus, H. (1977). Self-schemata and processing information about the self. *Journal of Personality and Social Psychology, 35,* 63–78.

Martin, E. (1989). *The woman in the body: A cultural analysis of reproduction.* Milton Keynes, UK: Open University Press.

Martini, C. J., Allan, G. J., Davison, J., & Backett, E. M. (1979). Health indexes sensitive to medical care variation. In J. Elinson et al. (Eds.), *Socio-medical health indicators* (p. 145). Farmingdale, NJ: Baywood.

McFarlane, J., Martin, C. L., & Williams, T. M. (1988). Mood fluctuations: Women versus men and menstrual versus other cycles. *Psychology of Women Quarterly, 12*(2), 201–223.

McGhee, P. (1996). *Exploring decision making. Project notes from D317 a third-level social science course*. Buckingham, UK: Open University Press.

McGraw, M. (1963). *The neuromuscular maturation of the human infant*. New York: Harper. [Cited in Bush, J. P. (1987). Pain in children: A review of the literature from a developmental perspective. *Psychology and Health, 1*(3), 215–236.]

McKenna, S. P., Hunt, S., & McEwen, J. (1981). Weighting the seriousness of perceived health problems using Thurstone's method of paired comparisons. *International Journal of Epidemiology, 10*, 93–97.

McKeown, T. (1979). *The role of medicine: Dream, mirage or nemesis*. London: Nuffield Provincial Hospital Trust.

McManus, I. C., Kidd, J. M., & Aldus, I. R. (1997). Self-perception of communicative ability: Evaluation of a questionnaire completed by medical students and general practitioners. *British Journal of Health Psychology, 2*(4), 301–316.

McNeil, B. J., Parker, S. G., Sox, H. C. Jnr., & Tversky, A. (1982). On the elicitation of preferences for alternative therapies. *New England Journal of Medicine, 306*, 1259–1262.

McNicol, D. (1972). *A primer of signal detection theory*. London: Allen & Unwin.

Mechanic, D. (1980). The experience and reporting of common physical complaints. *Journal of Health and Social Behaviour, 21*, 146–155.

Meeuwesen L., Schaap, C., & van der Staak, C. (1991). Verbal analysis of doctor–patient communication. *Social Science and Medicine, 32*(10), 1143–1150.

Meininger, J. C. (1986). Sex differences in factors associated with use of medical care and alternative illness behavours. *Social Science and Medicine, 22*(3), 285–292.

Melzack, R., & Katz, J. (1992). The McGill Pain Questionnaire: Appraisal and current status. In D. C. Turk & R. Melzack (Eds.), *Handbook of pain assessment*. New York: Guilford Press.

Melzack, R., & Torgerson, W. S. (1971). On the language of pain. *Anesthesiology, 34*, 50–59.

Melzack, R., & Wall, P. (1988). *The challenge of pain*. London: Penguin.

Mercer, J. (1973). *Labelling the mentally retarded*. University of California Press.

Merksey, H., Albe-Fessard, D. G., Bonica, J. J., Carmen, A., Dubner, R., Kerr, F. W. L. et al. (1979). IASP sub-committee on taxonomy. *Pain, 6*(3), 249–252.

Miell, D., & Dallos, R. (1996). Introduction: Exploring interactions and relationships. In D. Miell & R. Dallos (Eds.), *Social interaction and personal relationships* (pp. 1–22). London: Sage, in association with the Open University.

Milne, S., Sheeran, P., & Orbell, S. (2000). Prediction and intervention in health-related behaviour: A meta-analytic review of protection motivation theory. *Journal of Applied Social Psychology, 30,* 106–143.

Minuchin, S. (1974). *Families and family therapy.* Cambridge, MA: Harvard University Press.

Moebius (undated). [Cited in Ehrenreich B., & English, D. (1978). The "sick" women of the upper classes. In J. Ehrenreich (Ed.), *The cultural crisis of modern medicine* (p. 131). New York: Monthly Review Press.]

Molleman, E., Pruyn, J., & van Knippenberg, A. (1986). Social comparison processes among cancer patients. *British Journal of Social Psychology, 25,* 1–13.

Montgomery, M. (1986). *An introduction to language and society.* London & New York: Methuen.

Morgan, M. (1997). The doctor–patient relationship. In G. Scambler (Ed.), *Sociology as applied to medicine* (pp. 41–62). London: Saunders.

Moscovici, S. (1981). On social representations. In J. P. Forgas (Ed.), *Social cognition: Perspectives on everyday understanding* (pp. 181–209). London: Academic Press.

Moss-Morris, R., Petrie, K. J., & Weinman, J. (1996). Functioning in chronic fatigue syndrome: Do illness perceptions play a regulatory role? *British Journal of Health Psychology, 1,* 15–25.

Motsiou, A. (1999). *The effects of doctors' communication skills on cancer patients' perceptions of power and social distance: A retrospective study.* MSc research project, Department of Experimental Psychology, University of Bristol, UK.

Murphy, J. (1996). *Trigger unit for Social psychology: Personal lives, social worlds. A third level social sciences course.* Milton Keynes, UK: Open University Press.

Neugarten, B. L., Wood, V., Kraines, R. J., & Loomis, B. (1968). Women's attitudes toward menopause. In B. L Neugartenn (Ed.), *Middle age and aging* (pp. 195–200). Chicago: University of Chicago Press. [Cited in Golub, S. (1992). *Periods: From menarche to menopause.* New York: Sage International Edition.]

Noller, P. (1980). Misunderstandings in marital communication: A study of couples' nonverbal communication. *Journal of Personality and Social Psychology, 39,* 1135–1148.

Norfolk, D. (1990). *Think well, feel great: Seven b-attitudes that will change your life.* London: Michael Joseph.

Norman, P., & Bennett, P. (1996). Health locus of control. In M. Conner & P. Norman (Eds.), *Predicting health behaviour* (pp. 62–94). Buckingham, UK: Open University Press.

Norman, P. & Conner, M. (1996). The role of social cognition models in predicting health behavours: Future directions. In M. Conner & P. Norman (Eds.) *Predicting health behaviour* (pp. 197–225). Buckingham, UK: Open University Press.

Norretranders, T. (1998). *The user illusion* (Trans Johathan Sydenham). London: Penguin Press.

Oakes, P., & Turner, J. (1980). Social categorisation and intergroup behaviour: Does minimal intergroup discrimination make social identity more positive? *European Journal of Social Psychology*, *10*, 295–301.

O'Brien, B. (1984). *Patterns of European diagnosis and prescribing*. London: Office of Health Economics. [Cited in Helman, C. G. (1994). *Culture, health and illness* (3rd ed). London: Wright.]

Olasov, B., & Jackson, J. (1987). Effects of expectancies on women's reports of moods during the menstrual cycle. *Psychosomatic Medicine*, 49, 65–78.

Ong L. M. L., de Haes, J. C. J. M., Hoos, A. M. & Lammes, F. B. (1995). Doctor–patient communication: A review of the literature. *Social Science and Medicine*, *40*(7), 903–918.

O'Rourke, T., Smith B. J., & Nolte, A. E. (1984). Health risk attitudes, beliefs and behaviours of students grades 7–12. *Journal of School Health*, *15*, 8–17.

Osterweis, M., Bush, P. J., & Zuckerman, A. (1979). Family context as a predictor of individual medicine use. *Social Science and Medicine*, *13*A, 287–291.

Paige, K. E. (1973). Women learn to sing the menstrual blues. *Psychology Today*, *7*, 41–46.

Parsons, T. (1951). *The social system*. Glencoe, IL: Free Press.

Pendleton, D., & Hasler, J. (Eds). (1983). *Dr. patient communication*. London: Academic Press.

Pendleton, D., Schofield, T., Tate P., & Havelock, P. (1984). *The consultation*. Oxford: Oxford University Press.

Pennebaker, J. W. (1980). Perceptual and environmental determinants of coughing. *Basic and Applied Social Psychology*, *1*, 83–91.

Pennebaker, J. W. (1982). *The psychology of physical symptoms*. New York: Heidelberg.

Pennebaker, J. W. (1984). Accuracy of symptom perception. In A. Baum, S. E. Taylor, & J. E. Singer (Eds.) *Handbook of psychology and health IV*. Hove, UK: Lawrence Erlbaum Associates Ltd.

Pennebaker, J. W., & Brittingham, G. L. (1982). Environmental and sensory cues affecting the perception of physical symptoms. In A. Baum, S. E. Taylor, & J. E. Singer (Eds.), *Advances in environmental psychology IV* (pp. 115–136). Hillsdale, NJ: Lawrence Erlbaum Associates Inc.

Pennebaker, J. W., Kiecott-Glaser, J. K., & Glaser, R. (1988). Confronting traumatic experience and immunocompetence: A reply to Neale, Cox, Valdimarsdottir and Stone. *Journal of Consulting and Clinical Psychology*, *56*(4), 638–639.

Pennebaker, J. W., & Lightner, J. M. (1980). Competition of internal and external information in an exercise setting. *Journal of Personality and Social Psychology*, *39*, 165–174.

Pennebaker, J. W., & Skelton J. A. (1978). Psychological parameters of physical symptoms. *Personality and Social Psychology Bulletin*, *4*(4), 524–530.

Pennebaker, J. W., & Skelton, J. A. (1981). Selective monitoring of bodily sensations. *Journal of Personality and Social Psychology*, *41*, 213–223.

Perry J., & Felce, D. (1995). Objective assessments of quality of life: How much do they agree with each other? *Journal of Community and Applied Social Psychology*, *5*, 1–19.

Petersen, A. C. (1983). Menarche: Meaning of measures and measuring meaning. In S. Golub (Ed.), *Menarche* (pp. 63–76). Lexington, MA: Lexington Books.

Pill, R., & Stott, N. C. H. (1982). Concepts of illness causation and responsibility: Some preliminary data from a sample of working class mothers. *Social Science and Medicine*, *16*, 43–52.

Potter, J. (1996). Attitudes, social representations and discursive psychology. In M. Wetherell (Ed.), *Identities, Groups and Social Issues* (pp. 119–176). London: Sage, in association with the Open University.

Potter, J., & Wetherell, M. (1987). *Discourse and social psychology: Beyond attitudes and behaviour*. London: Sage.

Povey, R., Conner, M., Sparks, P., James, R., & Shepherd, R. (2000). Application of the Theory of Planned Behaviour to two dietary behaviours: Roles of perceived control and self-efficacy. *British Journal of Health Psychology*, *5*(2), 121–140.

Prochaska, J. O., DiClemente, C. C., & Norcross, J. C. (1992). In search of how people change: Applications to addictive behaviors. *American Psychologist*, *47*, 1102–1114.

Prochaska, J. O., Velicer, W. F., Guidagnoli, E., Rossi, J. S., & DiClemente, C. C. (1991). Patterns of change: Dynamic typology applied to smoking cessation. *Multivariate Behavioral Research*, *26*, 83–107.

Quadrel, M. J., & Lau, R. R. (1990). A multivariate analysis of adolescents' orientations toward physician use. *Health Psychology*, *9*(6), 750–773.

Radley, A. (1996). Relationships in detail: The study of social interaction. In D. Miell & R. Dallos (Eds.), *Social interaction and personal relationships* (pp. 23–101). London: Sage, in association with the Open University.

Ragland, D. R., & Brand, R. J. (1988). Type A behaviour and mortality from CHD. *New England Journal of Medicine*, *318*, 65–69.

Rains, A. J. H., & Capper, W. M. (1968). *Bailey and Love's short practice of surgery* (14th ed). London: Lewis.

Ray, C., Wier, W. R. C., Cullen, S., & Phillips, S. (1991). Illness perception and symptom components in chronic fatigue syndrome. *Journal of Psychosomatic Research*, *36*(3), 243–256.

Redlich, F. C. (1949). The patient's language. *Yale Journal of Biology and Medicine*, *17*, 427–453. [Cited in Ley, P. (1990). *Communicating with patients*. London: Chapman & Hall.]

Reiss, S., & Szysko, H. (1983). Diagnostic overshadowing and professional experience with mentally retarded persons. *American Journal of Mental Deficiency, 87*, 396–402.

Relton, P. (2000). New mentality. *Guardian*, 26th January, p. 6.

Richard, R., van der Pligt, J., & de Vries, N. (1995). Anticipated affective reactions and prevention of AIDS. *British Journal of Social Psychology, 34*, 9–21.

Robb, S. L., Nichols, R. J., Rutan, R. L., Bishop, B. L., & Parker, J. C. (1995). The effects of music assisted relaxation on preoperative anxiety. *Journal of Music Therapy, 32*, 2–21.

Roberts, H. (undated). *The practical way to keep fit*. London: Odhams Press.

Rogers, R. W. (1975). A protection motivation theory of fear appeals and attitude change. *Journal of Psychology, 91*, 93–114.

Rogers, R. W. (1983). Cognitive and physiological processes in fear appeals and attitude change: A revised theory of protection motivation. In J. T. Cacioppo & R. E. Petty (Eds.), *Social psychophysiology: A source book* (pp. 153–176). New York: Guilford Press.

Rosch, E. (1975). Cognitive representations of semantic categories. *Journal of Experimental Psychology: General, 104*(3), 192–233.

Rosenman, R. H. (1978). The interview method of assessment of the coronary prone behaviour pattern. In T. M. Dembroski et al. (Eds.), *Coronary-prone behaviour* (pp. 55–70). New York: Springer-Verlag.

Rosenman, R. H., Brand, R. J., Jenkins, D., Friedman, M., Straus, R., & Wurm, M. (1975). CHD in the Western collaborative heart study: Final follow-up experience of eight and a half years. *Journal of the American Medical Association, 233*, 872–877.

Roskies, E. (1991). Type A intervention: Where do we go from here? In M. J. Strube (Ed.), *Type A behaviour* (pp. 389–408). London: Sage.

Rosser, R., Cottee, M., Rabin, R., & Selai, C. (1991). *Index of health-related quality of life* (unpublished MS) Academic Department of Psychiatry, University College and Middlesex School of Medicine, The Middlesex Hospital, London.

Rossi, A. S., & Rossi, P. E. (1977). Body time and social time: Mood patterns by menstrual phase and day of the week. *Social Science Research, 6*, 273–308. [Cited in Golub, S. (1992). *Periods: From menarche to menopause*. New York: Sage International Edition.]

Roter, D., & Frankel, R. (1992). Quantitative and qualitative approaches to the evaluation of the medical dialogue. *Social Science and Medicine, 34*(10), 1097–1103.

Roter, D. & Hall, J. A. (1987). Physician interviewing styles and medical information obtained from patients. *Journal of General Internal Medicine, 2*, 326.

Roth, I., & Bruce, V. (1996). *Perception and representation: Current issues* (2nd ed). Buckingham, UK: Open University Press.

Rotter, J. B. (1966). Generalised expectancies for internal versus external control of reinforcement. *Psychological Monographs, 80*(1).

Rowling, J. K. (1997). *Harry Potter and the philosopher's stone*. London: Bloomsbury.

Ruble, D. (1977). Premenstrual symptoms: A reinterpretation. *Science, 197*, 291–292.

Rutter, D. R. (2000). Attendance and reattendance for breast cancer screening: A prospective 3-year test of the Theory of Planned Behaviour. *British Journal of Health Psychology, 5*(1), 1–14.

Safer, M. A., Tharps, Q. J., Jackson, T. C., & Leventhal, H. (1979). Determinants of three stages of delay in seeking care at a medical clinic. *Medical Care, 17*, 11–29.

Salovey, P., Rothman, A. J., & Rodin, J. (1998). Health behaviour. In D. T. Gilbert, S. Fiske, & G. Lindzey (Eds.), *The handbook of social psychology* (4th ed, pp. 633–683). Boston: McGraw-Hill.

Sampson, G. A. (1979). Premenstrual syndrome: A double-blind controlled trial of progesterone and placebo. *British Journal of Psychiatry, 135*, 209–215.

Sanders, G. S. (1982). Social comparison and perceptions of health and illness. In G. S. Sanders, & J. Suls (Eds.), *The social psychology of health and illness* (Ch. 5). Hillsdale, NJ: Lawrence Erlbaum Associates Inc.

Sapsford, R. (1996). Domains of analysis. In R. Sapsford (Ed.), *Issues for social psychology* (pp. 67–76). London: Sage, in association with the Open University.

Sapsford, R., & Dallos, R. (1996). Resisting social psychology. In R. Sapsford (Ed.), *Issues for social psychology* (pp. 191–208). London: Sage, in association with the Open University.

Sarafino, E. P. (1994). *Health psychology: Biopsychosocial interactions* (Second International Edition). Chichester, UK: Wiley.

Sarafino, E. P. (1998). *Health psychology: Biopsychosocial interactions* (Third International Edition). Chichester, UK: Wiley.

Sarason, I. G., Levine, H. M., Basham, R. B., & Sarason, B. R. (1983). Assessing social support: The social support questionnaire. *Journal of Personality and Social Psychology, 44*, 127–139.

Scambler, A., & Scambler, G. (1985). Menstrual symptoms, attitudes and consulting behaviour. *Social Science and Medicine, 20*, 1065–1068.

Scambler, A., & Scambler, G. (1993). *Menstrual disorders*. London & New York: Tavistock/Routledge.

Scambler, A., Scambler, G., & Craig, D. (1981). Kinship and friendship networks and women's demand for primary care. *Journal of the Royal College of General Practitioners, 26*, 746–750.

Schacter, S., & Singer, J. E. (1962). Cognitive, social and physiological determinants of emotional state. *Psychological Review, 69*, 379–399.

Scherer, K. R. (2001). Emotion. In M. Hewstone & W. Stroebe (Eds.), *Introduction to social psychology* (3rd ed., pp. 151–196). Oxford: Blackwell.

Schifter, D. E., & Ajzen, I. (1985). Intention, perceived control and weight loss:

An application of the theory of planned behaviour. *Journal of Personality and Social Psychology, 49*, 843–851.

Schipper, H., Clinch, J., & Powell, V. (1990). Definitions and conceptual issues. In B. Spiker (Ed.), *Quality of life assessments in clinical trials*. New York: Raven Press. [Cited in Hyland, M. E., Finnios, S., & Irvine, S. H. (1991). A scale for assessing quality of life in adult asthma sufferers. *Journal of Psychosomatic Research, 35*(1) 99–110.]

Scott, J., & Huskisson, E. C. (1976). Accuracy of subjective measurements made with or without previous scores—an important source of error in social measurement of subjective states. *Annals of the Rheumatic Diseases, 38*, 558–559. [Cited in Skevington, S. (1995). *Psychology of pain*. Chichester, UK: Wiley.]

Sedgwick, P. (1982). *Psychopolitics*. London: Pluto. [Cited in Stainton Rogers, W. (1991). *Explaining health and illness*. Hemel Hempstead, UK: Harvester Wheatsheaf.]

Segovia, J., Bartlett, R. F., & Edwards, A. C. (1989). An empirical analysis of the dimension of health status measures. *Social Science and Medicine, 29*(6), 761–768.

Selye, H. (1956). *The stress of life*. New York: McGraw Hill.

Selye, H. (1974). *Stress without distress*. London: Hodder & Stoughton.

Sheeran, P., & Abraham, C. (1996). The health belief model. In M. Conner, & P. Norman (Eds.), *Predicting health behaviour* (pp. 23–61). Buckingham, UK: Open University Press.

Shelvin, B. (1981) Painful patients and happy doctors. In G. Edwards (Ed.), *Psychiatry in general practice*. Southampton: Southampton University Press.

Sheridan, C. L., & Radmacher, S. A. (1992). *Health Psychology: Challenging the biomedical model*. Chichester, UK: Wiley International Edition.

Sherif, M. (1936). *The psychology of social norms*. New York: Harper & Row.

Siminoff, L. A. (1992). Improving communication with cancer patients. *Oncology, 6*(10), 83–87.

Siminoff, L. A., & Fetting, J. H. (1991). Factors affecting treatment decisions for a life-threatening illness. *Social Science and Medicine, 32*(7), 813–881.

Singer, J. E., & Lord, D. (1984). The role of social support in coping with chronic or life-threatening illness. In A. Baum, S. E. Taylor, & J. E. Singer (Eds.), *Handbook of psychology and health IV*. London: Lawrence Erlbaum Associates Ltd.

Skevington, S. (1994). Social comparisons in cross-cultural QOL assessment. *International Journal of Mental Health, 23*(2), 29–47.

Skevington, S. (1995). *Psychology of pain*. Chichester, UK: Wiley.

Skevington, S. M. (1998). Investigating the relationship between pain and discomfort and quality of life, using the WHOQUAL. *Pain, 76*, 395–406.

Smith, A. J. (1950). Menstruation and industrial efficiency, I: Absenteeism and activity level: II: Quality and quantity of production. *Journal of Applied Psychology, 34*(1), 15, 148–152.

Smits, A. J. A., Meyboom, W. A., Mokkink H. G. A., Van Son, J. A. J., & Van Eijk, J. (1991). Medical versus behavioural skills: An observation study of 75 general practitioners. *Family Practice, 8*(1), 14–18.

Somerville, G. (undated) Nervous illnesses in women. In Sir W. Arbuthnot Lane (Ed.), *The Modern Woman's Home Doctor* (pp. 35–42). London: Odhams Press Ltd.

Sparks, P., & Guthrie, C. A. (1998). Self-identity and the theory of planned behaviour: A useful addition or an unhelpful artifice? *Journal of Applied Social Psychology, 28*, 1393–1410.

Spencer, C. (1998a). Personality—The individual and society. In P. Scott & C. Spencer (Eds.), *Psychology. A contemporary introduction* (pp. 549–582). Oxford: Blackwell.

Spencer, C. (1998b). Social processes—from the dyad to the small group to the crowd. In P. Scott, & C. Spencer (Eds.), *Psychology: A contemporary introduction* (pp. 467–508). Oxford: Blackwell.

Stacey, M. (1977). *Concepts of health and illness: A working paper on the concepts and their relevance to research. Appendix 3. Health and Health Policy: Priorities for research*. Social Science Research Council Document. London: Social Science Research Council.

Stahlberg, D., & Frey, D. (1996). Attitudes, structure, measurement and functions. In M. Hewstone, W. Stroebe, & G. M. Stephenson (Eds.), *Introduction to social psychology* (2nd ed, pp. 205–239). Oxford: Blackwell.

Stainton Rogers, W. (1991). *Explaining health and illness*. Hemel Hempstead, UK: Harvester Wheatsheaf.

St. Claire, L. (1986a). Mental retardation: Impairment or handicap? *Disability, Handicap and Society, 1*(3), 233–243.

St. Claire, L. (1986b). *Measuring the health status of teenagers. Report to The Health Promotion Trust*. Department of Child Health, Bristol University, UK.

St. Claire, L. (1989). A multi-dimensional model of mental retardation impairment, subnormal behaviour, role failures and socially constructed retardation. *American Journal on Mental Retardation, 94*(1), 88–96.

St. Claire, L. (1993). Does medics' social identification increase handicap for mentally retarded patients? *Journal of Community and Applied Social Psychology, 3*, 183–195.

St. Claire, L. (2000). Measuring communication skills of medical students to patients with cancer. *British Journal of Medical Psychology, 73*, 99–116.

St. Claire, L., & Clift, A. (2003). *The experience of cold-relevant symptoms and the saliency of a "cold sufferer" social identification*. Manuscript in submission.

St. Claire, L., & Turner, D. (1995). *"Still Tickin'" Report on Weston's Cardiac Rehabilitation Programme*. Unpublished MS.

St. Claire, L., Watkins, C. J., & Billinghurst, B. (1996). Differences in meanings of health. A preliminary study of doctors and their patients. *Family Practice, 13*(6), 511–516.

Steinem, G. (1978, October) If men could menstruate. *Ms Magazine*, *110*. [Cited in Golub, S. (1992). *Periods: From menarche to menopause*. New York: Sage International Edition.]

Stevens, R. (1996a). Introduction: Making sense of the person in a social world. In R. Stevens (Ed.), *Understanding the self* (pp. 1–35). London: Sage, in association with the Open University.

Stevens, R. (1996b). The reflexive self: An experiential perspective. In R. Stevens (Ed.), *Understanding the self* (pp. 147–218). London: Sage, in association with the Open University.

Stevens, R. (1996c). Trimodal theory as a model for interrelating perspectives in psychology. In R. Sapsford (Ed.), *Issues for social psychology* (pp. 77–84). London: Sage, in association with the Open University.

Still, A. (1996a). Historical origins of social psychology. In R. Sapsford (Ed.), *Issues for social psychology* (pp. 19–40). London: Sage, in association with the Open University.

Still, A. (1996b). Theories of meaning. In R. Sapsford (Ed.), *Issues for social psychology* (pp. 85–98). London: Sage, in association with the Open University.

Stimson, G. V., & Webb, B. (1975). *Going to see the doctor: The consultation process in general practice*. London: Routledge & Kegan Paul.

Stockwell, F. (1972). *The unpopular patient*. London: Royal College of Nursing.

Stroebe, W., & Jonas, K. (1996). Principles of attitude formation and strategies of change. In M. Hewstone, W. Stroebe, & G. M. Stephenson (Eds.), *Introduction to social psychology* (2nd ed, pp. 240–276). Oxford: Blackwell.

Stroebe W., & Jonas, K. (2001). Health psychology: a social psychological perspective. In M. Hewstone, & W. Stroebe (Eds.), *Introduction to social psychology* (3rd Ed, pp. 519–558). Oxford: Blackwell.

Stroebe W., & Stroebe, M. (1995). *Social psychology and health*. Buckingham, UK: Open University Press.

Strube, M. J. (Ed.) (1991). *Type A behaviour*. London: Sage.

Suchman, E. A. (1972). Social patterns of illness and medical care. In E. G. Jaco (Ed.), *Patients, physicians and illness* (2nd ed, pp. 262–297). New York: The Free Press.

Sugarbaker, P. H., Barofsky, I., Rosenberg, S. A., & Gianola, P. A. C. (1982). Quality of life assessment of patients in extremity sarcoma clinical trials *Surgery, January*, 17–23.

Suls, J., & Fletcher, B. (1985). The efficacy of avoidant and non-avoidant coping: A meta-analysis. *Health Psychology*, *4*, 249–288.

Suls, J., Martin, R., & Leventhal, H. (1997). Social comparison, lay referral and the decision to seek medical care. In B. P. Buunk & F. X. Gibbons (Eds.), *Health, coping and wellbeing* (pp. 195–226). Mahwah, NJ: Lawrence Erlbaum Associates Inc.

Suls, J. M. (1977). Social comparison theory and research: An overview from 1954. In J. M. Suls, & R. L. Miller (Eds.), *Social comparison processes* (pp. 1–20). Washington: Hemisphere.

Sutherland R., & Cooper G. L. (1992). *Understanding stress: A psychological perspective for health professionals*. London: Chapman & Hall.

Sutton, S. (1998). Predicting and explaining intentions and behaviour: How well are we doing? *Journal of Applied Social Psychology, 28*, 1317–1338.

Svarstad, B. L. (1976). Physician–patient communication and patient conformity with medical advice. In D. Mechanic (Ed.), *The growth of bureaucratic medicine* (pp. 220–238). New York: Wiley. [Cited in Skevington, S. (1995). *Psychology of pain*. Chichester, UK: Wiley.]

Tajfel, H. (1970). Experiments in intergroup discrimination. *Scientific American, 223*(5).

Tajfel, H. (1972). Social categorisation. In S. Moscovici (Ed.), *Introduction à la psychologie sociale*. Paris: Larousse.

Tajfel, H. (1978a). *Differentiation between social groups: Studies in the social psychology of intergroup relations*. London: Academic Press.

Tajfel, H. (1978b). *The social psychology of minorities. Report No. 38*. London: Minority Rights Group.

Tajfel, H. (1981). *Human groups and social categories: Studies in social psychology*. Cambridge: Cambridge University Press.

Tajfel, H., Flament, L., Billig, M., & Bundy, R. P. (1971). Social categorisation and intergroup behaviour. *European Journal of Social Psychology, 1*, 149–178.

Tajfel, H., & Turner, J. (1979). An integrative theory of intergroup conflict. In W. G. Austin, & S. Worchel (Eds.), *The social psychology of intergroup relations*. Monterey, CA: Brooks Cole.

Tajfel, H., & Wilkes, A. L (1963). Classification and quantitative judgement. *British Journal of Psychology, 54*, 101–114.

Tampax Report (1981). New York: Ruder, Finn, & Rotman. [Cited in Golub, S. (1992). *Periods: From menarche to menopause*. New York: Sage International Edition].

Tapp, J. T., & Warner R. (1985). The multisystems view of health and disease. In N. Schneiderman, & J. T. Tapp (Eds.), *Behavioural medicine: The biopsychosocial approach*. Hillsdale, NJ: Lawrence Erlbaum Associates Inc.

Taylor, S. E. (1983). Adjustment to threatening events, a theory of cognitive adaption. *American Psychologist, 817*, 1161–1173.

Taylor, S. E. (1995). *Health psychology* (3rd ed). New York: McGraw Hill.

Taylor, S. E., & Brown J. D. (1988). Illusion and well-being: A social psychological perspective on mental health. *Psychological Bulletin, 103*, 193–210.

Taylor, S. E., & Clark L. F. (1986). Does information improve adjustment to noxious events? In M. J. Saks & L. Saks (Eds.), *Advances in applied social psychology*. Hillsdale, NJ: Lawrence Erlbaum Associates Inc.

Telles, J. L., & Pollack, M. H. (1981). Feeling sick—the experience and legitimation of illness. *Social Science and Medicine, 15*A, 243–251.

Temoshok, L., Sweet, D. M., & Zich, J. (1987) A three city comparison of the public's knowledge and attitudes about AIDS. *Psychology and Health, 1*(1), 43–60.

Tennen, H., & Affleck, G. (1997). Social comparison as a coping process: A critical review and application to chronic pain disorders. In B. P. Buunk & F. X. Gibbons (Eds.), *Health, coping and wellbeing* (pp. 263–298). Mahwah, NJ: Lawrence Erlbaum Associates Inc.

Tew, M. (1990). *Safer childbirth?* London: Chapman & Hall.

Thoits, P. A. (1982). Conceptual, methodological and theoretical problems in studying social support as a buffer against life stress. *Journal of Health and Social Behaviour, June*, 145–159.

Thompson, S. C. (1981). Will it hurt less if I can control it? A complex answer to a simple question. *Psychological Bulletin, 90*(1), 89–101.

Tissue, T. (1972). Another look at self-rated health among the elderly. *Journal of Gerontology, 27*(1), 91–94.

Toates, F. (1996). The embodied self: A biological perspective. In R. Stevens (Ed.), *Understanding the self* (pp. 35–89). London: Sage, in association with the Open University.

Townsend, P., & Yeo, S. (1979). *Poverty in the UK*. Harmondsworth, UK: Penguin.

Trabin, T., Rader, C., & Cummings, C. (1987). A comparison of pain management outcomes for disability compensation and non-compensation patients groups. *Psychology and Health, 1*(4), 303–424.

Tuckett, D. A., Boulton, M., & Olsen, C. (1985). A new approach to the measurement of patients' understanding of what they are told in medical consultations. *Journal of Health and Social Behaviour, 26*, 27–38.

Turner, J. (1981). Towards a cognitive redefinition of the social group. *Cahiers de Psychologie Cognitive, 1*(2), 93–118.

Turner, J. C. (1975). Social categorisation and social identity: Some prospects for intergroup behaviour. *European Journal of Social Psychology, 5*, 5–34.

Turner, J. C. (1991). *Social influence*. Milton Keynes, UK: Open University Press.

Turner, J. C. (2000). Preface. In S. A. Haslam (2001). *Psychology in organizations. The social identity approach*. London: Sage.

Turner, J. C., & Brown, R. (1978). Social status, cognitive alternatives and intergroup relations. In H. Tajfel (Ed.), *Differentiation between social groups*. London: Academic Press.

Turner, J. C., Hogg, M. A., Oakes, P. J., Reicher, S. D., & Wetherell, M. S. (1987). *Rediscovering the social group: A self-categorisation theory*. Oxford: Blackwells.

Turpin, G., & Slade, P. (1998). Clinical and health psychology. In P. Scott & C. Spencer (Eds.), *Psychology: A contemporary introduction* (pp. 618–659). Oxford: Blackwell.

Tversky, A., & Kahneman, D. (1981). The framing of decisions and the psychology of choice. *Science, 211*, 453–458.

Twaddle, A. (1974). The concept of health status. *Social Science and Medicine, 8*, 29–38.

Ussher, J. (1991). *Women's madness*. Hemel Hempstead, UK: Harvester Wheatsheaf.

Valins, S. (1966). Cognitive effects of false heart-rate feedback. *Journal of Personality and Social Psychology*, 4(4), 400–408.

Valpey, D. D. (1982). The psychological impact of 18 years in a board and care home. *Journal of Community Psychology*, 10(1), 95–97.

van Dam, F. S. A. M., Linssen, A. C. G., Englesman E., van Benthem, J., & Hanewald, G. J. F. P. (1980). Life with cytostatic drugs. *European Journal of Cancer Supplement*, 1, 229–233.

Viner, E. D. (1985). Life at the other end of the endotracheal tube: A physician's personal view of critical illness. *Progress in Critical Care Medicine*, 2, 3–13. [Cited in Murphy, J. (1996). *Trigger unit for social psychology: Personal lives, social worlds. A third level social sciences course*. Buckingham, UK: Open University Press.]

Waddell, G., McCullock, J. A., Kummel, E., & Venner, R. M. (1980). Nonorganic physical signs in low-back pain. *Spine*, 5, 117–125. [Cited in Helman, C. G. (1994). *Culture, Health and Illness* (3rd ed). London: Wright.]

Walker, A. E. (1997). *The menstrual cycle*. London: Routledge.

Wallen, J., Waitzkin, H., & Stroeckle, J. D. (1979). Physician stereotypes about female health and illness. *Women and Health*, 4, 135–146.

Wallston, K. A., Wallston, B. S., & De Vellis, R. (1978). Development of multidimensional health locus of control scales. *Health Education Monographs*, 6, 160–170.

Walters, A. (1961). Psychogenic regional pain alias hysterical pain. *Brain*, 84, 1–18. [Cited in Helman, C. G. (1994). *Culture, health and illness* (3rd ed). London: Wright.

Warburton, D. M. (1978). Poisoned people: Internal pollution. *Journal of Biosocial Science*, 10, 309–319. [Cited in Helman, C. G. (1994). *Culture, health and illness* (3rd ed). London: Wright.

Ware, J. (1984). Conceptualising disease impact and treatment. *Cancer, May 15*, 2316–2326.

Watson, D. (1988). Intraindividual and interindividual analyses of positive and negative affect: Their relation to health complaints, perceived stress and daily activities. *Journal of Personality and Social Psychology*, 54(6), 1020–1030.

Weideger, P. (1975). *Female cycles*. London: The Women's Press.

Weinberger, M., Tierney, W. M., Booker, P., & Katz, B. P. (1989). Can the provision of information to patients with osteoarthritis improve functional status? A randomised controlled trial. *Arthritis and Rheumatism*, 32(12), 1577. [Cited in Skevington,. S. (1995). *Psychology of pain*. Chichester, UK: Wiley.]

Weinstein, N. D. (1987). Unrealistic optimism about susceptibility to health problems: Conclusions from a community-wide sample. *Journal of Behavioural Medicine*, 10, 481–500.

Weinstein, N. D., & Sandman, P. M. (1992). A model of the precaution adoption process: Evidence from home radon testing. *Health Psychology*, 11, 170–180.

West, C., & Frankel, R. (1991). Miscommunication in medicine. In N. Coupland,

H. Giles, & J. M. Wiemann (Eds.), *Miscommunication and problematic talk.* Newbury Park, CA: Sage.

Wetherell, M. (1996a). Defining social psychology. In R. Sapsford (Ed.), *Issues for social psychology* (pp. 5–18). London: Sage, in association with the Open University.

Wetherell, M. (1996b) Life histories and social histories. In M. Wetherell (Ed.), *Identities, groups and social issues* (pp. 229–361). London: Sage, in association with the Open University.

Wetherell M., & Still, A. (1996). Realism and relativism. In R. Sapsford (Ed.), *Issues for social psychology* (pp. 99–116). London: Sage, in association with the Open University.

Whisnant, L., & Zegans, L. (1975). A study of attitudes toward menarche in white middle class American adolescent girls. *American Journal of Psychiatry, 132*(8), 809–814. [Cited in Golub, S. (1992). *Periods: From menarche to menopause.* New York: Sage International Edition.]

Whitehead, W. E., Busch, C. M., Heller, B. R., & Costa, P. T. Jr. (1986). Social learning influences on menstrual symptoms and illness behaviour. *Health Psychology, 5*(1), 13–23.

WHOQUAL Group (1993). Study protocol for the World Health Organisation project to develop a quality of life assessment instrument (WHOQUAL). *Quality of Life Research, 2*, 153–159.

WHOQUAL Group (1995). The World Health Organisation Quality of Life assessment (WHOQUAL): Position paper from the World Health Organisation. *Social Science and Medicine, 41*, 1403–1409.

WHOQUAL Group (1998). Development of the World Health Organisation WHOOQOL-BREF Quality of Life Assessment. *Psychological Medicine, 28*, 551–558.

Wiemann, J. M., & Giles, H. (1996). Communication in interpersonal and social relationships. In M. Hewstone, W. Stroebe and G. M. Stephenson (Eds.), *Introduction to social psychology* (2nd ed). Oxford: Blackwell.

Wilcoxon, L. A., Schrader, S. L., & Sherif, C. W. (1976). Daily self reports on activities, life events, moods and somatic changes during the menstrual cycle. *Psychosomatic Medicine, 38*(6), 399–417. [Cited in Golub, S. (1992). *Periods: From menarche to menopause.* New York: Sage International Edition.]

Williams, A., Whitfield, M., Bucks, R., & St. Claire, L. (1991). Differences in the attitudes of men and women practitioners to responsibility and competence. *British Journal of General Practice, 41*, 327–329.

Williams, L. R. (1983). Beliefs and attitudes of young girls regarding menstruation. In S. Golub (Ed.), *Menarche* (pp. 139–148). Lexington, MA: Lexington Books.

Williams, R. (1983). Concepts of health: An analysis of lay logic. *Sociology, 17*(2), 185–205.

Wills, T. A. (1981). Downward comparison principles in social psychology. *Psychological Bulletin, 90*(2), 245–271.

Wilson D., Kaplan, R. M., & Schneiderman, L. J. (1987). Framing of decisions and selections of alternatives in health care. *Social Behaviour, 2*, 51–59.

Wood, J. V., Taylor, S. E., & Lichtman, R. R. (1985). Social comparison in adjustment to breast cancer. *Journal of Personality and Social Psychology, 49*(5), 1169–1183.

Wood, J. V., & Vanderzee, K. (1997). Social comparisons among cancer patients: Under what conditions are comparisons upward and downward? In B. P. Buunk & F. X. Gibbons (Eds.), *Health, coping and wellbeing* (pp. 299–328). Mahwah, NJ: Lawrence Erlbaum Associates Inc.

Wood, P. H. N., & Badley, E. M. (1980). *People with disabilities. Toward acquiring information which reflects more sensitivity to their problems and needs*. New York: World Rehabilitation Fund, Inc.

Woods, N., Kramer Dery, G., & Most, A. (1982). Recollections of menarche, current menstrual attitudes and premenstrual symptoms. *Psychosomatic Medicine, 44*, 285–293.

Worchel, S., Iuzzini, J., Coutant, D., & Ivaldi, M. (2000). A multidimensional model of identity: Relating individual and group identities to intergroup behaviour. In D. Capozza & R. Brown (Eds.), *Social identity processes* (pp. 15–32). London: Sage.

World Health Organization (1948). Constitution of the World Health Organisation. Geneva: WHO Basic Documents.

World Health Organization (1958). The First 10 years. The Health Organization. Geneva: World Health Organization.

Ybema, J. F., & Buunk, B. P. (1995). Affective responses to social comparisons: A study among disabled individuals. *British Journal of Social Psychology, 34*(3).

Young, G. (1981). A woman in medicine: Reflections from the inside. In H. Roberts (Ed.), *Women, health and reproduction*. London: Routledge.

Zachary Cope (undated). [Cited in Rains, A. J. H., & Capper, W. M. (1968). *Bailey and Love's short practice of surgery* (14th ed). London: Lewis.]

Zeldow, P. B., & Daugherty, S. R. (1987). The stability and attitudinal correlations of warmth and caring in medical students. *Medical Education, 21*, 353–357.

Zillmann, D., Johnson, R. C., & Day, K. D. (1974). Attribution of apparent arousal and proficiency of recovery from sympathetic activation affecting excitation transfer to aggressive behaviour. *Journal of Experimental Social Psychology, 10*, 503–515.

Zola, I. K. (1966). Culture and symptoms—an analysis of patients' presenting complaints. *American Sociological Review, 31*, 615–630.

Author index

Subject index

Note: page numbers in *italics* refer to diagrams, page numbers in **bold** refer to information presented in tables.